Operative Dictations in Urologic Surgery

Operative Dictations in Urologic Surgery

Noel A. Armenakas, M.D.
Clinical Professor of Urology
Weill Cornell Medical College
Attending Surgeon
New York Presbyterian Hospital
Lenox Hill Hospital

John A. Fracchia, M.D.
Clinical Professor of Urology
Weill Cornell Medical College
Attending Surgeon
New York Presbyterian Hospital
Lenox Hill Hospital
Chairman Emeritus
Department of Urology
Lenox Hill Hospital

Ron Golan, M.D.
Chief Resident
Department of Urology
Weill Cornell Medical College
New York Presbyterian Hospital

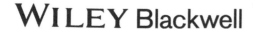

WILEY Blackwell

Registered Office(s)
John Wiley & Sons, Inc., 111 River Street, Hoboken, NJ 07030, USA
John Wiley & Sons Ltd, The Atrium, Southern Gate, Chichester, West Sussex, PO19 8SQ, UK

Editorial Office
9600 Garsington Road, Oxford, OX4 2DQ, UK

For details of our global editorial offices, customer services, and more information about Wiley products visit us at www.wiley.com.

Wiley also publishes its books in a variety of electronic formats and by print-on-demand. Some content that appears in standard print versions of this book may not be available in other formats.

Library of Congress Cataloging-in-Publication Data

Names: Armenakas, Noel, author. | Fracchia, John A., author. | Golan, Ron, author.
Title: Operative dictations in urologic surgery [electronic resource] / Noel A. Armenakas,
    John A. Fracchia, Ron Golan.
Description: Hoboken, NJ : Wiley Blackwell, 2019. | Includes bibliographical references and index. |
Identifiers: LCCN 2019003282 (print) | LCCN 2019004182 (ebook) | ISBN 9781119524304 (Adobe PDF) |
    ISBN 9781119524335 (ePub) | ISBN 9781119524311 (pbk.)
Subjects: | MESH: Urologic Surgical Procedures—methods
Classification: LCC RD572 (ebook) | LCC RD572 (print) | NLM WJ 168 | DDC 617.460597—dc23
LC record available at https://lccn.loc.gov/2019003282

Cover Design: Wiley
Cover Image: © Blend Images - ERproductions Ltd/Getty Images

Set in 10/12pt Warnock by SPi Global, Pondicherry, India

To all the past, present, and future residents who continue to inspire us and from whom we never cease to learn.

Contents

Foreword

This is an essential book for all urological surgeons. It should be studied by urological residents as well as mature urological surgeons to enhance the knowledge of information needed in an operative report.

The details of the necessary information in an operative report are provided for virtually all urological procedures that I can think of, including open surgery as well as endoscopic, percutaneous, laparoscopic, and robotics. Each procedure has a template that serves as a valuable guide for the detailed information to be included in the operative record so it provides essential information should the surgeon need to recall what was done if complications occur or the procedure fails, and it is available for review years later if necessary.

In addition, the operative record is a legal document, and detailed procedures are necessary should a medico-legal issue arise. In my review of operative dictations in medico-legal issues, I find operative reports are frequently inadequate and deficient in details of the operation. A sound operative report can address many issues that can potentially arise, and this book provides the necessary guidance in a format that will result in an excellent, comprehensive report even in the most complex procedures.

Another wonderful aspect of this book is that it serves as a verbal atlas for the 126 surgical procedures provided. A surgeon can read the examples of each procedure and, with previous understanding of anatomy and pathology, can know in detail, from start to finish, how the procedure is done. I find this a rewarding feature.

The authors, Professors Armenakas and Fracchia, are outstanding surgeons who have successfully demonstrated in this book the detailed methodology of composing an operative dictation. They have included Dr. Golan, the chief urology resident at Cornell, to have input and insight from a young surgeon, which adds diversity and completeness to the project.

This is a unique book and a "must" for every urologist.

Jack W. McAninch M.D, FACS, FRCS (Eng)(Hon)
Emeritus Professor of Urological Surgery
University of California San Francisco

Foreword

Preface

Teaching is the highest form of understanding.
——Aristotle——

The impetus for writing *Operative Dictations in Urologic Surgery* arose from the need for a dedicated operative dictation text that describes each surgical procedure in a stepwise, methodical, and detailed format. The available urologic surgical atlases, which are exceptional, provide a hybrid operative description combining high-level illustrations with a narrative. Our objective was to focus and expand on the narrative and create a step-by-step "cookbook"-type description in a comprehensive, all-inclusive operative dictation format. In addition, for each procedure we have included the indications, essential steps, variations and complications. Space is provided after each section to allow for user notes.

It was not possible to describe every operation with their infinite variations. Instead, we have chosen 126 of the most relevant adult and pediatric urologic surgical procedures, and included both open and minimally invasive techniques. Although there are many technical options for each procedure, ranging from the sutures used to the details of each surgical step, we have attempted to incorporate a comprehensive operative description that is accurate, informative, and universally applicable. Details including types of retractors, sutures, dressings, etc. are meant only as a guide and will understandably vary from surgeon to surgeon.

In undertaking the preparation of this textbook, we have referenced multiple texts and atlases, including *Hinman's Atlas of Urologic Surgery*, *Glenn's Urologic Surgery*, *Atlas of Urologic Clinics*, and *Campbell-Walsh Urology*. These valuable resources, coupled with our personal surgical experiences totaling more than 75 years in aggregate, provide the basis of this book. Each of us separately and independently reviewed and critiqued all of the material. For this reason, we decided not to assign authorship to any of the individual chapters.

We acknowledge and thank all our teachers and residents who have educated, guided, and inspired us throughout the years. It is our hope and expectation that *Operative Dictations in Urologic Surgery* will serve preoperatively as a valuable and informative resource in preparation for surgery and will assist postoperatively in creating a dictation that is comprehensive, accurate, and medico-legally sound. We are grateful for the opportunity to share these operative dictations with you and welcome your comments and suggestions.

Please send email communications to: operativedictations@gmail.com

SECTION I OPEN SURGERY

- *Adrenal*
- *Bladder*
- *Kidney*
- *Lymphatics*
- *Penis*
- *Prostate*
- *Testis and Scrotum*
- *Ureter*
- *Urethra*
- *Urinary Diversion*

Adrenal

1

Adrenalectomy

Indications

- Select adrenal tumors or metastases

Essential Steps

1) Perform the appropriate preoperative catecholamine blockade in patients with suspected pheochromocytoma.
2) Expose the adrenal gland and identify, dissect, and ligate the adrenal vein and inferior adrenal artery. With pheochromocytomas, this should be done initially prior to any adrenal manipulation in order to limit hemodynamic instability from blood pressure changes caused by catecholamine release. The anesthesiologist should be informed prior to any adrenal manipulation in these instances.
3) Gently mobilize the adrenal gland cranially and divide its superior vascular supply.
4) Using lateral and upward traction on the adrenal gland, divide the remaining medial vascular attachments.
5) Dissect the adrenal gland caudally off the kidney.
6) After removing the adrenal gland, inspect for renal or vascular bleeding and pleural tears.

Note These Variations

- The choice of incision is dependent on the anatomic characteristics of the tumor (including size, extension, and histology), the patient's body habitus, and the surgeon's preference and comfort. Large tumors, or locally invasive tumors extending superomedially, and bilateral tumors can be managed with a thoracoabdominal or transabdominal (e.g. Chevron) approach, respectively. Alternatively, a posterior approach may be considered in patients with small localized tumors.
- In cases of renal invasion by large adrenal carcinomas, *en bloc* resection of the adrenal gland and kidney should be performed.

Operative Dictations in Urologic Surgery, First Edition. Noel A. Armenakas, John A. Fracchia, and Ron Golan.
© 2019 John Wiley & Sons Ltd. Published 2019 by John Wiley & Sons Ltd.

- If there is any suspicion of lymphatic invasion, after removal of the adrenal gland a regional lymphadenectomy should be performed from the level of the renal vessels to the diaphragmatic crus.

Complications

- Bleeding
- Infection
- Hemodynamic instability
- Intraabdominal organ injury
- Pneumothorax
- Ileus
- Adrenal Insufficiency

Template Operative Dictation

Preoperative diagnosis: Adrenal tumor
Postoperative diagnosis: Same
Procedure: *Right/Left* adrenalectomy
Indications: The patient is a _____-year-old *male/female* with a ____cm *right/left* adrenal tumor presenting for an adrenalectomy.

> ***For pheochromocytoma*:** The biochemical evaluation was consistent with a pheochromocytoma and the appropriate preoperative medical management completed.

Description of Procedure: The indications, alternatives, benefits, and risks were discussed with the patient and informed consent was obtained.

The patient was brought onto the operating room table, positioned supine, and secured with a safety strap. Pneumatic compression devices were placed on the lower extremities.

After the administration of intravenous antibiotics and general endotracheal anesthesia, a 16 Fr urethral catheter was inserted into the bladder and connected to a drainage bag.

The patient was placed in the lateral decubitus position at a 45° angle with the lower leg flexed 90° and the upper leg extended. An axillary roll was positioned to protect the brachial plexus and a gel pad placed to support the back. Multiple pillows were used to pad beneath and between both the upper and lower extremities to ensure adequate cushioning. The kidney rest was elevated and the table flexed and adjusted horizontally, obtaining optimal flank exposure. The patient was secured to the table with 3 in. surgical tape and safety straps, and was prepped and draped in the standard sterile manner.

The radiographic images were in the room.

A time-out was completed, verifying the correct patient, surgical procedure, site, and positioning, prior to beginning the procedure.

The space between the 10th and 11th ribs was palpated and an incision made at this level from the mid-axillary line and extended medially to the lateral border of the rectus abdominis muscle. Using electrocautery, the latissimus dorsi and external oblique muscles were incised, exposing the underlying ribs. The intercostal attachments were transected, taking care to avoid injury to the pleura and neurovascular bundle on the inferior surface of the rib. The internal oblique muscle was divided with cautery and the transversus abdominis carefully split in the direction of its fibers, avoiding entry into the peritoneum. A generous paranephric space was created by sweeping the peritoneum medially and the retroperitoneal connective tissue superiorly and inferiorly. A self-retaining retractor (e.g. Bookwalter, Omni-Tract) was appropriately positioned to optimize exposure, using padding on each retractor blade.

The parietal peritoneum was incised on the white line of Toldt and the colon reflected medially, exposing Gerota's fascia.

> *On the right*: The hepatic flexure and duodenum were mobilized, freeing the kidney and adrenal gland within Gerota's fascia superiorly and medially. The hepatorenal ligament was divided sharply and the liver lifted cranially off the anterior surface of the adrenal gland. Gerota's fascia was incised, exposing the anterior surface of the kidney and adrenal gland. The lateral wall of the inferior vena cava was dissected and the insertion of the right adrenal vein identified posterolaterally. The right adrenal vein was carefully dissected, doubly ligated with 2-0 silk ties and divided. The inferior adrenal artery was then secured and similarly divided.
>
> *On the left*: The splenorenal ligament was mobilized and divided sharply freeing the kidney and adrenal gland within Gerota's fascia superiorly, and the spleen and pancreatic tail which was lifted cranially off the anterior surface of the adrenal gland. Gerota's fascia was incised exposing the anterior surface of the kidney and adrenal gland. The insertion of the left adrenal vein into the left renal vein was identified. The left adrenal vein was carefully dissected, doubly ligated with 2-0 silk ties, and divided. The inferior adrenal artery was then secured and similarly divided.

The dissection was continued cranially, using gentle downward traction from lateral to medial. Multiple small adrenal branches were ligated using *an electrothermal bipolar tissue sealing device (LigaSure)/surgical clips*, freeing all apical adrenal attachments. (*Alternatively, these vessels can be clamped, divided, and ligated with chromic or silk ties*). The adrenal gland was retracted laterally exposing the remaining medial vascular and lymphatic attachments, which were divided between surgical clips. Finally, the inferior surface of the adrenal gland was dissected off the renal capsule using sharp and blunt dissection, and meticulous hemostasis obtained with electrocautery.

Once the specimen was completely freed, it was removed and sent to pathology for evaluation. The retroperitoneum was irrigated with warm sterile saline and hemostasis was again confirmed. Prior to closure, the vascular stumps, visceral organs and pleura were inspected and found to be intact. The self-retaining retractor was removed, the kidney rest lowered, and the table taken out of flexion.

The incision was closed using running 1-0 polydioxanone (PDS) to approximate the three muscle layers individually, taking care not to entrap the neurovascular bundle. 3-0

chromic sutures were used on Scarpa's fascia and the skin approximated with a subcuticular 4-0 poliglecaprone (Monocryl) suture. A sterile dressing was applied and the patient repositioned supine.

At the end of the procedure, all counts were correct.

The patient tolerated the procedure well and was taken to the recovery room in satisfactory condition.

Estimated blood loss: Approximately _____ml

Bladder

2

Augmentation Cystoplasty

Indications

- Medically refractory neurogenic detrusor overactivity
- Poorly compliant bladder
- Idiopathic detrusor overactivity
- Inflammatory bladder conditions (e.g. interstitial cystitis, schistosomiasis, tuberculosis) with a resultant small, noncompliant bladder
- Previously diverted patients suitable for undiversion
- Intractable autonomic dysreflexia

Suitable candidates must be willing and able to catheterize and have normal renal function. They should be free of any small (if using ileum) or large (if using colon) bowel disease.

Essential Steps

1) Distend the bladder with normal saline through a urethral catheter.
2) Incise the posterior bladder wall from the level of the trigone toward the dome creating an anterior bladder flap.
3) Isolate and divide a segment of ileum (usually 20–25 cm) sufficient to reach the bladder comfortably and to allow an approximate four-hour interval between catheterizations after the bladder is "stretched" over the postoperative period. Use transillumination to identify the vascular arcades.
4) Perform a functional end-to-end ileo-ileal anastomosis, restoring bowel continuity.
5) Fold the posterior segment of opened ileum and close its posterior wall.
6) Suture the open segment of isolated ileum to the previously opened bladder wall.
7) Place a drain.

Note These Variations

- A preoperative bowel prep is optional.
- A colocystoplasty or, rarely, a ureterocystoplasty can be used in select patients.

Operative Dictations in Urologic Surgery, First Edition. Noel A. Armenakas, John A. Fracchia, and Ron Golan.
© 2019 John Wiley & Sons Ltd. Published 2019 by John Wiley & Sons Ltd.

- The patient may be positioned with their legs in universal (Allen) stirrups and placed in modified Trendelenburg to enhance exposure.
- Alternatively, a suprapubic longitudinal incision (modified Pfannenstiel) may be used.
- In select cases, ureteral reimplantation and/or a continent catheterizable stoma may need to be performed.
- The ileo-ileal anastomosis may be hand-sewn, using a two-layer technique.
- A suprapubic tube with or without a urethral catheter can be used for drainage.

Complications

- Bleeding
- Infection
- Ileus/bowel obstruction
- Bowel injury/leak
- Urine leak (enterocystoplasty)
- Urinary incontinence
- Stone formation
- Spontaneous perforation

Template Operative Dictation

Preoperative diagnosis: Neurogenic bladder
Postoperative diagnosis: Same
Procedure: Augmentation cystoplasty
Indications: The patient is a ____-year-old *male/female* with a severely debilitating poorly compliant bladder presenting for augmentation cystoplasty.
Description of Procedure: The indications, alternatives, benefits, and risks were discussed with the *patient/patient's family* and informed consent was obtained.

The patient was brought onto the operating room table, positioned supine, and secured with a safety strap. All pressure points were carefully padded and pneumatic compression devices were placed on the lower extremities.

After the administration of intravenous antibiotics and general endotracheal anesthesia, the lower abdomen and external genitalia were prepped and draped in the standard sterile manner.

A time-out was completed, verifying the correct patient, surgical procedure, and positioning, prior to beginning the procedure.

A ___Fr urethral catheter was inserted into the bladder and the bladder distended with sterile normal saline to aid in dissection of the bladder wall from the peritoneum.

A midline abdominal incision was made from the umbilicus to the pubic symphysis. The subcutaneous tissue was incised with electrocautery, exposing the underlying rectus abdominis aponeurosis. This was incised at the linea alba and the rectus abdominis muscles separated at the midline and retracted laterally, taking care not to injure the underlying inferior epigastric vessels.

The peritoneum was freed posteriorly to the level of the trigone and the bowel was thoroughly packed into the upper abdomen. A self-retaining retractor (e.g. Bookwalter,

Omni-Tract, Balfour) was appropriately positioned to optimize exposure, using padding on each retractor blade. The bladder wall was identified and four 2-0 polyglactin (Vicryl) sutures were used to outline a wide U-shaped posterior incision extending from the bladder dome to an area just superior to where the ureters enter the bladder; this created a large, anteriorly based bladder flap with a posteriorly facing opening.

The bowel packing was removed and attention was focused on isolating an appropriate ileal segment. The distal ileum was inspected and a 25 cm segment of ileum was chosen, 15–20 cm from the ileocecal valve and marked with a silk suture. With the aid of transillumination, the ileocolic and right colic arteries were identified. An avascular mesenteric window was opened on each side of the desired ileal segment using an electrothermal bipolar tissue sealing device (LigaSure) to incise and ligate the mesentery on both sides, avoiding injury to the main intestinal vasculature. *(Alternatively, the mesentery can be incised and its blood vessels individually clamped, divided and doubly ligated with chromic or silk ties.)* Additional hemostasis was achieved using 3-0 *chromic/ silk* ties. The isolated ileal segment was transected at its proximal and distal antimesenteric borders, using a GIA60 stapler.

The continuity of the distal ileum was restored using a stapled technique as follows: The antimesenteric corners of the proximal and distal ileal segments were identified, and a small segment of tissue was resected off each end of the stapled suture lines. One limb of the GIA60 stapler was inserted into the proximal and the other into the distal ileal segment with care taken not to injure the bowel mesentery. The ileal segments were rotated ensuring that the antimesenteric bowel walls faced each other prior to firing the stapler. Four small clamps were then placed on the ends of the transected bowel. The two clamps on the lines of the original bowel transection were held together, while the others were spread apart, creating a wide opening. A TA55 stapler was used to complete the functional end-to-end ileoileal anastomosis. The staple line was checked confirming its integrity, and additionally reinforced with interrupted 3-0 silk sutures. The mesenteric window was closed with a running 4-0 chromic to avoid internal herniation. The ileoileal anastomosis was returned to its natural position in the abdomen with the isolated ileal segment placed caudal to it.

Attention was then turned to the isolated ileal segment, which was opened at its antimesenteric border. Both staple lines were resected to avoid subsequent stone formation. The bladder mucosa was copiously irrigated with sterile normal saline. The posterior wall of the ileal segment was folded back on itself and sutured together with running, locking 3-0 Vicryl sutures, creating a bowel cup to be anastomosed to the bladder.

The augmentation opening in the bladder was measured and the superoanterior wall of the ileal segment was closed with interrupted 3-0 Vicryl sutures to match this opening. The configured ileal segment was sewn onto the opened bladder using running, locking 3-0 Vicryl sutures, proceeding from the most inferoposterior aspect cephalad.

An 18 Fr urethral catheter was inserted into the bladder and the bladder distended with 300 ml sterile normal saline confirming a watertight reconstruction. *(Note: If a suprapubic tube is desired for drainage, it can be placed through the lateral bladder wall, not through the ileal segment.)*

Having completed the enterocystoplasty, the abdomen was irrigated with warm sterile normal saline and examined for any bleeding. Meticulous hemostasis was obtained. A surgical drain (e.g. Jackson-Pratt) was placed in the retroperitoneum and brought out at the skin through a separate stab incision, where it was secured with a 2-0 silk suture.

Prior to closure, the ureters, bladder, bowel, mesentery and abdominal wall were inspected and found to be intact without any evidence of devascularization or injury.

The self-retaining retractor was removed and the abdominal incision was closed using a running 2-0 chromic to approximate the rectus muscles and 1-0 polydioxanone (PDS) for the rectus aponeurosis. 3-0 chromic sutures were used on Scarpa's fascia and the skin approximated with a subcuticular 4-0 poliglecaprone (Monocryl) suture. The incision was reinforced with sterile adhesive strips and a sterile dressing applied. The urethral catheter was connected to a drainage bag.

At the end of the procedure, all counts were correct.

The patient tolerated the procedure well and was taken to the recovery room in satisfactory condition.

Estimated blood loss: Approximately _____ml

3

Bladder Diverticulectomy

Indications

- Symptomatic bladder diverticulum (recurrent infections, irritative or obstructive voiding symptoms, hematuria, bladder calculi, etc.)
- Select intradiverticular bladder tumors

Essential Steps

1) Partially fill the bladder through a urethral catheter.
2) Expose the bladder, sweep the peritoneum superiorly and make a vertical mid-anterior cystotomy.
3) Resect the diverticulum using a combined intra- and extravesical approach.
4) Close the diverticular rent and the midline cystotomy in two layers using absorbable sutures.
5) Place a urethral catheter and a drain.

Note These Variations

- Alternatively, a suprapubic longitudinal incision (modified Pfannenstiel) may be used.
- If the procedure is performed for an intradiverticular tumor, it is important to isolate the diverticulum. Laparotomy pads can be used and the mouth of the diverticulum occluded with a sponge to avoid tumor spillage.
- Small diverticula often can be managed with an entirely intravesical approach by eversion and resection.
- For paraureteral diverticula, the patency of the ureter can be further evaluated with the intravenous injection of dye (methylene blue or indigo carmine). If there has been suspected compromise to the ureter, it should be repaired and a double-J stent placed.
- Diverticula located laterally or posteriorly may require concomitant ureteral reimplantation. In such cases bladder mobilization can be facilitated by ligating the superior vesical pedicle.

Operative Dictations in Urologic Surgery, First Edition. Noel A. Armenakas, John A. Fracchia, and Ron Golan.
© 2019 John Wiley & Sons Ltd. Published 2019 by John Wiley & Sons Ltd.

Complications

- Bleeding
- Infection
- Ureteral injury/obstruction
- Urine leak/urinoma
- Bowel/vascular injury
- Lymphocele
- Recurrent diverticulum

Template Operative Dictation

Preoperative diagnosis: *Symptomatic bladder diverticulum/Intradiverticular bladder tumor*
Postoperative diagnosis: Same
Procedure: Bladder diverticulectomy
Indications: The patient is a _____ -year-old *male/female* with *a symptomatic bladder diverticulum/an intradiverticular bladder tumor* presenting for a diverticulectomy.
Description of Procedure: The indications, alternatives, benefits, and risks were discussed with the patient and informed consent was obtained.

The patient was brought onto the operating room table, positioned supine, and secured with a safety strap. All pressure points were carefully padded and pneumatic compression devices were placed on the lower extremities.

After the administration of intravenous antibiotics and *general endotracheal/regional* anesthesia, the entire abdomen and genitalia were prepped and draped in the standard sterile manner.

A time-out was completed, verifying the correct patient, surgical procedure, and positioning, prior to beginning the procedure.

The radiographic images were in the room.

An 18 Fr urethral catheter was inserted into the bladder and filled with 200 ml sterile normal saline.

A midline abdominal incision was made from just below the umbilicus to the pubic symphysis. The subcutaneous tissue was incised with electrocautery, exposing the underlying rectus abdominis aponeurosis. This was incised at the linea alba and the rectus abdominis muscles separated at the midline and retracted laterally, taking care not to injure the underlying inferior epigastric vessels. A self-retaining retractor (e.g. Bookwalter, Omni-Tract, Balfour) was appropriately positioned to optimize exposure, using padding on each retractor blade.

The peritoneum was swept superiorly after incising the perivesical fat just below the peritoneal reflection, and two 2-0 chromic stay sutures were placed into the mid-anterior bladder wall. A 1 cm full-thickness vertical stab incision was made between these using electrocautery. The partially filled bladder was drained using suction. Allis clamps were placed on both edges of the cystotomy, which was extended cranially and caudally, exposing the entire bladder.

The urethral catheter was removed and the bladder was thoroughly inspected confirming the absence of any tumors or foreign bodies. The bladder wall was

minimally/moderately/significantly/not trabeculated, with a normal appearing mucosa. Both ureteral orifices were in the normal anatomic position with clear urinary efflux noted bilaterally. The diverticulum was identified on the _____*(location)*_____ wall.

The *right/left* ureteral orifice was intubated with a *5 Fr open-ended catheter/infant feeding tube*.

An index finger was placed within the mouth of the diverticulum and lifted anteriorly. With intravesical finger control, using blunt and sharp dissection, the diverticular neck was carefully mobilized extravesically. The dissection was continued circumferentially, freeing the diverticulum from the adjacent tissues. The neck of the diverticulum was completely transected and the specimen was removed and sent to pathology for evaluation. Meticulous hemostasis was achieved with electrocautery. The resulting rent in the bladder was closed in two layers with running 3-0 and 2-0 polyglactin (Vicryl) sutures on the mucosal and muscularis/adventitial layers, respectively.

The distal *right/left* ureter was noted to be intact and the *open-ended catheter/infant feeding tube* removed. A new 18 Fr urethral catheter was inserted into the bladder and connected to a drainage bag.

The midline cystotomy was similarly closed in two layers with Vicryl sutures.

The patency of the repair was confirmed by irrigating the urethral catheter with 300 ml sterile normal saline.

> **If a lymphadenectomy is performed:** A bilateral pelvic lymph node dissection was performed beginning on the *left/right*. The iliac vessels were exposed from just above the common iliac bifurcation to the femoral canal. The ureters were identified anteriorly at the bifurcation of the external and internal iliac vessels and protected. The lymph nodes appeared *unremarkable/enlarged/matted* on palpation. The nodal dissection was started at the medial aspect of the *left/right* external iliac artery by incising the perivascular fibroareolar sheath. Using gentle medial traction, the obturator neurovascular bundle was identified posteriorly and preserved. The dissection was carried laterally to the genitofemoral nerve and medially to the ipsilateral ureter. The cranial and caudal limits of dissection were the common iliac bifurcation and femoral canal (node of Cloquet), respectively. Small vessels and lymphatic branches were fulgurated or ligated with surgical clips to maintain meticulous hemo- and lymphostasis. A large surgical clip was used to individually secure the distal and proximal extents of lymph node packet. The nodal packet was removed and sent to pathology for evaluation.
>
> The contralateral lymph node dissection was performed in a similar manner and the nodal packet sent to pathology for evaluation.

Prior to closure, the operative field was inspected for bleeding or injury, and the pelvis was irrigated with warm sterile water. A surgical drain (e.g. Jackson-Pratt) was placed in the pelvis and brought out at the skin through a separate stab incision, where it was secured with a 2-0 silk suture.

The self-retaining retractor was removed and the abdominal incision was closed using a running 2-0 chromic to approximate the rectus muscles and 1-0 polydioxanone (PDS) for the rectus aponeurosis. 3-0 chromic sutures were used on Scarpa's fascia

and the skin approximated with a subcuticular 4-0 poliglecaprone (Monocryl) suture. A sterile dressing was applied.

At the end of the procedure, all counts were correct.

The patient tolerated the procedure well and was taken to the recovery room in satisfactory condition.

Estimated blood loss: Approximately _____ml

4

Cystolithotomy

Indications

- Select bladder stones (e.g. > 6 cm, hard consistency, multiple bladder stones, failed cystolithotripsy, stone(s) within a diverticulum, procedure performed in conjunction with an open prostatectomy or diverticulectomy)

Essential Steps

1) Partially fill the bladder through a urethral catheter.
2) Expose the bladder, sweep the peritoneum superiorly, and make a vertical mid-anterior cystotomy.
3) Remove all stones and inspect the bladder.
4) Close the midline cystotomy in two layers with absorbable sutures.
5) Maintain a urethral catheter.

Note these Variations

- Alternatively, an infraumbilical midline abdominal incision may be used.
- The use of a suprapubic tube and a drain are optional.

Complications

- Bleeding
- Infection
- Urine leak/urinoma
- Urinary retention

Operative Dictations in Urologic Surgery, First Edition. Noel A. Armenakas, John A. Fracchia, and Ron Golan.
© 2019 John Wiley & Sons Ltd. Published 2019 by John Wiley & Sons Ltd.

Template Operative Dictation

Preoperative diagnosis: Bladder calculus(i)
Postoperative diagnosis: Same
Procedure: Cystolithotomy
Indications: The patient is a _____ -year-old *male/female* with *a ____cm/multiple* bladder stone(s) presenting for a cystolithotomy.
Description of Procedure: The indications, alternatives, benefits, and risks were discussed with the patient and informed consent was obtained.

The patient was brought onto the operating room table, positioned supine, and secured with a safety strap. All pressure points were carefully padded and pneumatic compression devices were placed on the lower extremities.

After the administration of intravenous antibiotics and *general/regional* anesthesia, the abdomen and genitalia were prepped and draped in the standard sterile manner.

A time-out was completed, verifying the correct patient, surgical procedure, and positioning, prior to beginning the procedure.

An 18 Fr urethral catheter was inserted into the bladder and filled with 200 ml sterile normal saline.

An 8 cm longitudinal incision was made 2 cm above the pubic symphysis *(modified Pfannenstiel)*. The subcutaneous tissue was incised with electrocautery, exposing the underlying rectus abdominis aponeurosis. This was incised at the linea alba and the rectus abdominis muscles separated at the midline and retracted laterally, taking care not to injure the underlying inferior epigastric vessels. A self-retaining retractor (e.g. Balfour) was appropriately positioned to optimize exposure, using padding on each retractor blade.

The perivesical fat was incised just below the peritoneal reflection and the perito-neum swept superiorly. Two, 2-0 chromic stay sutures were placed into the mid-anterior bladder wall. A 1 cm full-thickness vertical stab incision was made between these using electrocautery. The partially filled bladder was drained using suction and Allis clamps placed on both edges of the cystotomy, which was extended cranially and caudally for a total distance of 5 cm. The bladder stone(s) *was/were* visualized at the base, removed using Randall forceps and sent for chemical analysis. The bladder was thoroughly inspected confirming the absence of any tumors, foreign bodies, or diverticula. The bladder wall was *minimally/moderately/significantly/not* trabecu-lated, with a normal appearing mucosa. Both ureteral orifices were in the normal anatomic position with clear urinary efflux noted bilaterally.

The cystotomy was closed in two layers using 3-0 and 2-0 polyglactin (Vicryl) sutures on the mucosal and muscularis/adventitial layers, respectively. Meticulous hemostasis was achieved using electrocautery. The patency of the repair was confirmed by irrigating the urethral catheter with 300 ml sterile normal saline, and the catheter connected to a drainage bag. A surgical drain (e.g. Jackson-Pratt, 0.25 in. Penrose) was placed in the space of Retzius away from the cystotomy and brought out through a separate stab incision, where it was secured at the skin with a 2-0 silk suture. Prior to closure, the operative field was inspected and found to be intact without evidence of bleeding or injury.

The self-retaining retractor was removed and the abdominal incision closed using a running 2-0 chromic to approximate the rectus muscles and a running 1-0 polydioxanone (PDS) for the rectus aponeurosis. 3-0 chromic sutures were used on Scarpa's fascia and

the skin approximated with a subcuticular 4-0 poliglecaprone (Monocryl) suture. A sterile dressing was applied.

At the end of the procedure, all counts were correct.

The patient tolerated the procedure well and was taken to the recovery room in satisfactory condition.

Estimated blood loss: Approximately _____ml

5

Enterovesical Fistula Repair (with Omental Flap)

Indications

- Enterovesical fistula

Essential Steps

1) Identify the fistulous area and separate the adherent enteric segment from the bladder.
2) Resect the diseased bowel and perform a functional end-to-end enteric anastomosis.
3) Debride the fistulous tract and close the bladder in two layers using absorbable sutures.
4) Cover the repair with an omental flap.
5) Place a drain and maintain a urethral catheter.

Note These Variations

- A preoperative bowel prep is optional.
- The enteric anastomosis can be hand sewn using a two-layer technique.
- A multistage procedure may be required, depending on the clinical situation.

Complications

- Bleeding
- Infection
- Ileus/bowel obstruction
- Bowel injury/leak
- Urine leak/urinoma
- Recurrent fistula

Operative Dictations in Urologic Surgery, First Edition. Noel A. Armenakas, John A. Fracchia, and Ron Golan.
© 2019 John Wiley & Sons Ltd. Published 2019 by John Wiley & Sons Ltd.

Template Operative Dictation

Preoperative diagnosis: Enterovesical fistula
Postoperative diagnosis: Same
Procedure: Resection of enterovesical fistula
Indication: The patient is a _____ -year-old *male/female* presenting for resection of an enterovesical fistula.
Description of Procedure: The indications, alternatives, benefits, and risks were discussed with the. patient and informed consent was obtained.

The patient was brought onto the operating room table, positioned supine and secured with a safety strap. All pressure points were carefully padded and pneumatic compression devices were placed on the lower extremities.

After the administration of intravenous antibiotics and general endotracheal anesthesia, the patient's entire abdomen was prepped and draped in the standard sterile manner.

A time-out was completedn verifying the correct patient, surgical procedure, and positioning, prior to beginning the procedure.

A 20 Fr urethral catheter was inserted into the bladder and connected to a drainage bag.

A midline abdominal incision was made starting just above the umbilicus and carried down to the pubic symphysis. The subcutaneous tissue was incised with electrocautery, exposing the underlying rectus abdominis aponeurosis. This was incised at the linea alba and the rectus abdominis muscles separated at the midline and retracted laterally, taking care not to injure the underlying inferior epigastric vessels.

The peritoneal cavity was entered sharply and several intestinal adhesions were carefully lysed, avoiding injury to the bowel. A self-retaining retractor (e.g. Bookwalter, Omni-Tract, Balfour) was appropriately positioned to optimize exposure, using padding one each retractor blade. The peritoneal contents were examined and there was no evidence of any inflammatory disease outside of the pelvis, where the *sigmoid/descending/ascending colon//ileum* was noted to be adherent to the *dome/posterior wall* of the urinary bladder. The fistulous tract was identified and the adherent bowel segment separated from the bladder wall using sharp and blunt dissection.

The diseased enteric segment measured approximately _____cm. The mesentery on both sides of the diseased segment was incised using an electrothermal bipolar tissue sealing device (LigaSure), and the bowel transected using a GIA60 stapler. The entire specimen was sent to pathology for evaluation.

The continuity of the bowel was restored with a stapled anastomosis as follows: The antimesenteric corners of the proximal and distal *colonic/ileal* segments were identified and a small segment of tissue was resected off each end of the stapled suture lines. One limb of the GIA60 stapler was inserted into the proximal and the other into the distal segment with care taken not to injure the bowel mesentery. The bowel segments were rotated ensuring that the antimesenteric walls faced each other prior to firing the stapler. Four small clamps were then placed on the ends of the transected bowel. The two clamps on the lines of the original bowel transection were held together, while the others were spread apart, creating a wide opening. A TA55 stapler was used to complete the functional end-to-end *colonic/ileal* anastomosis. The staple line was checked, confirming its integrity, and additionally reinforced with interrupted 3-0 silk sutures. The mesenteric window was closed with a running 4-0 chromic suture to avoid internal herniation. Meticulous hemostasis was obtained throughout the procedure.

Having completed the bowel resection and anastomosis, attention was focused on the bladder. The fistulous tract was thoroughly debrided and the bladder inspected. There was no additional intravesical pathology, and both ureters were identified with clear efflux seen bilaterally.

The bladder wall was closed in two layers using 3-0 and 2-0 polyglactin (Vicryl) sutures on the mucosal and muscularis/adventitial layers, respectively. The patency of the repair was confirmed by irrigating the urethral catheter with 300 ml sterile normal saline.

An omental flap was created by mobilizing the greater omentum off the stomach, preserving the right gastroepiploic artery. The left gastroepiploic artery was ligated using 2-0 silk ties and divided close to its origin at the splenic artery. The short gastric arteries were individually ligated with 3-0 silk ties and the omentum was dissected off the greater gastric curvature. The well-vascularized omental flap was brought down to the pelvis to cover the cystorrhaphy and sutured to the bladder wall with interrupted 3-0 chromic sutures.

A surgical drain (e.g. Jackson-Pratt, 0.25 in. Penrose) was placed in the space of Retzius and brought out through a separate cutaneous incision where it was secured at the skin with a 2-0 silk suture. The wound was irrigated with warm sterile saline and hemostasis again confirmed. Prior to closure, the abdominal vessels and visceral organs were inspected and found to be intact without evidence of devascularization or injury.

The self-retaining retractor was removed and the abdominal incision was closed using a running 2-0 chromic to approximate the rectus muscles and 1-0 polydioxanone (PDS) for the rectus aponeurosis. 3-0 chromic sutures were used on Scarpa's fascia and the skin approximated with a subcuticular 4-0 poliglecaprone (Monocryl) suture. A sterile dressing was applied.

At the end of the procedure, all counts were correct.

The patient tolerated the procedure well and was taken to the recovery room in satisfactory condition.

Estimated blood loss: Approximately _____ml.

6

Insertion of a Sacral Neuromodulation Device

Indications

- Medically refractory overactive bladder
- Urge urinary incontinence
- Nonobstructive urinary retention

Essential Steps

1) Identify and mark the S3 foramen utilizing anatomic landmarks and fluoroscopy.
2) Insert the tined lead under fluoroscopic guidance adjacent to the S3 sacral nerve root, confirming placement by ipsilateral great toe flexion or pelvic floor contractions ("bellows").
3) Tunnel the lead to a subcutaneous pocket and connect it to the neuromodulation device.

Note These Variations

- A percutaneous peripheral nerve evaluation may be undertaken to assess the anticipated therapeutic response. This is commonly performed in the office/outpatient setting under local anesthesia, after which time the patient is instructed to maintain a voiding diary over a period of 72 hours with the temporary test stimulation leads in position. If the patient experiences a favorable response, the surgeon may proceed to implantation of a sacral neuromodulation device (full implant).
- If there is no response following Stage 1, the test stimulation lead may be removed in the office/outpatient setting. If there is an appropriate response following Stage 1, a Stage 2 may be performed whereby the pulse generator is implanted.

Operative Dictations in Urologic Surgery, First Edition. Noel A. Armenakas, John A. Fracchia, and Ron Golan.
© 2019 John Wiley & Sons Ltd. Published 2019 by John Wiley & Sons Ltd.

Complications

- Bleeding
- Infection
- Persistent voiding symptoms
- Neuropathic pain
- Nerve injury

Template Operative Dictation

Preoperative diagnosis: Overactive bladder
Postoperative diagnosis: Same
Procedure: Stage ___ insertion of a sacral neuromodulation device (i.e. InterStim)
Indications: The patient is a ___ -year-old *male/female* with *medically refractory overactive bladder/nonobstructive urinary retention* presenting for insertion of a sacral neuromodulation device.

Description of Procedure

Stage 1

The indications, alternatives, benefits, and risks were discussed with the patient and informed consent was obtained.

The patient was brought onto the operating room table, placed prone, and secured with a safety strap. Care was taken to ensure that all pressure points were carefully padded and the toes left visible and free beyond the table.

After delivery of preoperative intravenous antibiotics and intravenous sedating agents, the patient was prepped and draped in the standard sterile manner including the lower back, buttocks, gluteal cleft, and anus.

A time-out was completed, verifying the correct patient, surgical procedure, and positioning, prior to beginning the procedure.

Fluoroscopy was used to identify the position of the S3 foramen and the overlying skin was marked. The patient was administered __ ml of local anesthetic *(specify)* subcutaneously. A ___ inch foramen needle was inserted into the superior, medial aspect of the S3 foramen with placement confirmed by fluoroscopy. Appropriate positioning was confirmed by eliciting the plantar flexion of the great toes as well as bellowing of the perineum using the external neurostimulator. A 1 cm incision was made in the skin. The foramen needle was removed from the sheath and a guidewire inserted through the lumen. A dilator was passed over the wire and fluoroscopy used to confirm its position within the canal. The dilator and guidewire were removed and replaced with the tined lead through the sheath. The stimulation lead was advanced under fluoroscopy until the first two electrodes had cleared the anterior sacrum and the third was approximately at the distal border. The four electrodes were tested utilizing the external stimulator, with the desired response elicited on all four electrodes. The sheath was removed under fluoroscopy with the tines remaining in the appropriate position.

A 3 cm incision for the subcutaneous pocket was made below the *right/left* iliac crest and lateral to the sacrum after administration of __ ml of local anesthetic *(specify)*. The space

was bluntly dissected to create a small pocket, and hemostasis was obtained using electrocautery. A tunneling sheath was passed from the site of the stimulation lead incision to the subcutaneous pocket, with the stimulation lead threaded through the sheath. The sheath was withdrawn with the stimulation lead exiting from the subcutaneous pocket. The stimulation lead was cleaned and dried prior to securing to the temporary external percutaneous extension. The connection components were placed into the subcutaneous pocket and the percutaneous extension was further tunneled and externalized.

The subcutaneous pouch was irrigated with antibiotic solution and excellent hemostasis obtained. The deep dermal layer was reapproximated with 2-0 interrupted polyglactin (Vicryl) sutures. The skin was closed with a 4-0 subcuticular poliglecaprone (Monocryl) suture and reinforced with sterile adhesive strips. A sterile dressing was applied and the patient was repositioned supine on the stretcher.

At the end of the procedure, all counts were correct.

The patient tolerated the procedure well and was taken to the recovery room in satisfactory condition.

The patient was instructed to complete a voiding diary during the follow-up period.

Estimated blood loss: Approximately _____ml

Stage 2

The indications, alternatives, benefits, and risks were discussed with the patient and informed consent was obtained.

The patient was brought onto the operating room table, placed prone, and secured with a safety strap. Care was taken to ensure that all pressure points were carefully padded and the toes left visible and free beyond the table.

After delivery of preoperative intravenous antibiotics and intravenous sedating agents, the patient was prepped and draped in the standard sterile manner, incorporating the temporary extension, lower back, buttocks, gluteal cleft, and anus. An iodine-impregnated incision drape (e.g. Ioban) was placed over the prepped field.

A time-out was completed, verifying the correct patient, surgical procedure, and positioning, prior to beginning the procedure.

The previous incision overlying the subcutaneous pocket was opened with a combination of sharp and blunt dissection and the connection components exposed. The temporary percutaneous extension was disconnected from the stimulation lead and removed from the field. The stimulation lead was cleaned and dried, and connected to the pulse generator. The subcutaneous pocket was bluntly dilated to accommodate the pulse generator, and the components were buried within the pocket. The pouch was irrigated with antibiotic solution and excellent hemostasis obtained.

The deep dermal layer was reapproximated with 2-0 interrupted polyglactin (Vicryl) sutures. The skin was closed with a 4-0 subcuticular poliglecaprone (Monocryl) suture and reinforced with sterile adhesive strips. A sterile dressing was applied and the patient was repositioned supine on the stretcher.

At the end of the procedure, all counts were correct.

The patient tolerated the procedure well and was taken to the recovery room in satisfactory condition.

Estimated blood loss: Approximately _____ml

7

Partial Cystectomy

Indications

- Select solitary urothelial cell carcinomas without associated carcinoma in situ, where an adequate surgical margin can be obtained
- Urachal adenocarcinoma

Essential Steps

1) Explore the pelvis to assess bladder mobility and the abdominal contents for visible or palpable metastatic disease.
2) Properly pack the bowel to optimize the operative field and mobilize the bladder.
3) Perform a bilateral pelvic lymph node dissection.
4) *For urothelial cell carcinoma*: Ligate and divide the urachus and use this for traction. Resect the bladder tumor with a 1 cm margin of normal bladder and remove the entire specimen with its overlying perivesical fat and peritoneum. Send the normal bladder wound edges for frozen section.
   For urachal adenocarcinoma: Excise the umbilicus and follow the course of the urachus to the bladder dome. Resect a segment of the bladder dome and remove the entire specimen (umbilicus, urachus, and bladder dome) *en bloc*, avoiding tumor spillage.
5) Close the bladder in two layers.
6) Place a urethral catheter and drain.

Note these Variations

- The patient may be positioned with his or her legs in (Allen) universal stirrups and placed in modified Trendelenburg to enhance exposure.
- Cystoscopy may be performed at the start of the case to delineate the extent of the tumor.
- Tumors located laterally or posteriorly may require concomitant ureteral reimplantation. In such cases, bladder mobilization can be facilitated by ligating the superior vesical pedicle.

Operative Dictations in Urologic Surgery, First Edition. Noel A. Armenakas, John A. Fracchia, and Ron Golan.
© 2019 John Wiley & Sons Ltd. Published 2019 by John Wiley & Sons Ltd.

- An extended or standard pelvic lymph node dissection can be performed prior to or following the partial cystectomy, depending on surgeon preference.
- The lymph nodes may be removed and sent separately based on their anatomic origin rather than as one packet from each side. This may allow for a more thorough histologic lymph node evaluation.

Complications

- Bleeding
- Infection
- Ureteral injury/obstruction
- Urine leak/urinoma
- Bowel/vascular injury
- Tumor spillage/implantation

Template Operative Dictation

Preoperative diagnosis: *Invasive localized bladder cancer/Urachal adenocarcinoma*
Postoperative diagnosis: Same
Procedure: Partial cystectomy
Indications: The patient is a ____ -year-old *male/female* with a *clinical stage T* ___ *urothelial cell carcinoma/urachal adeno*carcinoma presenting for a partial cystectomy.
Description of Procedure: The indications, alternatives, benefits, and risks were discussed with the patient and informed consent was obtained.

The patient was brought onto the operating room table, positioned supine, and secured with a safety strap. Pneumatic compression devices were placed on the lower extremities.

After the administration of intravenous antibiotics and initiation of general endotracheal anesthesia, the patient was positioned with the break just above the anterosuperior iliac spine, and the operating table flexed 15°. The entire abdomen and genitalia were prepped and draped in the standard sterile manner.

The radiographic images were in the room.

A time-out was completed, verifying the correct patient, surgical procedure, and positioning, prior to beginning the procedure.

A 16 Fr urethral catheter was inserted into the bladder and connected to a drainage bag.

A midline abdominal incision was made from the umbilicus to the pubic symphysis. The subcutaneous tissue was incised with electrocautery, exposing the underlying rectus abdominis aponeurosis. This was incised at the linea alba and the rectus abdominis muscles separated at the midline and retracted laterally, taking care not to injure the underlying inferior epigastric vessels.

The space of Retzius was developed by sweeping the infrapubic space posterolaterally and mobilizing the peritoneum cranially on both sides along the pelvic sidewall. Blunt dissection was used to expose the endopelvic fascia inferiorly and the obturator nerve and vessels posteriorly. The bladder was carefully palpated and noted to be mobile without fixation to the pelvic sidewall or adjacent organs. The *vas deferens/round ligaments*

were ligated and divided to facilitate mobilization of the peritoneal sac, and the perito-neum was entered above the umbilicus. A systematic intraabdominal exploration was performed, confirming the absence of hepatic metastases or retroperitoneal lymphadenopathy.

> ***For urothelial cell carcinoma***: The urachus was ligated with a 2-0 silk tie, divided, and traced caudally to the bladder dome.

> ***For urachal adenocarcinoma***: The urachus was identified and traced to the umbilicus cranially and the bladder caudally. The umbilicus was circumferentially excised, maintaining its continuity with the urachus. An Allis clamp was placed on the umbilicus for traction.

The ascending and descending colon were mobilized along the white line of Toldt. The root of the small bowel mesentery was dissected off the retroperitoneum, provid-ing sufficient cephalad bowel mobility. The bowel was thoroughly packed and a self-retaining retractor (e.g. Bookwalter, Omni-Tract, Balfour) was appropriately positioned to optimize exposure, using padding one each retractor blade.

A bilateral pelvic lymph node dissection was performed, beginning on the *left/right*. The iliac vessels were exposed from just above the common iliac bifurcation to the femo-ral canal. The ureters were identified anteriorly at the bifurcation of the external and internal iliac vessels and protected. The lymph nodes appeared *unremarkable/enlarged/matted* on palpation. The nodal dissection was started at the medial aspect of the *left/right* external iliac artery by incising the perivascular fibroareolar sheath. Using gentle medial traction, the obturator neurovascular bundle was identified posteriorly and pre-served. The dissection was carried laterally to the genitofemoral and medially to the ipsilateral ureter. The cranial and caudal limits of dissection were the common iliac bifurcation and femoral canal (node of Cloquet), respectively. Small vessels and lym-phatic branches were fulgurated or ligated with surgical clips to maintain meticulous hemo- and lymphostasis. A large surgical clip was used to individually secure the distal and proximal extents of the lymph node packet. The nodal packet was removed and sent to pathology for evaluation.

The contralateral lymph node dissection was performed in a similar manner and the nodal packet sent to pathology for evaluation.

> ***For urothelial carcinoma***: The bladder tumor was palpated at the *dome//posterior/lateral wall* and, using electrocautery, the tumor was superficially circumscribed leaving a 1 cm margin of surrounding normal bladder. 2-0 chromic stay sutures were placed lateral to the marked area for traction. The entire segment with its overlying perivesical fat was removed *en bloc* and sent to pathology for evaluation. Additionally, biopsies of the adjacent normal bladder wall were sent for frozen section evaluation, confirming a clear surgical margin.

> ***For urachal adenocarcinoma***: A 3 cm area at the bladder dome corresponding to the urachal remnant was circumscribed using electrocautery. 2-0 chromic stay sutures were placed lateral to the marked area for traction. A circumferential full-thickness 3 cm segment of bladder wall was excised and removed en *bloc* with the urachus and umbilicus and sent to pathology for evaluation.

The bladder was closed in two layers using 3-0 and 2-0 polyglactin (Vicryl) sutures on the mucosal and muscularis/adventitial layers, respectively. The patency of the repair was confirmed by irrigating the urethral catheter with 300 ml sterile normal saline.

A surgical drain (e.g. Jackson-Pratt, 0.25 in. Penrose) was placed in the space of Retzius, and brought out through a separate cutaneous incision where it was secured at the skin with a 2-0 silk suture. The pelvis was irrigated with warm sterile saline. Prior to closure, the iliac vessels, colon and intraabdominal and pelvic structures were inspected and found to be intact.

The self-retaining retractor was removed and the abdominal incision was closed using a running 2-0 chromic to approximate the rectus muscles and 1-0 polydioxanone (PDS) for the rectus aponeurosis. 3-0 chromic sutures were used on Scarpa's fascia and the skin approximated with a subcuticular 4-0 poliglecaprone (Monocryl) suture. A sterile dressing was applied.

At the end of the procedure, all counts were correct.

The patient tolerated the procedure well and was taken to the recovery room in satisfactory condition.

Estimated blood loss: Approximately _____ ml

8

Radical Cystectomy (Female)

Indications

- Invasive urothelial cell carcinoma, primary intravesical squamous cell, bladder adenocarcinoma or sarcoma, refractory bladder carcinoma in situ
- Intravesical extension of tumors from adjacent organs precluding bladder preservation
- Persistent refractory intravesical bleeding (rare)

Essential Steps

1) Explore the pelvis to assess bladder mobility, and the abdominal contents for visible or palpable metastatic disease.
2) Properly pack the bowel to optimize exposure.
3) Perform a thorough bilateral pelvic lymph node dissection.
4) Identify the ureters at their crossing over the common iliac arteries and carefully dissect them distally, preserving the periureteral tissue.
5) Ligate the lateral and posterior vascular pedicles to the bladder and mobilize the bladder caudally.
6) Incise the posterior vaginal wall and develop a plane between the vagina and anterior rectum. During dissection of the anterior vaginal wall, it is important to achieve meticulous hemostasis to avoid bleeding from its rich vascular plexus.
7) Dissect the entire urethra (transvaginally). In patients undergoing an orthotopic diversion, the anterior vaginal wall and urethra should be preserved and dissection in those areas limited to avoid injury to the rhabdosphincteric mechanism.
8) Remove the bladder, uterus, cervix, anterior vaginal wall, and urethra *en bloc* and obtain meticulous hemostasis.
9) Perform a urinary diversion.

Operative Dictations in Urologic Surgery, First Edition. Noel A. Armenakas, John A. Fracchia, and Ron Golan.
© 2019 John Wiley & Sons Ltd. Published 2019 by John Wiley & Sons Ltd.

Note These Variations

- Preoperative bowel preparation and oral antibiotics varies by surgeon preference and institutional guidelines.
- The timing of the lymph node dissection within the procedure, and extent of the dissection, may vary by surgeon preference and patient disease.
- If the reason for the cystectomy is refractory vesical bleeding, a pelvic lymphadenectomy is not routinely performed.
- The lymph nodes may be removed and sent separately based on their anatomic origin, rather than as one packet from each side. This will allow for a more thorough histologic lymph node evaluation.
- In the case of an invasive posterior bladder wall tumor involving the vagina, the anterior vaginal wall should be removed *en bloc* with the bladder. This may restrict appropriate vaginal reconstruction and subsequent sexual function.

Complications

- Bleeding
- Infection
- Ileus/bowel obstruction/leak
- Ureteral injury/obstruction
- Urine leak/urinoma
- Intraabdominal organ injury
- Nerve injury
- Lymphocele

Template Operative Dictation

Preoperative diagnosis: Bladder cancer
Postoperative diagnosis: Same
Procedure: Anterior pelvic exenteration
Indications: The patient is a ＿＿＿ -year-old female with clinical stage T＿＿ *urothelial cell/squamous cell/adeno* carcinoma of the bladder presenting for an anterior pelvic exenteration.
Description of Procedure: The indications, alternatives, benefits, and risks were discussed with the patient and informed consent was obtained.

The patient was brought onto the operating room table, positioned supine, and secured with a safety strap. Pneumatic compression devices were placed on the lower extremities.

After the administration of intravenous antibiotics and initiation of general endotracheal anesthesia, the patient was positioned with the break just above the anterosuperior iliac spine, and the operating table flexed 15°. The lower extremities were placed in low (Allen) universal stirrups. The lower chest, abdomen, genitalia, and upper thighs were prepped and draped in the standard sterile manner.

The radiographic images were in the room.

A time-out was completed, verifying the correct patient, surgical procedure, and positioning, prior to beginning the procedure.

A 20 Fr urethral catheter was inserted into the bladder and connected to a drainage bag.

A midline abdominal incision was made 3 cm above the umbilicus and carried down to the pubic symphysis. The subcutaneous tissue was incised with electrocautery, exposing the underlying rectus abdominis aponeurosis. This was incised at the linea alba and the rectus abdominis muscles separated at the midline and retracted laterally, taking care not to injure the underlying inferior epigastric vessels.

The space of Retzius was developed by sweeping the infrapubic space posterolaterally and mobilizing the peritoneum cranially on both sides along the pelvic sidewall. Blunt dissection was used to expose the endopelvic fascia inferiorly and the obturator nerve and vessels, posteriorly. The bladder was carefully palpated and noted to be mobile without any fixation to the pelvic sidewall or adjacent organs. The round ligaments were ligated and divided to facilitate mobilization of the peritoneal sac, and the peritoneum was entered above the umbilicus. A systematic intraabdominal exploration was performed. There was no evidence of hepatic metastases or retroperitoneal lymphadenopathy.

The urachus was ligated with a 2-0 silk tie and divided, and the peritoneum incised obliquely on both sides of the bladder in a V-configuration, lateral to the medial umbilical ligaments. The ascending and descending colon were mobilized along the white line of Toldt, and the root of the small bowel mesentery dissected off the retroperitoneum providing sufficient cephalad bowel mobility. The bowel was thoroughly covered with three moistened open laparotomy pads, and a moist rolled towel placed horizontally at the base of the covered bowel. A self-retaining retractor (e.g. Bookwalter, Omni-Tract, Balfour) was appropriately positioned to optimize exposure, using padding on each retractor blade.

The iliac vessels were exposed from just above the common iliac bifurcation to the femoral canal, and the perivascular fibroareolar sheath carefully opened over the external iliacs. The lymph nodes appeared *unremarkable/enlarged/matted* on palpation. The nodal tissue was circumferentially swept off the *left/right* external iliac vessels, using electrocautery and surgical clips to secure the lymphatic channels. The *left-/right*-sided lymphadenectomy was completed with the limits of dissection being the genitofemoral nerve laterally, the ureter medially, the common iliac artery bifurcation cranially, the endopelvic fascia caudally (node of Cloquet) and the obturator nerve inferiorly. The entire nodal package was removed *en bloc* and sent to pathology for evaluation. Meticulous hemo- and lymphostasis were achieved with surgical clips and electrocautery.

An identical lymph node dissection was performed on the contralateral side, completing the lymphadenectomy.

The ureters were identified bilaterally at the common iliac bifurcation, circumferentially dissected and encircled with vessel loops. Ureteral dissection was continued distally to the ureterovesical junction, ligating the obliterated umbilical artery and superior vesical pedicle. Each ureter was mobilized cephalad, leaving the lateral periureteral tissue intact to avoid vascular compromise. Hemostasis was achieved with electrocautery.

The ureters were individually clipped and divided at the level of the ureterovesical junction, and the distal stumps ligated with a 2-0 silk suture. The distal ureteral margins were sent for frozen section section. Each ureter was tagged with a long 3-0 chromic suture, covered with a moist sponge and placed craniolaterally in the retroperitoneal space.

Using gentle anterior traction on the cut urachus for exposure, the *right/left* lateral vascular pedicles to the bladder were sequentially ligated and divided using an endovascular stapler. The identical procedure was performed on the contralteral side.

The infundibulopelvic ligaments were identified, clamped, suture ligated with 1-0 polyglactin (Vicryl) and divided, freeing the fallopian tubes and ovaries. An Allis clamp was placed on the uterine fundus, which was retracted anterocaudally, exposing the peritoneum posterior to the bladder. This was incised transversely and a plane developed within the pouch of Douglas, using sharp and blunt dissection to separate the bladder from the rectum. The bladder was further mobilized caudally exposing the posterior vascular bladder pedicles and cardinal ligaments on each side, which were individually ligated and divided with the endovascular stapler.

An intravaginally placed povidone–iodine (Betadine)-soaked sponge stick was used to identify the apex of the vagina, which was opened posteriorly distal to the cervix. The anterior vaginal wall was sharply dissected off the bladder to the level of the bladder neck and circumferentially excised from its cervical attachments. Vaginal reconstruction was accomplished with a horizontal closure using a running 1-0 Vicryl suture, and the vaginal wall was suspended from Cooper's ligament to prevent subsequent prolapse.

The bladder was displaced posteriorly and the pubourethral suspensory ligaments identified, carefully dissected and divided, exposing the dorsal vein complex. This was ligated with a running 2-0 Vicryl suture and the underlying urethra freed.

Attention was directed at the external genitalia. A weighted vaginal speculum and labial traction sutures were placed to facilitate exposure. A circumferential full-thickness perimeatal incision was made maintaining a 1 cm margin of tissue. Using sharp and blunt dissection, the urethra was carefully dissected into the pelvis, avoiding bladder entry.

Having freed the entire specimen, the urethra, bladder, uterus, fallopian tubes, and ovaries were removed *en bloc* and sent to pathology for evaluation. The pelvis was irrigated with warm sterile water and hemostasis was again confirmed.

Add the appropriate urinary diversion; see Section I, subsection Urinary Diversion

Estimated blood loss: Approximately _____ml

9

Radical Cystectomy (Male)

Indications

- Invasive urothelial cell carcinoma, primary intravesical squamous cell carcinoma, adenocarcinoma or sarcoma
- Recurrent/residual bladder carcinoma in situ, refractory to medical therapy.
- Intravesical extension of tumors from adjacent organs precluding bladder preservation
- Persistent refractory intravesical bleeding (rare)

Essential Steps

1) Explore the pelvis to assess bladder mobility and the abdominal contents for visible or palpable metastatic disease.
2) Properly pack the bowel to optimize exposure.
3) Perform a thorough bilateral pelvic lymph node dissection.
4) Identify the ureters at their crossing over the common iliac arteries and carefully dissect them distally, leaving the periureteral tissue intact to avoid devascularization. Send the distal ureteral margins for frozen section.
5) Expose the plane between the bladder and rectum.
6) Ligate the lateral and posterior vascular pedicles to the bladder.
7) Begin the prostatic dissection by opening the endopelvic fascia, ligating the dorsal vein complex, transecting the urethra, and dividing the rectourethralis muscles. If an orthotopic diversion is being created, preserve as much striated urethral sphincter length as possible.
8) Free the neurovascular bundles and dissect the prostate laterally.
9) Remove the bladder, prostate, and seminal vesicles *en bloc* and achieve meticulous hemostasis.
10) Perform a urinary diversion.

Operative Dictations in Urologic Surgery, First Edition. Noel A. Armenakas, John A. Fracchia, and Ron Golan.
© 2019 John Wiley & Sons Ltd. Published 2019 by John Wiley & Sons Ltd.

Note These Variations

- The patient may be positioned with his legs in (Allen) universal stirrups and placed in modified Trendelenburg to enhance exposure.
- When dissecting the distal portion of the external iliac vein, care must be taken to avoid injury to the accessory obturator vein, found in 25% of patients.
- Pelvic lymph node dissection, which may be extended or standard, can be performed prior to or following the cystectomy, depending on surgeon preference.
- The lymph nodes may be removed and sent separately based on their anatomic origin, rather than as one packet from each side. This will allow for a more thorough histologic lymph node evaluation.
- If the reason of the cystectomy is refractory vesical bleeding, a pelvic lymphadenectomy is not routinely performed.
- A non-nerve-sparing technique may be performed that incorporates the neurovascular bundles.

Complications

- Bleeding
- Infection
- Ileus/bowel obstruction/leak
- Ureteral injury/obstruction
- Urine leak/urinoma
- Intraabdominal organ injury
- Nerve injury
- Lymphocele

Template Operative Dictation

Preoperative diagnosis: Invasive bladder cancer
Postoperative diagnosis: Same
Procedure: Radical cystoprostatectomy
Indications: The patient is a ____-year-old male with clinical stage T____ *urothelial cell/squamous cell/adeno* carcinoma of the bladder presenting for a radical cystoprostatectomy.
Description of Procedure: The indications, alternatives, benefits, and risks were discussed with the patient and informed consent was obtained.

The patient was brought onto the operating room table, positioned supine, and secured with a safety strap. Pneumatic compression devices were placed on the lower extremities.

After the administration of intravenous antibiotics and initiation of general endotracheal anesthesia, the patient was positioned with the break just above the anterosuperior iliac spine, and the operating table flexed 15°. The lower chest, abdomen, genitalia, and upper thighs were prepped and draped in the standard sterile manner.

The radiographic images were in the room.

A time-out was completed, verifying the correct patient, surgical procedure, and positioning, prior to beginning the procedure.

A 20 Fr urethral catheter was inserted into the bladder and connected to a drainage bag.

A midline abdominal incision was made 3 cm above the umbilicus and carried down to the pubic symphysis. The subcutaneous tissue was incised with electrocautery, exposing the underlying rectus abdominis aponeurosis. This was incised at the linea alba and the rectus abdominis muscles separated at the midline and retracted laterally, taking care not to injure the underlying inferior epigastric vessels.

The space of Retzius was developed by sweeping the infrapubic space posterolaterally and mobilizing the peritoneum cranially on both sides along the pelvic sidewall. Blunt dissection was used to expose the endopelvic fascia inferiorly and the obturator nerve and vessels, posteriorly. The bladder was carefully palpated and noted to be mobile without fixation to the pelvic sidewall or adjacent organs. The vas deferens were ligated and divided to facilitate mobilization of the peritoneal sac, and the peritoneum was entered above the umbilicus. A systematic intraabdominal exploration was performed. There was no evidence of hepatic metastases or retroperitoneal lymphadenopathy.

The urachus was ligated with a 2-0 silk tie and divided, and the peritoneum incised obliquely on both sides of the bladder in a V-configuration, lateral to the medial umbilical ligaments. The ascending and descending colon were mobilized along the white line of Toldt, and the root of the small bowel mesentery dissected off the retroperitoneum providing sufficient cephalad bowel mobility. The bowel was thoroughly covered with three moistened open laparotomy pads, and a moist rolled towel placed horizontally at the base of the covered bowel. A self-retaining retractor (e.g. Bookwalter, Omni-Tract, Balfour) was appropriately positioned to optimize exposure, using padding on each retractor blade.

The iliac vessels were exposed from just above the common iliac bifurcation to the femoral canal, and the perivascular fibroareolar sheath carefully opened over the external iliacs. The lymph nodes appeared *unremarkable/enlarged/matted* on palpation. The nodal tissue was circumferentially swept off the *left/right* external iliac vessels, using electrocautery and surgical clips to secure the lymphatic channels. The *left-/right*-sided lymphadenectomy was completed with the limits of dissection being the genitofemoral nerve laterally, the ureter medially, the common iliac artery bifurcation cranially, the endopelvic fascia caudally (node of Cloquet) and the obturator nerve inferiorly. The entire nodal package was removed *en bloc* and sent to pathology for evaluation. Meticulous hemo- and lymphostasis were achieved with surgical clips and electrocautery.

The identical lymph node dissection was performed on the contralateral side, completing the lymphadenectomy.

The ureters were identified bilaterally at the common iliac bifurcation, circumferentially dissected and encircled with vessel loops. Ureteral dissection was continued distally to the ureterovesical junction, ligating the obliterated umbilical artery and superior vesical pedicle. Each ureter was mobilized cephalad, leaving the lateral periureteral tissue intact to avoid vascular compromise. Hemostasis was achieved with electrocautery.

The ureters were individually clipped and divided at the level of the ureterovesical junction, and the distal stumps ligated with a 2-0 silk suture. The distal ureteral margins were sent for frozen section evaluation. Each ureter was tagged with a long 3-0 chromic suture, covered with a moist sponge and placed craniolaterally in the retroperitoneal space.

Using gentle anterior traction on the cut urachus for exposure, the *right/left* lateral vascular pedicles to the bladder were sequentially ligated and divided using an

endovascular stapler. The identical procedure was performed on the contralateral side. Having achieved adequate lateral bladder mobilization, the peritoneum posterior to the bladder was incised transversely. Sharp and blunt dissection was used to develop an avascular plane, separating the bladder and prostate from the rectum. The bladder was further mobilized caudally, exposing the posterior vascular bladder pedicles on each side, which were individually ligated and divided with the endovascular stapler.

Attention was then directed at the prostate. The superficial branch of the dorsal vein was coagulated and divided. The endopelvic fascia was incised bilaterally from the lateral edge of the puboprostatic ligaments to the medial prostatic fascia, using gentle lateral traction on the bladder and prostate. The puboprostatic ligaments were sharply divided superficially at the inferior border of the pubic symphysis and a plane developed below the dorsal vein complex staying above the urethra. A right-angle clamp was passed anterior to the urethra through the opening in the endopelvic fascia, encompassing the dorsal vein complex distal to the prostatic apex. The dorsal vein complex was ligated at this level using two 2-0 *polyglactin (Vicryl)/poliglecaprone (Monocryl)* sutures and divided between these exposing the urethra. Residual bleeding was controlled with a similar *running/figure-of-eight Vicryl/Monocryl* suture.

Using sharp and blunt dissection, the neurovascular bundles lateral to the urethra were carefully separated on each side. The urethra was mobilized circumferentially with a right-angle clamp and its anterior wall transected transversely close to the bladder neck. The urethral catheter was grasped with a Kelly clamp and transected. The distal portion was removed through the urethral meatus and the proximal clamped end was used for cephalad traction on the prostate. The posterior urethral wall was then transected.

The posterior striated urethral sphincter was divided midway between the apex of the prostate and the urethra while displacing the neurovascular bundles posteriorly. The superficial layers of the levator fascia were carefully dissected from the bladder neck to the apex, releasing the neurovascular bundles laterally. The dissection was extended caudally and residual layers of the striated sphincter divided at the midline exposing the anterior rectal wall. Hemostasis was achieved with small clips, avoiding the use of electrocautery in this area.

Using blunt and sharp dissection, a plane was developed between the anterior rectum and Denonvilliers' fascia. The lateral aspects of the prostate were dissected parallel to the neurovascular bundles to the junction of the seminal vesicles and bladder, carefully dividing the lateral pedicles in layers using clips.

Denonvilliers' fascia covering the ampullae of the vasa and the seminal vesicles was incised, and each vas deferens dissected and divided near the ampulla. The seminal vesicles were individually mobilized from their attachments. The apical seminal vesicle arteries were clipped prior to dividing the seminal vesicles. The remaining vascular pedicles to the prostate and bladder were ligated and divided, lateral to the seminal vesicles.

Having freed the entire specimen, the bladder, prostate, and seminal vesicles were removed *en bloc* and sent to pathology for evaluation. The pelvis was irrigated with warm sterile water and hemostasis was again confirmed.

Add the appropriate urinary diversion; see Section I, subsection Urinary Diversion

Estimated blood loss: Approximately _____ml

10

Suprapubic Cystostomy

Indications

- Urinary retention where a urethral catheter cannot or should not be utilized.
- Postoperative temporary urinary diversion (e.g. after suprapubic prostatectomy or select urethral or transvaginal surgeries)

Essential Steps

1) Partially fill the bladder through a urethral catheter, when possible.
2) Expose the bladder, sweep the peritoneum superiorly, and make a stab cystotomy in the mid-anterior wall.
3) Place a Foley catheter into the bladder and ensure that the tip does not rest on the trigone.
4) Close the cystotomy securely around the catheter.

Note These Variations

- Alternatively, a suprapubic longitudinal incision (modified Pfannenstiel) may be used.
- A Malecot catheter can be utilized instead of a Foley catheter. Its insertion can be facilitated by using a curved clamp to stretch its tip. In addition, two of the four wings can be removed to facilitate any subsequent tube change.
- The catheter can be brought out through a separate cutaneous stab incision.

Complications

- Bleeding
- Infection
- Peri-catheter urinary leakage

Operative Dictations in Urologic Surgery, First Edition. Noel A. Armenakas, John A. Fracchia, and Ron Golan.
© 2019 John Wiley & Sons Ltd. Published 2019 by John Wiley & Sons Ltd.

Template Operative Dictation

Preoperative diagnosis: Urinary retention
Postoperative diagnosis: Same
Procedure: Suprapubic cystostomy
Indications: The patient is a _____ -year-old *male/female* with urinary retention *secondary to* _____ presenting for an open suprapubic cystostomy.
Description of Procedure: The indications, alternatives, benefits, and risks were discussed with the patient and informed consent was obtained.

The patient was brought onto the operating room table, positioned supine, and secured with a safety strap. All pressure points were carefully padded and pneumatic compression devices were placed on the lower extremities.

After the administration of intravenous antibiotics and *general/regional* anesthesia, the entire abdomen and genitalia were prepped and draped in the standard sterile manner.

A time-out was completed, verifying the correct patient, surgical procedure, and positioning, prior to beginning the procedure.

An 18 Fr urethral catheter was inserted into the bladder and filled with 200 cc sterile normal saline.

An 5 cm midline abdominal incision was made between the umbilicus and the symphysis pubis, and carried down through the subcutaneous tissue using electrocautery. The underlying rectus abdominis aponeurosis was identified and incised at the linea alba. The rectus abdominis muscles were separated at the midline and retracted laterally, taking care not to injure the underlying inferior epigastric vessels. A self-retaining retractor (e.g. Balfour) was appropriately positioned to optimize exposure, using padding on each retractor blade.

The peritoneum was swept superiorly after incising the perivesical fat just below the peritoneal reflection, and two 2-0 polyglactin (Vicryl) stay sutures were placed into the mid-anterior bladder wall. A 1 cm full-thickness vertical stab incision was made between these using electrocautery. A *20/22/24* Fr Foley catheter was inserted into the bladder and the balloon inflated with 5 ml sterile water.

The cystotomy was closed around the catheter, using interrupted 3-0 Vicryl sutures. The catheter was brought out through the abdominal incision superiorly and secured to the skin with a 2-0 silk suture. The patency of the closure was confirmed by irrigating the urethral catheter with 300 ml sterile normal saline.

The self-retaining retractor was removed and the abdominal incision was closed using a running 2-0 chromic to approximate the rectus muscles and a 1-0 polydioxanone (PDS) for the rectus aponeurosis. 3-0 chromic sutures were used on Scarpa's fascia and the skin approximated with a subcuticular 4-0 poliglecaprone (Monocryl) suture. A sterile dressing was applied.

At the end of the procedure, all counts were correct.

The patient tolerated the procedure well and was taken to the recovery room in satisfactory condition.

Estimated blood loss: Approximately _____ml

Kidney

11

Anatrophic Nephrolithotomy

Indications

- Staghorn calculus

Essential Steps

1) Consider obtaining a three-dimensional CT reconstruction of the kidney to identify the specific anatomic characteristics.
2) Fully mobilize the kidney using sharp and blunt dissection and isolate the renal pedicle.
3) Temporarily occlude the posterior segmental artery to identify Brödel's line.
4) Occlude the main renal artery and cool the kidney with ice slush.
5) Dissect the renal parenchyma on Brödel's line and incise the collecting system.
6) Incise and appropriately suture or reconstruct any stenotic infundibulum using the Heinecke-Mikulicz approach, in order to prevent recurrent stone formation.
7) Remove all stones and perform flexible nephroscopy for confirmation.
8) Reconstruct the collecting system and approximate the renal parenchyma hemostatically.
9) Place a drain.

Note These Variations

- The ureteropelvic junction can be temporarily occluded to avoid distal migration of fragments.
- Identification of Brödel's line may be facilitated by injecting intravenous methylene blue or indigo carmine after clamping the posterior segmental renal arterial branch.
- The main renal vein can be occluded if significant bleeding impedes visualization, but this is usually not necessary.
- A radial nephrotomy can be used to extract a stone fragment lodged in a calyx with a narrowed infundibulum.

Operative Dictations in Urologic Surgery, First Edition. Noel A. Armenakas, John A. Fracchia, and Ron Golan.
© 2019 John Wiley & Sons Ltd. Published 2019 by John Wiley & Sons Ltd.

- If Gerota's fascia is not available for renal coverage, perirenal fat or an omental flap brought out through a small peritoneal window can be used to protect the reconstructed kidney.
- Intraoperative fluoroscopy may be used to confirm removal of all densely radiopaque stone fragments prior to completing the renal reconstruction.
- The use of a nephrostomy tube (Malecot or Foley catheter) may be considered, depending on the characteristics of the repair and the surgeon's preference.
- The role of mannitol in limiting acute tubular injury is somewhat controversial.

Complications

- Bleeding
- Infection
- Intraabdominal organ injury
- Pneumothorax
- Urine leak/urinoma
- Ileus
- Retained stone fragments
- Renal infarct/loss of renal function
- Arteriovenous fistula

Template Operative Dictation

Preoperative diagnosis: Staghorn calculus
Postoperative diagnosis: Same
Procedure: *Right/Left* anatrophic nephrolithotomy
Indications: The patient is a _____ -year-old *male/female* with a _____cm *right/left* renal staghorn calculus presenting for an anatrophic nephrolithotomy.
Description of Procedure: The indications, alternatives, benefits, and risks were discussed with the patient and informed consent was obtained.

The patient was brought onto the operating room table, positioned supine, and secured with a safety strap. Pneumatic compression devices were placed on the lower extremities.

After the administration of intravenous antibiotics and general endotracheal anesthesia, a 16 Fr urethral catheter was inserted into the bladder and connected to a leg bag.

The patient was placed in the lateral decubitus position at a 90° angle with the lower leg flexed 90° and the upper leg extended. An axillary roll was positioned to protect the brachial plexus and a gel pad placed to support the back. Multiple pillows were used to pad beneath and between both the upper and lower extremities to ensure adequate cushioning. The kidney rest was elevated and the table flexed and adjusted horizontally, obtaining optimal flank exposure. The patient was secured to the table with 3 in. surgical tape and safety straps, and prepped and draped in the standard sterile manner.

The radiographic images were in the room.

A time-out was completed, verifying the correct patient, surgical procedure, site, and positioning, prior to beginning the procedure.

The space between the 11th and 12th ribs was palpated and an incision made at this level from the mid-axillary line and extended medially to the lateral border of the rectus abdominis muscle. Using electrocautery, the latissimus dorsi and external oblique muscles were incised exposing the underlying ribs. The intercostal attachments were transected taking care to avoid injury to the pleura and neurovascular bundle on the inferior surface of the 11th rib. The internal oblique muscle was divided with cautery and the transversus abdominis carefully split in the direction of its fibers, avoiding entry into the peritoneum. The pararenal space was entered by sweeping the peritoneum medially and the retroperitoneal connective tissue superiorly and inferiorly. A self-retaining retractor (e.g. Bookwalter, Omni-Tract, Finochietto) was appropriately positioned to optimize exposure, using padding on each retractor blade.

The parietal peritoneum was incised on the white line of Toldt and the colon reflected medially, exposing Gerota's fascia. Using sharp dissection, Gerota's fascia was incised posteriorly and the underlying kidney and renal pelvis identified. The renal pelvis and proximal ureter were carefully dissected, preserving the periureteral tissues. Next, the entire kidney was thoroughly mobilized, using blunt and sharp dissection.

Attention was then turned to the renal pedicle anteromedially. The retroperitoneal fascia overlying the renal vessels was separated exposing the underlying renal vein, which was carefully dissected, mobilized, and encircled with a vessel loop. Using gentle retraction on the renal vein, the main renal artery was identified deep to this, dissected, and surrounded with a vessel loop.

After isolating the renal pedicle, the posterior segmental artery was identified as the first branch of the main renal artery and dissected. This artery was briefly clamped to precisely identify the avascular plane on the posterior renal surface, and Brödel's line was superficially marked with electrocautery.

The kidney was suspended using narrow umbilical tape carefully placed around each pole as a sling to facilitate its mobility. 25 g of mannitol were administered intravenously and a barrier drape was placed around the kidney. The main renal artery was gently occluded with a *bulldog clamp/Rummel*. Renal hypothermia was accomplished using ice slush to cool the kidney for 15 minutes.

A capsulotomy was made on the posterior surface of the kidney, along Brödel's line, and extended up to the apical and basilar segments. Care was taken to preserve the capsule for subsequent closure. Using the back of a scalpel handle, the renal parenchyma was bluntly dissected and the collecting system carefully incised poste-rolaterally over the staghorn calculus. A *malleable brain retractor/Penfield dissector* was used to gently retract the parenchyma. Transverse incisions were made exposing the posterior and anterior calyces. Visible bleeders were ligated with figure-of-eight 4-0 chromic sutures. The stone(s) *was/were* carefully extracted in *its/their* entirety using Randall stone forceps and sent for chemical analysis. Each calyx was thoroughly inspected and the renal pelvis and calyces copiously irrigated with warm sterile normal saline.

The main renal artery was unclamped and renal hemostasis achieved with 4-0 chromic sutures. The kidney was noted to rapidly regain its dark pink color and turgor. The barrier drape, remaining ice slush, and vascular loops were removed.

The total cold ischemia time was _____ minutes.

Nephroscopy was performed using a flexible *cystoscope/ureteroscope* to ensure removal of all stone fragments.

A 6 Fr ____cm double-J stent was advanced over a guidewire, with the proximal end positioned in the renal pelvis and the distal end within the bladder, and the wire removed.

Renal reconstruction was initiated by systematically closing the collecting system with 4-0 chromic sutures. Absorbable gelatin sponge (Gelfoam) bolsters were placed between the dissected renal parenchyma, and the renal capsule reapproximated over bolsters using interrupted 2-0 polydioxanone (PDS) sutures. A hemostatic sealant ____*(specify brand)*____ was used to further reinforce the repair. The kidney was repositioned within Gerota's fascia, which was closed with 2-0 chromic sutures.

A surgical drain (e.g. Jackson-Pratt) was placed in the perirenal space, away from the repair, and brought out through a separate, more caudal cutaneous incision where it was secured at the skin with a 2-0 silk suture. Meticulous hemostasis was achieved throughout the procedure. Prior to closure, the renal vessels, visceral organs, and pleura were inspected and found to be intact. The self-retaining retractor was removed, the kidney rest lowered, and the table taken out of flexion.

The incision was closed using running 1-0 PDS to approximate the three muscle layers individually, taking care not to entrap the intercostal neurovascular bundle. 3-0 chromic sutures were used on Scarpa's fascia and the skin approximated with a subcuticular 4-0 poliglecaprone (Monocryl) suture. A sterile dressing was applied and the patient repositioned supine.

At the end of the procedure, all counts were correct.

The patient tolerated the procedure well and was taken to the recovery room in satisfactory condition.

Estimated blood loss: Approximately _____ml

12

Nephroureterectomy

Indications

- Carcinoma of the upper urinary tract

Essential Steps

1) Mobilize the colon and incise the anterior renal fascia medially.
2) Obtain early vascular control.
3) Ligate and divide the renal artery, then the vein.
4) Dissect the kidney circumferentially.
5) Dissect the ureter caudally along its entire length.
6) Excise the entire intramural ureter with a 5 mm bladder cuff.
7) Remove the specimen *en bloc*.
8) Place a drain.

Note These Variations

- A single intravesical instillation of Mitomycin C may be given immediately prior to surgery to decrease the risk of bladder recurrence.
- The choice of incision is dependent on the anatomic characteristics of the kidney and tumor (including location, size, and extension), the patient's body habitus, and the surgeon's preference. Although an intercostal incision between the 10th and 11th ribs provides adequate exposure for most tumors, with large tumors, or if only one incision is used, a thoracoabdominal approach may be considered.
- The pelvic ureter with a bladder cuff can be removed through a modified Pfannenstiel or midline incision using an intra- or extravesical approach, or purely endoscopically. These approaches often require repositioning the patient supine and re-prepping and draping.
- A lymph node dissection is at the discretion of the surgeon and can include retroperitoneal and/or pelvic lymph nodes.

Operative Dictations in Urologic Surgery, First Edition. Noel A. Armenakas, John A. Fracchia, and Ron Golan.
© 2019 John Wiley & Sons Ltd. Published 2019 by John Wiley & Sons Ltd.

Complications

- Bleeding
- Infection
- Intraabdominal organ injury
- Pneumothorax
- Urine leak/urinoma
- Ileus
- Lymphocele

Template Operative Dictation

Preoperative diagnosis: Upper urinary tract carcinoma
Postoperative diagnosis: Same
Procedure: *Right/Left* nephroureterectomy
Indications: The patient is a _____ -year-old *male/female* with a _____ cm *pelvis/calyceal/ureteral* mass presenting for a *right/left* nephroureterectomy.
Description of Procedure: The indications, alternatives, benefits, and risks were discussed with the patient and informed consent was obtained.

The patient was brought onto the operating room table, positioned supine, and secured with a safety strap. Pneumatic compression devices were placed on the lower extremities.

After the administration of intravenous antibiotics and general endotracheal anesthesia, a 16 Fr urethral catheter was inserted into the bladder and connected to a drainage bag.

The patient was placed in the lateral decubitus position at a 30° angle with the pelvis rotated posteriorly. The lower leg was flexed 90° and the upper leg extended. An axillary roll was positioned to protect the brachial plexus and a gel pad placed to support the back. Multiple pillows were used to pad beneath and between both the upper and lower extremities ensuring adequate cushioning. The kidney rest was elevated and the table flexed and adjusted horizontally, obtaining optimal flank exposure. The patient was secured to the table with 3 in. surgical tape and safety straps, and the abdomen and flank were prepped and draped in the standard sterile manner.

The radiographic images were in the room.

A time-out was completed, verifying the correct patient, surgical procedure, site and positioning, prior to beginning the procedure.

The space between the 10th and 11th ribs was palpated and an incision made at this level from the mid-axillary line and extended medially to the lateral border of the rectus abdominis muscle. Using electrocautery, the latissimus dorsi and external oblique muscles were incised exposing the underlying ribs. The intercostal attachments were transected taking care to avoid injury to the pleura and neurovascular bundle on the inferior surface of the rib. The internal oblique muscle was divided with cautery and the transversus abdominis carefully split in the direction of its fibers, avoiding entry into the peritoneum. A generous paranephric space was created by sweeping the peritoneum medially and the retroperitoneal connective tissue superiorly and inferiorly. A self-retaining retractor (e.g. Bookwalter, Omni-Tract, Finochietto) was appropriately positioned to optimize exposure, using padding on each retractor blade.

The parietal peritoneum was incised on the white line of Toldt and the colon reflected medially, exposing Gerota's fascia.

> **On the right**: The hepatic flexure and duodenum were mobilized, freeing the kidney superiorly and medially.
> **On the left**: The splenorenal ligament was mobilized, freeing the kidney superiorly.

Using sharp and blunt dissection, the retroperitoneal fascia overlying the renal vessels was separated, exposing the underlying main renal vein, which was carefully dissected, mobilized, and encircled with a vessel loop. The gonadal vein was doubly ligated with 3-0 silk ties and divided.

> **On the left**: The adrenal branch was similarly ligated at its insertion into the renal vein.

With gentle retraction on the renal vein, the main renal artery was identified deep to this and dissected for a distance of 2 cm. It was doubly ligated with 2-0 silk and a 3-0 silk suture ligature, and sharply divided. Having interrupted the renal vascular inflow, the renal vein was similarly ligated and divided and the vessel loop removed.

Using both sharp and blunt dissection, Gerota's fascia was mobilized circumferentially, obtaining meticulous hemostasis with surgical clips and electrocautery. Attention was directed to the cranial attachments with the adrenal gland, which were carefully divided using *an electrothermal bipolar tissue sealing device (LigaSure)/surgical clips*, completely freeing the adrenal off the superior pole of the kidney. Inferiorly, the ureter was identified and dissected down to the common iliac bifurcation.

A regional lymphadenectomy was performed using a "split and roll" technique starting just above the renal hilum and continuing caudally to the mesenteric vein. The entire nodal package was removed and sent to pathology for evaluation. Meticulous hemo- and lymphostasis were achieved with surgical clips and electrocautery.

The kidney was placed in a specimen retrieval bag and pushed caudally into the wound. The retroperitoneum was irrigated with warm sterile water and thoroughly inspected, confirming the absence of bleeding or injury to the renal vessels, visceral organs, and pleura. The self-retaining retractor was removed, the kidney rest lowered, and the table taken out of flexion.

The flank incision was closed using running 1-0 polydioxanone (PDS) to approximate the three muscle layers individually, taking care not to entrap the intercostal neurovascular bundle.

3-0 chromic sutures were used on Scarpa's fascia and the skin approximated with a subcuticular 4-0 poliglecaprone (Monocryl) suture.

Attention was turned to the ipsilateral lower abdomen where a Gibson incision was made. This was taken down through the external, internal, and transversus abdominis muscles exposing the space of Retzius, which was developed using blunt dissection. A self-retaining retractor (e.g. Balfour, Bookwalter) was appropriately placed to optimize exposure. The peritoneum was mobilized superomedially off the iliac vessels, and the attached ureter identified at the iliac bifurcation. The pelvic ureter was dissected distally to its insertion into the bladder. The intramural ureter with a 5 mm full-thickness bladder cuff was dissected from its orifice, and the entirely freed specimen was removed *en bloc* and sent to pathology for evaluation.

The bladder wall was closed in two layers using running 2-0 polyglactin (Vicryl) sutures. A surgical drain (e.g. Jackson-Pratt) was placed in the space of Retzius away from the cystotomy and brought out through a separate cutaneous incision, where it was secured at the skin with a 2-0 silk suture. Prior to closure, the pelvis was inspected and noted to be intact without evidence of bleeding or injury.

The self-retaining retractor was removed and the abdominal wall closed by individually approximating the internal and external oblique aponeuroses with a running 1-0 PDS suture. Scarpa's fascia was closed with interrupted 3-0 chromic sutures and the skin approximated with a subcuticular 4-0 Monocryl suture. Sterile dressings were applied to both incisions and the patient repositioned supine.

At the end of the procedure, all counts were correct.

The patient tolerated the procedure well and was taken to the recovery room in satisfactory condition.

Estimated blood loss: Approximately _____ml

13

Partial Nephrectomy

Indications

- Localized tumor (usually ≤ 7 cm) that does not invade the renal hilum and is amenable to a partial nephrectomy
- Bilateral renal tumors
- Tumor in a solitary kidney

Essential Steps

1) Expose and thoroughly mobilize the kidney.
2) Obtain control of the renal pedicle.
3) Cool the kidney with ice slush.
4) Excise the tumor with a rim of normal renal parenchyma.
5) Perform the appropriate renal reconstruction and obtain hemostasis within the resection bed.
6) Cover the repair with perirenal fat, Gerota's fascia, or omentum.
7) Place a drain.

Note These Variations

- The choice of incision is dependent on the anatomic characteristics of the kidney and tumor (including location, size, and extension), the patient's body habitus, and the surgeon's preference. An intercostal incision provides adequate exposure for most tumors. This can be made either between the 10th and 11th or the 11th and 12th ribs, depending on the kidney's location in the retroperitoneum and the renal vasculature (e.g. presence of supernumery or aberrant vessels). Alternatively, a transcostal incision can be performed by removing either the 11th or 12th rib. Large upper pole tumors and locally invasive tumors extending superomedially, or bilateral tumors can be managed with a thoracoabdominal or transabdominal (e.g. Chevron) approach, respectively.
- Intraoperative ultrasonography can be used to facilitate identification of the tumor and its margins.

Operative Dictations in Urologic Surgery, First Edition. Noel A. Armenakas, John A. Fracchia, and Ron Golan.
© 2019 John Wiley & Sons Ltd. Published 2019 by John Wiley & Sons Ltd.

- Renal cooling may not be necessary for small or exophytic tumors where warm ischemia time is limited.
- The role of mannitol in limiting acute tubular injury is somewhat controversial.
- Upper and lower pole tumors may be managed with a polar nephrectomy.
- There are a number of ways to obtain renal hemostasis within the resection bed, including the use of electrocauterization, argon beam coagulation, absorbable bolsters, hemostatic agents, and tissue sealants.

Complications

- Bleeding
- Infection
- Intraabdominal organ injury
- Pneumothorax
- Urine leak/urinoma
- Renal infarct/loss of renal function
- Pseudoaneurysm

Template Operative Dictation

Preoperative diagnosis: Renal tumor
Postoperative diagnosis: Same
Procedure: *Right/Left* partial nephrectomy
Indications: The patient is a _____ -year-old *male/female* with a _____cm *right/left* renal mass presenting for a partial nephrectomy.
Description of Procedure: The indications, alternatives, benefits, and risks were discussed with the patient and informed consent was obtained.

The patient was brought onto the operating room table, positioned supine, and secured with a safety strap. Pneumatic compression devices were placed on the lower extremities.

After the administration of intravenous antibiotics and general endotracheal anesthesia, a 16 Fr urethral catheter was inserted into the bladder and connected to a drainage bag.

The patient was placed in the lateral decubitus position at a 45° angle with the lower leg flexed 90° and the upper leg extended. An axillary roll was positioned to protect the brachial plexus and a gel pad placed to support the back. Multiple pillows were used to pad beneath and between both the upper and lower extremities to ensure adequate cushioning. The kidney rest was elevated and the table flexed and adjusted horizontally, obtaining optimal flank exposure. The patient was secured to the table with 3 in. surgical tape and safety straps, and prepped and draped in the standard sterile manner.

The radiographic images were in the room.

A time-out was completed, verifying the correct patient, surgical procedure, site, and positioning, prior to beginning the procedure.

The space between the 10th and 11th ribs was palpated and an incision made from the mid-axillary line and extended medially to the lateral border of the rectus abdominis

muscle. Using electrocautery, the latissimus dorsi and external oblique muscles were incised exposing the underlying ribs. The intercostal attachments were transected taking care to avoid injury to the pleura and the neurovascular bundle on the inferior surface of the rib. The internal oblique muscle was divided with cautery and the transversus abdominis carefully split in the direction of its fibers, avoiding entry into the peritoneum. A generous paranephric space was created by sweeping the peritoneum medially and the retroperitoneal connective tissue superiorly and inferiorly. A self-retaining retractor (e.g. Bookwalter, Omni-Tract, Finochietto) was appropriately positioned to optimize exposure, using padding on each retractor blade.

The parietal peritoneum was incised on the white line of Toldt and the colon reflected medially, exposing Gerota's fascia.

> **On the right:** The hepatic flexure and duodenum were mobilized, freeing the kidney superiorly and medially.
>
> **On the left:** The splenorenal ligament was mobilized, freeing the kidney superiorly.

Using sharp and blunt dissection, the retroperitoneal fascia overlying the renal vessels was separated, exposing the underlying main renal vein, which was carefully dissected, mobilized, and encircled with a loop. Using gentle retraction on the renal vein, the main renal artery was identified deep to this, dissected, and surrounded with a vessel loop.

Having achieved control of the main renal vessels, attention was turned to the kidney. The renal tumor was identified at the ____(location)____. The overlying Gerota's fascia was defatted, leaving adequate perirenal fat over the tumor. 25 g of mannitol were administered intravenously and a barrier drape was placed around the kidney. The main renal artery was gently occluded with a *bulldog clamp/Rummel*. Renal hypothermia was accomplished using ice slush to cool the kidney for 15 minutes.

Using electrocautery, the tumor was circumscribed, leaving a 5 mm margin of surrounding normal parenchyma. The entire tumor was resected using a combination of sharp and blunt dissection, and was sent to pathology for evaluation. Additionally, a biopsy of the tumor bed was sent for frozen-section evaluation. All visible bleeding vessels were ligated with figure-of-eight 4-0 chromic sutures.

> **For collecting system violation:** The collecting system was closed with running 4-0 chromic sutures.

The main renal artery was unclamped and additional parenchymal bleeders were similarly ligated with figure-of-eight 4-0 chromic sutures, ensuring adequate hemostasis. The kidney was noted to rapidly regain its dark pink color and turgor.

The barrier drape, remaining ice slush and vascular loops were removed. The total cold ischemia time was _____ minutes.

Once the frozen section confirmed a clear surgical margin, the reconstructive procedure was initiated using absorbable gelatin sponge (Gelfoam) bolsters to fill the parenchymal defect. Interrupted 2-0 polydioxanone (PDS) sutures were placed to loosely re-approximate the renal capsule over an additional superficially placed bolster. A hemostatic sealant (*specify brand*) was used to further reinforce the repair. Available perirenal fat was secured over the defect and Gerota's fascia loosely approximated

covering the kidney. A surgical drain (e.g. Jackson-Pratt) was placed in the perirenal space, away from the repair, and brought out through a separate more caudal cutaneous incision where it was secured at the skin with a 2-0 silk suture.

The retroperitoneum was irrigated with warm sterile water. Prior to closure, the renal vessels, visceral organs, and pleura were inspected and found to be intact. The self-retaining retractor was removed, the kidney rest lowered, and the table taken out of flexion.

The incision was closed using running 1-0 PDS to approximate the three muscle layers individually, taking care not to entrap the intercostal neurovascular bundle. 3-0 chromic sutures were used on Scarpa's fascia and the skin approximated with a subcuticular 4-0 poliglecaprone (Monocryl) suture. A sterile dressing was applied and the patient repositioned supine.

At the end of the procedure, all counts were correct.

The patient tolerated the procedure well and was taken to the recovery room in satisfactory condition.

Estimated blood loss: Approximately _____ml

14

Pyelolithotomy

Indications

- Large renal pelvis stone burden or body habitus precluding percutaneous or ureteroscopic stone access and/or extraction.

Essential Steps

1) Mobilize the renal pelvis and proximal ureter, preserving the adventitial vessels.
2) Thoroughly expose the renal pelvis by dissecting the perinephric fat off the posterior surface of the kidney at the level of the renal sinus.
3) Make an incision in the posterior renal pelvis, avoiding the ureteropelvic junction.
4) Remove all stone fragments and perform flexible nephroscopy for confirmation.
5) Ensure a watertight renal pelvis closure.

Note These Variations

- A dorsal lumbotomy, rather than the standard flank incision, may be used for stones confined to the renal pelvis. This approach provides limited access in the event of stone migration.
- For stones extending into a calyx, the renal pelvis incision can be lengthened superiorly into an infundibulum.
- In cases where there are multiple scattered intrarenal stones, a coagulum (consisting of cryoprecipitate, thrombin, and calcium chloride) can be used to facilitate stone removal.
- Intraoperative fluoroscopy may be used to confirm removal of all densely radiopaque stone fragments.
- The use of a ureteral stent and/or a nephrostomy tube (Malecot or Foley catheter) is dependent on the characteristics of the repair and the surgeon's preference.

Operative Dictations in Urologic Surgery, First Edition. Noel A. Armenakas, John A. Fracchia, and Ron Golan.
© 2019 John Wiley & Sons Ltd. Published 2019 by John Wiley & Sons Ltd.

Complications

- Bleeding
- Infection
- Intraabdominal organ injury
- Urine leak/urinoma
- Retained calculus(i)
- Urinary obstruction

Template Operative Dictation

Preoperative diagnosis: Nephrolithiasis
Postoperative diagnosis: Same
Procedure: *Right/Left* pyelolithotomy
Indications: The patient is a ____-year-old *male/female* with a ____cm renal calculus presenting for a *right/left* pyelolithotomy.
Description of Procedure: The indications, alternatives, benefits, and risks were discussed with the patient and informed consent was obtained.

The patient was brought onto the operating room table, positioned supine, and secured with a safety strap. Pneumatic compression devices were placed on the lower extremities.

After the administration of intravenous antibiotics and general endotracheal anesthesia, a 16 Fr urethral catheter was inserted into the bladder and connected to a drainage bag. The patient was placed in the lateral decubitus position at a 90° angle with the lower leg flexed 90° and the upper leg extended. An axillary roll was positioned to protect the brachial plexus and a gel pad placed to support the back. Multiple pillows were used to pad beneath and between both the upper and lower extremities to ensure adequate cushioning. The kidney rest was elevated and the table flexed and adjusted horizontally, obtaining optimal flank exposure. The patient was secured to the table with 3 in. surgical tape and safety straps, and prepped and draped in the standard sterile manner.

The radiographic images were in the room.

A time-out was completed, verifying the correct patient, surgical procedure, site, and positioning, prior to beginning the procedure.

The space between the 11th and 12th ribs was palpated and an incision made at this level from the mid-axillary line and extended medially to the lateral border of the rectus abdominis muscle. Using electrocautery, the latissimus dorsi and external oblique muscles were incised, exposing the underlying ribs. The intercostal attachments were transected, taking care to avoid injury to the pleura and neurovascular bundle on the inferior surface of the 11th rib. The internal oblique muscle was divided with cautery and the transversus abdominis carefully split in the direction of its fibers, avoiding entry into the peritoneum. A generous paranephric space was created by sweeping the peritoneum medially and the retroperitoneal connective tissue superiorly and inferiorly. A self-retaining retractor (e.g. Bookwalter, Omni-Tract, Finochietto) was appropriately positioned to optimize exposure, using padding on each retractor blade.

The parietal peritoneum was incised on the white line of Toldt and the colon reflected medially, exposing Gerota's fascia. Using sharp dissection, Gerota's fascia was incised posteriorly and the underlying kidney and renal pelvis identified. The renal pelvis and proximal ureter were carefully dissected and thoroughly mobilized, preserving the periureteral tissues. A Gil-Vernet retractor was used to elevate the renal sinus perinephric fat, which was dissected providing optimal exposure of the renal pelvis.

A curvilinear incision was made in the renal pelvis, avoiding the ureteropelvic junction. 3-0 chromic stay sutures were placed at both ends of the incision and the underlying stone(s) *was/were* carefully dislodged and removed using Randall forceps, taking care not to disrupt the friable tissues. The stones were sent for chemical analysis. The collecting system was irrigated with warm normal saline and nephroscopy was performed using a flexible *cystoscope/ureteroscope* to ensure removal of all stone fragments.

A 6 Fr ____ cm double-J stent was advanced over a guidewire with the proximal end positioned in the renal pelvis and the distal end within the bladder, and the guidewire removed. The pyelotomy was closed using a running 5-0 *polyglactin (Vicryl)/polydioxanone (PDS)* suture.

A surgical drain (e.g. Jackson-Pratt, 0.25 in. Penrose) was placed in the perirenal space, away from the repair, and brought out through a separate more caudal cutaneous incision where it was secured at the skin with a 2-0 silk suture. Meticulous hemostasis was achieved throughout the procedure. Prior to closure, the kidney and adjacent organs were noted to be intact.

The self-retaining retractor was removed and the incision was closed, using running 1-0 PDS to approximate the three muscle layers, individually, taking care not to entrap the intercostal neurovascular bundle. 3-0 chromic sutures were used on Scarpa's fascia and the skin approximated with a subcuticular 4-0 poliglecaprone (Monocryl) suture. A sterile dressing was applied and the patient was repositioned supine.

At the end of the procedure, all counts were correct.

The patient tolerated the procedure well and was taken to the recovery room in satisfactory condition.

Estimated blood loss: Approximately _____ ml

15

Pyeloplasty (Dismembered)

Indications

- Ureteropelvic junction obstruction

Essential Steps

1) Mobilize the proximal ureter toward the renal pelvis with minimal manipulation and judicious use of electrocautery to preserve the adventitial vessels.
2) Expose the ureteropelvic junction and identify the etiology of the ureteropelvic junction obstruction (e.g. crossing aberrant vessel, intrinsic narrowing or scarring).
3) Spatulate the ureter and anastomose it to the most dependent portion of the renal pelvis.
4) Close the remaining renal pelvis with a running suture creating a watertight, tension-free anastomosis.
5) Place a drain.

Note These Variations

- A dorsal lumbotomy can be used to access the renal pelvis, avoiding musculofascial incisions.
- In cases of a high ureteropelvic junction insertion, such as in patients with a horseshoe kidney, a Y-V plasty may be used.
- Optical magnification can be used to facilitate suture placement.
- Flap techniques (such as the Scardino and Culp repairs) may be applied in cases of insufficient proximal ureteral length, such as in patients with failed prior repairs.
- For redo procedures, the ureter may be more easily identified distally and dissected proximally.
- The use of a nephrostomy tube (Malecot or Foley catheter) and/or ureteral stent is dependent on the characteristics of the repair and the surgeon's preference.

Operative Dictations in Urologic Surgery, First Edition. Noel A. Armenakas, John A. Fracchia, and Ron Golan.
© 2019 John Wiley & Sons Ltd. Published 2019 by John Wiley & Sons Ltd.

Complications

- Bleeding
- Infection
- Urine leak/urinoma
- Intraabdominal organ injury
- Pneumothorax
- Ileus
- Recurrent ureteropelvic junction obstruction/stricture

Template Operative Dictation

Preoperative diagnosis: Ureteropelvic junction obstruction
Postoperative diagnosis: Same
Procedure: *Right/left* dismembered pyeloplasty
Indication: The patient is a _____-year-old *male/female* presenting with a *right/left* ureteropelvic junction obstruction for a pyeloplasty.
Description of Procedure: The indications, alternatives, benefits, and risks were discussed with the patient and informed consent was obtained.

The patient was brought onto the operating room table, positioned supine, and secured with a safety strap. Pneumatic compression devices were placed on the lower extremities.

After the administration of intravenous antibiotics and general endotracheal anesthesia, a 16 Fr urethral catheter was inserted into the bladder and connected to a drainage bag. The patient was placed in the lateral decubitus position at a 45° angle with the lower leg flexed 90° and the upper leg extended. An axillary roll was positioned to protect the brachial plexus and a gel pad placed to support the back. Multiple pillows were used to pad beneath and between both the upper and lower extremities to ensure adequate cushioning.

The kidney rest was elevated and the table flexed and adjusted horizontally, obtaining optimal flank exposure. The patient was secured to the table with 3 in. surgical tape and safety straps and prepped and draped in the standard sterile manner.

The radiographic images were in the room.

A time-out was completed, verifying the correct patient, surgical procedure, site, and positioning, prior to beginning the procedure.

An anterior incision was made from the tip of the twelfth rib and extended medially for approximately 10 cm. The external and internal oblique muscles were incised using electrocautery and the transversus abdominis carefully split in the direction of its fibers, avoiding entry into the peritoneum. The paranephric space was created by sweeping the peritoneum medially and the retroperitoneal connective tissue superiorly and inferiorly. A self-retaining retractor (e.g. Bookwalter, Omni-Tract, or Finochietto) was appropriately positioned to optimize exposure, using padding on each retractor blade.

The parietal peritoneum was incised on the white line of Toldt and the colon reflected medially, exposing Gerota's fascia. Using sharp dissection, Gerota's was opened and the underlying kidney and distended renal pelvis identified. The renal pelvis and proximal ureter were carefully dissected and thoroughly mobilized, preserving the periureteral tissues.

***For a crossing vessel*:** The cause of obstruction was found to be an inferior pole anteriorly crossing vessel, which was carefully dissected and freed. The ureter was tagged with a 4-0 chromic suture, transected, and transposed anterior to the crossing vessel. It was then spatulated along its lateral border for 2 cm.

***For a stenotic ureteropelvic junction*:** The cause of obstruction was found to be an intrinsic narrowing of the ureteropelvic junction. The stenotic ureteral segment was excised and a 4-0 chromic traction suture placed on the severed distal end. It was then spatulated along its lateral border for 2 cm.

Attention was turned to the renal pelvis, where a 4-0 chromic traction suture was placed anteromedially, allowing anterior rotation of the pelvis. A marking pen was used to outline the proposed rhombus-shaped pelvis incision, making sure not to remove excessive tissue. Additional 4-0 chromic sutures were placed at each corner for traction. Using angled Pott's scissors, the redundant renal pelvis was excised along the delineated lines.

The ureter was pulled cranially and anastomosed to the most dependent portion of the renal pelvis using *running/interrupted* 6-0 polydioxanone (PDS) sutures on each side, taking care to avoid kinking. Prior to completion of the anastomosis, a 6 Fr ___cm double-J stent was advanced over a guidewire with the proximal end positioned in the renal pelvis and the distal end within the bladder, and the guidewire was removed. A third PDS suture was used to close the renal pelvis defect cranially, ensuring a watertight, tension-free reconstruction. Meticulous hemostasis was achieved throughout the procedure.

A surgical drain (e.g. Jackson-Pratt, 0.25 in. Penrose) was placed in the perirenal space, away from the repair, and brought out through a separate more caudal cutaneous incision, where it was secured at the skin with a 2-0 silk suture. Prior to closure, the kidney and colon were noted to be intact.

The self-retaining retractor was removed and the incision was closed using running 1-0 PDS to approximate the three muscle layers, individually, taking care not to entrap the intercostal neurovascular bundle. 3-0 chromic sutures were used on Scarpa's fascia and the skin approximated with a subcuticular 4-0 poliglecaprone (Monocryl) suture. A sterile dressing was applied and the patient repositioned supine.

At the end of the procedure, all counts were correct.

The patient tolerated the procedure well and was taken to the recovery room in satisfactory condition.

Estimated blood loss: Approximately _____ml

16

Radical Nephrectomy

Indications

- Select solid renal masses
- Renal tumors with local extension or intracaval tumors
- Cytoreductive surgery for metastatic disease

Essential Steps

1) Mobilize the colon and incise the anterior renal fascia medially.
2) Identify and dissect the renal vein and place a vessel loop around it.
3) Dissect the renal artery deep to the vein and surround it with a vessel loop.
4) Ligate and divide the renal artery, then the vein.
5) Dissect the kidney posteriorly and inferiorly, preserving Gerota's fascia.
6) Ligate and divide the ureter.
7) Free the kidney from its cranial attachments and remove the specimen *en bloc*.

Note These Variations

- The choice of incision is dependent on the anatomic characteristics of the kidney and tumor (including location, size and extension), the patient's body habitus, and the surgeon's preference. An intercostal incision provides adequate exposure for most tumors. This can be made either between the 10th and 11th or the 11th and 12th ribs, depending on the kidney's location in the retroperitoneum and the renal vasculature (e.g. presence of supernumerary or aberrant vessels). Alternatively, a transcostal incision can be performed by removing either the 11th or 12th rib. Large upper pole tumors and locally invasive tumors extending superomedially, or bilateral tumors can be managed with a thoracoabdominal or transabdominal (e.g. Chevron) approach, respectively.
- With upper pole tumors, tumors involving the adrenal or associated lymphadenopathy, the ipsilateral adrenal gland may be removed en *bloc*.

Operative Dictations in Urologic Surgery, First Edition. Noel A. Armenakas, John A. Fracchia, and Ron Golan.
© 2019 John Wiley & Sons Ltd. Published 2019 by John Wiley & Sons Ltd.

Complications

- Bleeding
- Infection
- Intraabdominal organ injury
- Pneumothorax
- Ileus

Template Operative Dictation

Preoperative diagnosis: Renal tumor
Postoperative diagnosis: Same
Procedure: *Right/Left* radical nephrectomy
Indications: The patient is a ____-year-old *male/female* with a ____cm *right/left* renal mass presenting for a radical nephrectomy
Description of Procedure: The indications, alternatives, benefits, and risks were discussed with the patient and informed consent was obtained.

The patient was brought onto the operating room table, positioned supine, and secured with a safety strap. Pneumatic compression devices were placed on the lower extremities.

After the administration of intravenous antibiotics and general endotracheal anesthesia, a 16 Fr urethral catheter was inserted into the bladder and connected to a drainage bag.

The patient was placed in the lateral decubitus position at a 45° angle with the lower leg flexed 90° and the upper leg extended. An axillary roll was positioned to protect the brachial plexus and a gel pad placed to support the back. Multiple pillows were used to pad beneath and between both the upper and lower extremities, ensuring adequate cushioning. The kidney rest was elevated and the table flexed and adjusted horizontally, obtaining optimal flank exposure. The patient was secured to the table with 3 in. surgical tape and safety straps and was prepped and draped in the standard sterile manner.

The radiographic images were in the room.

A time-out was completed, verifying the correct patient, surgical procedure, site, and positioning, prior to beginning the procedure.

The space between the 10th and 11th ribs was palpated and an incision made at this level from the mid-axillary line and extended medially to the lateral border of the rectus abdominis muscle. Using electrocautery, the latissimus dorsi and external oblique muscles were incised exposing the underlying ribs. The intercostal attachments were transected taking care to avoid injury to the pleura and neurovascular bundle on the inferior surface of the rib. The internal oblique muscle was divided with cautery and the transversus abdominis carefully split in the direction of its fibers, avoiding entry into the peritoneum. A generous paranephric space was created by sweeping the peritoneum medially and the retroperitoneal connective tissue superiorly and inferiorly. A self-retaining retractor (e.g. Bookwalter, Omni-Tract, Finochietto) was appropriately positioned to optimize exposure, using padding on each retractor blade.

The parietal peritoneum was incised on the white line of Toldt and the colon was reflected medially.

> ***On the right***: The hepatic flexure and duodenum were mobilized carefully, freeing the kidney superiorly and medially.
> ***On the left***: The splenorenal ligament and lower edge of the pancreas were mobilized carefully, freeing the kidney superiorly.

Using sharp and blunt dissection, the retroperitoneal fascia overlying the renal vessels was separated, exposing the underlying renal vein, which was carefully dissected, mobilized, and encircled with a vessel loop. The gonadal vein was doubly ligated with 3-0 silk ties and divided.

> ***On the left***: The adrenal branch was similarly ligated.

With gentle retraction on the renal vein, the main renal artery was identified deep to this and dissected for a distance of 2 cm. It was doubly ligated with 2-0 silk and a 3-0 silk suture ligature, and sharply divided. Having interrupted the renal vascular inflow, the renal vein was similarly ligated and divided and the vessel loop removed.

Using both sharp and blunt dissection, Gerota's fascia was mobilized circumferentially achieving meticulous hemostasis with surgical clips and electrocautery. Attention was directed to the cranial attachments with the adrenal gland, which were carefully divided using *an electrothermal bipolar tissue sealing device (LigaSure)/surgical clips*, completely freeing the adrenal off the superior pole of the kidney. Inferiorly, the ureter was ligated with chromic ties and divided.

Once the specimen was completely freed, it was removed and sent to pathology for evaluation. The retroperitoneum was irrigated with warm sterile water and hemostasis was again ensured. Prior to closure, the vascular stumps, visceral organs, and pleura were inspected and found to be intact. The self-retaining retractor was removed, the kidney rest lowered, and the table taken out of flexion.

The incision was closed using running 1-0 polydioxanone (PDS) to approximate the three muscle layers, individually, taking care not to entrap the intercostal neurovascular bundle. 3-0 chromic sutures were used on Scarpa's fascia and the skin approximated with a subcuticular 4-0 poliglecaprone (Monocryl) suture. A sterile dressing was applied and the patient was repositioned supine.

At the end of the procedure, all counts were correct.

The patient tolerated the procedure well and was taken to the recovery room in satisfactory condition.

Estimated blood loss: Approximately _____ml

17

Renal Exploration and Reconstruction for Trauma (Renorrhaphy)

Indications

- Hemodynamic instability from renal hemorrhage suggested by an expanding or pulsatile retroperitoneal hematoma
- Select renovascular injuries
- In limited cases where a laparotomy is being performed for significant associated injuries and there is incomplete radiographic staging of a renal injury

Essential Steps

1) Explore the kidney and intraabdominal contents through a midline transperitoneal approach.
2) Obtain early vascular control.
3) Completely expose the kidney.
4) Perform minimal parenchymal debridement and achieve meticulous hemostasis.
5) Close the collecting system.
6) Complete the appropriate reconstructive procedure and cover the defect with adjacent tissue (omental flap or perirenal fat).
7) Place a drain.

Note These Variations

- Renal exploration is usually performed in conjunction with an exploratory laparotomy by the trauma surgical team. In such cases the abdominal contents have been examined and often the retroperitoneum has been exposed.
- If the patient is unstable for cross-sectional imaging, a one-shot intravenous pyelogram should be performed (using 2 ml/kg nonionic contrast) to assess the presence and location of a contralateral kidney.
- In cases where an extensive retroperitoneal hematoma obscures visualization and/ or palpation of the aorta, the renal pedicle can be identified by incising the parietal peritoneum medial to the inferior mesenteric vein.

Operative Dictations in Urologic Surgery, First Edition. Noel A. Armenakas, John A. Fracchia, and Ron Golan.
© 2019 John Wiley & Sons Ltd. Published 2019 by John Wiley & Sons Ltd.

- The renal vessels are occluded only for significant renovascular bleeding. In most cases, manual compression alone is sufficient.
- Renal reconstruction is dependent on the location and extent of injury. Parenchymal lacerations can be managed with a renorrhaphy. Major injures to the upper or lower poles are best managed with a polar nephrectomy.

Complications

- Bleeding
- Infection/abscess
- Missed injury
- Intraabdominal organ injury
- Urine leak/urinoma
- Ileus
- Renal infarct/loss of renal function
- Arteriovenous fistula
- Post-traumatic hypertension

Template Operative Dictation

Preoperative diagnosis: Grade *IV/V* renal injury
Postoperative diagnosis: Same
Procedure: *Right/left* renal exploration and reconstruction
Indications: The patient is a _____-year-old *male/female* who sustained a Grade *IV/V blunt/penetrating* injury to the *right/left* kidney and is taken to the operating room for renal exploration and reconstruction.
Description of Procedure: The indications, alternatives, benefits, and risks were discussed with the *patient/patient's family* and informed consent was obtained.

The patient was brought onto the operating room table, positioned supine, and secured with a safety strap. Pneumatic compression devices were placed on the lower extremities.

After the administration of intravenous antibiotics and initiation of general endotracheal anesthesia, the chest, abdomen, genitalia, and upper thighs were prepped and draped in the standard sterile manner.

The radiographic images were in the room.

A time-out was completed, verifying the correct patient, surgical procedure, site, and positioning, prior to beginning the procedure.

A midline abdominal incision was made from just below the xiphoid to the pubic symphysis. The subcutaneous tissue was incised with electrocautery, exposing the underlying rectus abdominis aponeurosis. This was incised at the linea alba and the rectus abdominis muscles separated at the midline and retracted laterally, exposing the peritoneal cavity, which was entered sharply, taking care not the injure the underlying bowel. A self-retaining retractor (e.g. Bookwalter, Omni-Tract) was positioned to optimize exposure, using padding on each retractor blade.

If the trauma surgical team is not present: A thorough exploratory laparotomy was performed, confirming the absence of intraperitoneal blood or injury to the visceral organs and vasculature.

Attention was directed to the *right/left* retroperitoneum were a large, *nonexpanding/expanding* hematoma was identified.

The transverse colon was moved cranially and the small bowel craniolaterally to expose the parietal peritoneum at the level of the aorta. The posterior peritoneum was incised medial to the inferior mesenteric vein over the aorta from the ligament of Treitz superiorly to the inferior mesenteric artery, inferiorly. The duodenum was Kocherized and the small bowel exteriorized onto the chest wall and placed in an intestinal (Lahey) bag. The left renal vein was identified, carefully mobilized and encircled with a loop.

For injuries to the left kidney: Using gentle retraction on the left renal vein, the left renal artery was identified deep to this and surrounded with a vessel loop.

For injuries involving the right kidney: After looping the left renal vein, the inferior vena cava was exposed and the right renal vein was identified and dissected. The right renal artery was then isolated deep to this and a vessel loop placed individually around both renal vessels.

Once vascular control was achieved, the white line of Toldt was incised, the *ascending/descending* colon mobilized medially and Gerota's fascia opened. All of the perirenal hematoma was removed and extracapsular mobilization of the entire kidney was performed using blunt and sharp dissection. The entire surface of the kidney, renal pelvis, and proximal ureter were inspected for any injuries.

A ___cm laceration was identified on the *anterior/posterior/lateral/medial* surface of the kidney. This was debrided of any nonviable parenchyma and visible bleeding vessels were ligated with figure-of-eight 4-0 chromic sutures. The collecting system was approximated with running 4-0 chromics. Absorbable gelatin sponge (Gelfoam) bolsters were inserted to fill the parenchymal defect. The renorrhaphy was completed with interrupted 2-0 polydioxanone (PDS) sutures, loosely reapproximating the renal capsule over an additional superficially placed gelatin bolster. A hemostatic sealant ____*(specify brand)*____ was used to further reinforce the repair. The defect was covered with *an omental flap/perirenal fat* and secured with 3-0 chromic sutures.

The wound was irrigated with warm sterile saline and hemostasis was confirmed. A surgical drain (e.g. Jackson-Pratt) was placed in the perinephric space and brought out through a separate stab incision, where it was secured at the skin with a 2-0 silk suture. The vessel loops were removed and the bowel was repositioned intraabdominally. The abdominal contents were again carefully inspected for any injury prior to removing the self-retaining retractor.

The abdominal incision was closed using a running 2-0 chromic suture to approximate the rectus muscles and 1-0 PDS suture for the rectus aponeurosis. Scarpa's fascia was closed with 3-0 chromic sutures and staples were used on the skin. A sterile dressing was applied.

At the end of the procedure, all counts were correct.

The patient tolerated the procedure well and was taken to the recovery room in *guarded/satisfactory* condition.

Estimated blood loss: Approximately _____ml

18

Simple Nephrectomy

Indications

- Nonmalignant renal disease (e.g. infection, nonfunctioning kidney, medically refractory renovascular hypertension, end-stage renal disease)

Essential Steps

1) Mobilize the colon and incise the anterior renal fascia medially.
2) Identify and dissect the renal vein and place a vessel loop around it.
3) Dissect the renal artery deep to the vein and surround it with a vessel loop.
4) Ligate and divide the renal artery, then the vein.
5) Dissect the kidney posteriorly and inferiorly.
6) Ligate and divide the ureter.
7) Free the kidney from its cranial attachments and remove the specimen.

Note These Variations

- The choice of incision is dependent on the reason for the nephrectomy, the anatomic characteristics of the kidney, the patient's body habitus, and the surgeon's preference. Although the standard flank incision is versatile, alternate options include anterior subcostal (e.g. Chevron) and midline abdominal incisions, which are preferred for very large tumors requiring more direct access to the renal pedicle and for renal trauma, respectively.
- With severe renal scarring and/or inflammation, subcapsular renal dissection may be required.
- In cases where the renal vein and artery cannot be safely dissected separately, they can be ligated en-masse using a vascular stapler.
- With acute or chronic infection, drainage of the surgical site is advised.

Operative Dictations in Urologic Surgery, First Edition. Noel A. Armenakas, John A. Fracchia, and Ron Golan.
© 2019 John Wiley & Sons Ltd. Published 2019 by John Wiley & Sons Ltd.

Complications

- Bleeding
- Infection
- Intraabdominal organ injury
- Pneumothorax
- Ileus

Template Operative Dictation

Preoperative diagnosis: _____
Postoperative diagnosis: Same
Procedure: *Right/left* simple nephrectomy
Indications: The patient is a _____-year-old *male/female* with _____
presenting for a *right/left* simple nephrectomy.
Description of Procedure: The indications, alternatives, benefits, and risks were discussed with the patient and informed consent was obtained.

The patient was brought onto the operating room table, positioned supine, and secured with a safety strap. Pneumatic compression devices were placed on the lower extremities.

After the administration of intravenous antibiotics and general endotracheal anesthesia, a 16 Fr urethral catheter was inserted into the bladder and connected to a drainage bag. The patient was placed in the lateral decubitus position at a 45° angle with the lower leg flexed 90° and the upper leg extended. An axillary roll was positioned to protect the brachial plexus and a gel pad placed to support the back. Multiple pillows were used to pad beneath and between both the upper and lower extremities to ensure adequate cushioning. The kidney rest was elevated and the table flexed and adjusted horizontally, obtaining optimal flank exposure. The patient was secured to the table with 3 in. surgical tape and safety straps, and was prepped and draped in the standard sterile manner.

The radiographic images were in the room.

A time-out was completed, verifying the correct patient, surgical procedure, site, and positioning, prior to beginning the procedure.

An anterior incision was made from the tip of the twelfth rib extending medially to the lateral border of the rectus abdominis muscle. The external and internal oblique muscles were incised using electrocautery, and the transversus abdominis carefully split in the direction of its fibers avoiding entry into the peritoneum. The paranephric space was created by sweeping the peritoneum medially and the retroperitoneal connective tissue superiorly and inferiorly. A self-retaining retractor (e.g. Bookwalter, Omni-Tract, or Finochietto) was appropriately positioned to optimize exposure, using padding on each retractor blade.

The parietal peritoneum was incised on the white line of Toldt and the colon reflected medially, exposing Gerota's fascia.

> ***On the right:*** The hepatic flexure and duodenum were mobilized carefully, freeing the kidney superiorly and medially.

On the left: The splenorenal ligament and lower edge of the pancreas were mobilized carefully, freeing the kidney superiorly.

Using sharp and blunt dissection, the retroperitoneal fascia overlying the renal vessels was separated, exposing the underlying renal vein, which was carefully dissected, mobilized, and encircled with a loop. The gonadal vein was doubly ligated with 3-0 silk ties and divided.

On the left: The adrenal branch was similarly ligated.

Using gentle retraction on the renal vein, the main renal artery was identified deep to this and dissected for a distance of 2 cm. It was doubly ligated with 2-0 silk and a 3-0 silk suture ligature, and sharply divided. Having interrupted the renal vascular inflow, the renal vein was similarly ligated and divided and the vessel loop was removed.

Gerota's fascia was incised and mobilized circumferentially, using sharp and blunt dissection, exposing the underlying *right/left* kidney. Attention was directed to the cranial attachments with the adrenal gland, which were carefully divided using surgical clips, completely freeing the adrenal off the superior pole of the kidney. Inferiorly, the ureter was ligated with chromic ties and divided. Meticulous hemostasis was achieved with surgical clips and electrocautery.

Once the extracapsular dissection was completed and the kidney was completely freed, it was removed and sent to pathology for evaluation. The retroperitoneum was copiously irrigated with warm sterile saline and hemostasis again was ensured. Prior to closure, the vascular stumps, visceral organs, and pleura were inspected and found to be intact. The self-retaining retractor was removed, the kidney rest lowered and the table was taken out of flexion.

The incision was closed using running 1-0 polydioxanone (PDS) to approximate the three muscle layers, individually, taking care not to entrap the intercostal neurovascular bundle. 3-0 chromic sutures were used on Scarpa's fascia, and the skin approximated with a subcuticular 4-0 poliglecaprone (Monocryl) suture. A sterile dressing was applied and the patient repositioned supine.

At the end of the procedure, all counts were correct.

The patient tolerated the procedure well and was taken to the recovery room in satisfactory condition.

Estimated blood loss: Approximately _____ml

19

Transplant Nephrectomy

Indications

- Failed renal allograft (usually rupture due to acute rejection, renal vein thrombosis, or acute tubular necrosis)

Essential Steps

1) Review the renal transplant operative report prior to surgery to be aware of the vascular anatomy.
2) Free the allograft circumferentially prior to addressing the renal hilum.
3) Ligate the renal vessels, either individually or en masse, taking care not to injure the iliac vessels.
4) Dissect, ligate, and divide the ureter, and remove the kidney.
5) Avoid using a surgical drain as it may increase the risk of infection.

Note These Variations

- In cases of extensive renal scarring from infection, previous surgery or biopsies, consider extending the incision laterally and approaching the renal allograft superiorly.
- Extracapsular renal dissection may be feasible in cases of early allograft failure with limited inflammation.
- A Satinsky clamp can be used to ligate the renal artery and vein en-masse, in cases of severe hilar scarring.

Complications

- Bleeding
- Infection
- Intraabdominal or pelvic organ injury
- Ileus

Operative Dictations in Urologic Surgery, First Edition. Noel A. Armenakas, John A. Fracchia, and Ron Golan.
© 2019 John Wiley & Sons Ltd. Published 2019 by John Wiley & Sons Ltd.

Template Operative Dictation

Preoperative diagnosis: Failed renal allograft
Postoperative diagnosis: Failed renal allograft
Procedure: Transplant nephrectomy
Indications: The patient is a _____-year-old *male/female* with a failed renal allograft due to _____ presenting for transplant nephrectomy.
Description of Procedure: The indications, alternatives, benefits, and risks were discussed with the patient and informed consent was obtained.

The patient was brought onto the operating room table, positioned supine, and secured with a safety strap. Pneumatic compression devices were placed on the lower extremities.

After the administration of intravenous antibiotics and general endotracheal anesthesia, the abdomen was prepped and draped in the standard sterile manner.

The radiographic images were in the room.

A time-out was completed, verifying the correct patient, surgical procedure, site, and positioning, prior to beginning the procedure.

A 16 Fr urethral catheter was inserted into the bladder and connected to a drainage bag.

An incision was made over the existing *right/left* lower quadrant scar and carried down through the subcutaneous tissue to the external oblique aponeurosis and muscle, which were incised using electrocautery. The underlying internal oblique was similarly opened, exposing the transversus abdominis, which was carefully separated using blunt dissection taking care not to injure the underlying transplant kidney. Additional medial exposure was obtained by transecting the lateral tendinous attachments of the rectus abdominis muscle to the pubis. The kidney was gently freed anteriorly from the undersurface of the muscle, superomedially from the peritoneum and laterally from the pelvic side wall. A self-retaining retractor (e.g. Balfour, Bookwalter, Omni-Tract) was appropriately positioned to optimize exposure, using padding on each retractor blade.

A small anterior renal capsulotomy was made and the renal parenchyma carefully enucleated subcapsularly, using sharp and blunt dissection. Once the kidney was mobilized circumferentially, attention was turned medially to the renal hilum. The minimal parenchymal bleeding encountered was controlled with manual compression. The renal artery and vein were identified, individually ligated with 2-0 silk ties, and sharply divided. The ureter was dissected, ligated with chromic ties and divided. The specimen was removed in its entirety and sent to pathology for evaluation. Meticulous hemostasis was ensured with electrocautery.

Prior to closure, the vascular stumps, iliac vessels, bowel, and bladder were inspected and found to be intact. The wound was irrigated with warm normal saline and the self-retaining retractor was removed.

The incision was closed using running 1-0 polydioxanone (PDS) sutures to approximate the internal and external oblique aponeuroses, individually. 3-0 chromic sutures were used on Scarpa's fascia and the skin approximated with a subcuticular 4-0 poliglecaprone (Monocryl) suture. A sterile dressing was applied.

At the end of the procedure, all counts were correct.

The patient tolerated the procedure well and was taken to the recovery room in satisfactory condition.

Estimated blood loss: Approximately _____ml

Lymphatics

20

Inguinal Lymph Node Dissection

Indications

- Penile or scrotal wall cancer

Essential Steps

1) Mark the area of dissection by drawing a line from the anterosuperior iliac spine to the pubic tubercle. Extend this caudally, both medially and laterally, and connect both inferior ends.
2) Incise the skin over the medial thigh approximately 3 cm below the inguinal ligament.
3) Create superior and inferior flaps, maintaining the superficial vasculature.
4) Incise the fascia lata to expose the sartorius and adductor longus muscles.
5) Begin the lymph node dissection inferiorly and continue superiorly along the saphenous vein and femoral vessels at the fossa ovalis to the node of Cloquet, removing both superficial and deep nodes. Lateral dissection of the femoral sheath should be avoided to prevent injury to the femoral nerve.
6) Mobilize the sartorius muscle laterally and rotate this medially to cover the femoral vessels. Avoid dissecting the sartorius medially to prevent compromise to its vasculature.
7) Ensure meticulous hemo- and lymphostasis throughout the procedure.
8) Prior to closing the incision, inspect the cutaneous flap for viability.
9) Place a drain.

Note These Variations

- A superficial or modified inguinal dissection may be considered in order to determine the presence of microscopic metastases.
- With massive lymphadenopathy, the saphenous vein should be ligated.
- Viability of the inferior and superior cutaneous thigh flaps can be assessed using intravenous fluorescein and a Wood's lamp.
- In cases of insufficient soft tissue coverage, a rectus abdominis myocutaneous flap can be used to close the defect.

Operative Dictations in Urologic Surgery, First Edition. Noel A. Armenakas, John A. Fracchia, and Ron Golan.
© 2019 John Wiley & Sons Ltd. Published 2019 by John Wiley & Sons Ltd.

Complications

- Bleeding
- Infection
- Vascular injury
- Flap necrosis
- Lymphocele
- Lymphedema

Template Operative Dictation

Preoperative diagnosis: Invasive *penile/scrotal wall* cancer
Postoperative diagnosis: Same
Procedure: Bilateral inguinal lymph node dissection
Indications: The patient is a _____-year-old male with clinical stage _____ penile cancer presenting for a bilateral inguinal lymph node dissection.
Description of Procedure: The indications, alternatives, benefits, and risks were discussed with the patient and informed consent was obtained.

The patient was brought onto the operating room table, positioned supine, and secured with a safety strap. Pneumatic compression devices were placed on the lower extremities.

After the administration of intravenous antibiotics and initiation of *general endotracheal/ regional* anesthesia, both hips were abducted and externally rotated with the knees flexed. Padding was used to prevent any pressure points. The abdomen, genitalia, and both thighs were prepped and draped in the standard sterile manner.

The radiographic images were in the room.

A time-out was completed, verifying the correct patient, surgical procedure, site, and positioning, prior to beginning the procedure.

A 16 Fr urethral catheter was inserted into the bladder and connected to a drainage bag.

The superior boundary of the dissection was carefully marked by drawing a line from the *right/left* anterosuperior iliac spine to the pubic tubercle. This was extended caudally for a distance of 15 cm medially and 20 cm laterally. The inferior limit of dissection was delineated by connecting the lateral and medial inferior margins.

An incision was made over the *right/left* medial thigh 3 cm below the inguinal ligament and carried down to Scarpa's fascia creating a plane for proper flap dissection. Using sharp and blunt dissection, superior and inferior skin flaps were developed below the subcutaneous tissue (Camper's fascia) to the marked boundaries of dissection. Skin hooks and well-padded Deaver retractors were used to protect the flaps and preserve their vascularity. The dissection was continued superiorly and medially, exposing the external oblique aponeurosis and spermatic cord, respectively.

A longitudinal incision was made in the fascia lata exposing the sartorius and adductor longus muscles, which served as the lateral and medial borders of the deep inguinal lymph node dissection, respectively.

The inferior portion of the lymphatic packet was dissected free, elevated off its deep margin, transected and ligated with *surgical clips/silk ties*. The dissection was continued superiorly to the level of the saphenous vein, which was identified medially and

preserved. Several tributaries of the saphenous vein were carefully dissected, ligated and the surrounding nodes dissected free.

The fossa ovalis was identified and the femoral sheath incised exposing the underlying femoral artery and vein. The dissection was continued medially isolating the node of Cloquet and the deep nodes located inferolateral to the femoral vein and between the femoral vessels. The lymph nodes appeared *unremarkable/enlarged/matted* on palpation. Upon completion of the dissection, the superficial and deep lymph node packet was ligated, transected, and removed *en bloc*. The entire packet was sent to pathology for evaluation.

Meticulous hemo- and lymphostasis were achieved throughout the dissection using surgical clips and electrocautery. The femoral artery and both the femoral and saphenous veins were carefully inspected, confirming the absence of any bleeding or trauma.

The exposed femoral vessels were covered by bluntly dissecting the sartorius muscle laterally, transecting it at its origin at the level of the anterosuperior iliac spine, rotating it medially, and suturing it to the external oblique aponeurosis and adductor longus edge using 3-0 interrupted polyglactin (Vicryl) sutures. Hemo- and lymphostasis were again confirmed and the wound irrigated with warm sterile water.

A surgical drain (e.g. Jackson Pratt) was placed beneath the cutaneous flap and brought out at the skin through a separate inferior stab incision, where it was secured with a 2-0 silk suture.

An identical lymph node dissection was performed on the contralateral side.

Prior to closure, both thigh flaps were inspected and noted to be intact without any evidence of vascular compromise. Each inguinal incision was closed in two layers, approximating Scarpa's fascia with 3-0 Vicryl sutures and the skin with staples. A sterile pressure dressing was applied bilaterally.

At the end of the procedure, all counts were correct.

The patient tolerated the procedure well and was taken to the recovery room in satisfactory condition.

Estimated blood loss: Approximately _____ml

21

Pelvic Lymph Node Dissection

Indications

- Bladder cancer
- Prostate cancer
- Urethral cancer
- Penile cancer with positive inguinal lymph nodes

Essential Steps

1) Expose the iliac vessels bilaterally from the bifurcation of the common iliac arteries to the femoral canal.
2) Identify and protect the ureters at their crossing over the common iliac arteries.
3) Perform a thorough bilateral pelvic lymph node dissection with the limits of dissection being the common iliac artery cranially, the genitofemoral nerve laterally, the ureter medially, the obturator nerve posteriorly, and the node of Cloquet caudally.
4) Achieve meticulous hemo- and lymphostasis using surgical clips and electrocautery.
5) Place a drain.

Note These Variations

- The patient may be positioned with his or her legs in (Allen) universal stirrups, and placed in modified Trendelenburg to enhance exposure.
- A lower abdominal (Pfannensteil) rather than of a midline abdominal incision can be used.
- An *extended* pelvic lymphadenectomy can be performed starting cranially at the aortic bifurcation, additionally incorporating paraaortic, presacral and presciatic lymph nodes.
- The lymph nodes may be removed and sent separately based on their anatomic origin, rather than as one packet from each side. This will allow for a more thorough histologic lymph node evaluation.

Operative Dictations in Urologic Surgery, First Edition. Noel A. Armenakas, John A. Fracchia, and Ron Golan.
© 2019 John Wiley & Sons Ltd. Published 2019 by John Wiley & Sons Ltd.

Complications

- Bleeding
- Infection
- Intraabdominal organ injury
- Nerve injury
- Ureteral injury
- Ileus
- Lymphocele

Template Operative Dictation

Preoperative diagnosis: *Bladder/Prostate/Urethral/Penile* cancer
Postoperative diagnosis: Same
Procedure: Pelvic lymph node dissection
Indications: The patient is a _____ -year-old *male/female* with clinical stage T_____ *bladder/prostate/urethral/penile* carcinoma presenting for a pelvic lymph node dissection.
Description of Procedure: The indications, alternatives, benefits, and risks were discussed with the patient and informed consent was obtained.

The patient was brought onto the operating room table, positioned supine, and secured with a safety strap. Pneumatic compression devices were placed on the lower extremities.

After the administration of intravenous antibiotics and initiation of general endotracheal anesthesia, the patient was positioned with the break just above the anterosuperior iliac spine, and the operating table flexed 15°. The entire abdomen and external genitalia were prepped and draped in the standard sterile manner.

The radiographic images were in the room.

A time-out was completed, verifying the correct patient, surgical procedure, and positioning, prior to beginning the procedure.

An 18 Fr urethral catheter was inserted into the bladder and connected to a drainage bag.

A midline abdominal incision was made 2 cm above the umbilicus and carried down to the pubic symphysis. The subcutaneous tissue was incised with electrocautery, exposing the underlying rectus abdominis aponeurosis. This was incised at the linea alba and the rectus abdominis muscles separated at the midline and retracted laterally, taking care not to injure the underlying inferior epigastric vessels.

The space of Retzius was developed by sweeping the infrapubic space posterolaterally and mobilizing the peritoneum cranially on both sides along the pelvic sidewall. The *vas deferens/round ligaments* were ligated and divided to facilitate mobilization of the peritoneal sac. A self-retaining retractor (e.g. Bookwalter, Omni-Tract, Balfour) was appropriately positioned to optimize exposure, using padding on each retractor blade.

The iliac vessels were exposed from just above the common iliac bifurcation to the femoral canal. The ureters were identified anteriorly at the bifurcation of the external and internal iliac vessels and protected. The lymph nodes appeared *unremarkable/ enlarged/matted* on palpation.

The nodal dissection was started at the medial aspect of the *left/right* external iliac artery by incising the perivascular fibroareolar sheath. Using gentle medial traction, the obturator neurovascular bundle was identified posteriorly and preserved. The dissection was carried laterally to the genitofemoral nerve and medially to the ipsilateral ureter. The cranial and caudal limits of dissection were the common iliac bifurcation and femoral canal (node of Cloquet), respectively. Small vessels and lymphatic branches were fulgurated or ligated with surgical clips to maintain meticulous hemo- and lymphostasis. A large surgical clip was used to individually secure the distal and proximal extents of lymph node packet. The nodal packet was removed and sent to pathology for evaluation.

The contralateral lymph node dissection was performed in a similar manner and the nodal packet sent to pathology for evaluation.

Upon completion of the lymphadenectomy bilaterally, the pelvis was irrigated with warm sterile water. A surgical drain (e.g. Jackson-Pratt) was placed in the pelvis and brought out at the skin through a separate stab incision, where it was secured with a 2-0 silk suture. Prior to closure, the iliac vessels, ureter, obturator neurovascular bundle, and pelvic structures were inspected and found to be intact.

The self-retaining retractor was removed and the abdominal incision was closed using a running 2-0 chromic to approximate the rectus muscles and 1-0 polydioxanone (PDS) for the rectus aponeurosis. 3-0 chromic sutures were used on Scarpa's fascia and the skin approximated with a subcuticular 4-0 poliglecaprone (Monocryl) suture. A sterile dressing was applied.

At the end of the procedure, all counts were correct.

The patient tolerated the procedure well and was taken to the recovery room in satisfactory condition.

Estimated blood loss: Approximately _____ml

22

Retroperitoneal Lymph Node Dissection

Indications

- Testis cancer

Essential Steps

1) Expose the retroperitoneum through a midline transperitoneal approach.
2) Apply the appropriate nodal template and perform the lymphadenectomy using a "split and roll" technique with delicate blunt and sharp dissection.
3) Carefully dissect and preserve the efferent sympathetic fibers, which run posterior to the vena cava on the right and posterolateral to the aorta on the left.
4) Lumbar vessels should be ligated and divided to expose the nerves and facilitate the nodal mobilization.
5) Accessory arteries to the kidney need to be identified and preserved.
6) Remove the appropriate nodal tissues and ipsilateral spermatic cord.
7) Achieve meticulous hemo- and lymphostasis using surgical clips and electrocautery.

Note These Variations

- Several "modified" surgical templates have been described.
- A thoracoabdominal incision can be utilized, limiting bowel manipulation. This is most applicable when employing a left-sided nodal template.
- With large retroperitoneal lymphadenopathy, exposure of the renal hilum may be facilitated by ligating and dividing the inferior mesenteric vein and/or artery.
- Care should be taken to avoid mistaking a retroaortic left renal vein for a lumbar vein and inadvertently ligating it. This aberrant anatomy occurs in up to 3% of patients.
- The lymph nodes may be removed and sent separately based on their anatomic origin, rather than *en bloc*. This will allow for a more thorough histologic lymph node evaluation.
- For extensive post-chemotherapy lymphadenopathy with adjacent organ involvement, a metastasectomy may be required, including nephrectomy, splenectomy, hepatectomy, lobectomy, and resection of the aorta or vena cava.

Operative Dictations in Urologic Surgery, First Edition. Noel A. Armenakas, John A. Fracchia, and Ron Golan.
© 2019 John Wiley & Sons Ltd. Published 2019 by John Wiley & Sons Ltd.

Complications

- Bleeding
- Infection
- Ileus/bowel obstruction
- Intraabdominal organ injury
- Loss of antegrade ejaculation
- Lymphocele

Template Operative Dictation

Preoperative diagnosis: Testis cancer
Postoperative diagnosis: Same
Procedure: Retroperitoneal lymph node dissection
Indications: The patient is a _____-year-old male with clinical stage T__ testis cancer, presenting for a retroperitoneal lymph node dissection.
Description of Procedure: The indications, alternatives, benefits, and risks were discussed with the patient and informed consent was obtained.

The patient was brought onto the operating room table, positioned supine, and secured with a safety strap. Pneumatic compression devices were placed on the lower extremities.

After the administration of intravenous antibiotics and initiation of general endotracheal anesthesia, the chest, abdomen, genitalia, and upper thighs were prepped and draped in the standard sterile manner.

The radiographic images were in the room.

A time-out was completed, verifying the correct patient, surgical procedure, and positioning, prior to beginning the procedure.

A 16 Fr urethral catheter was inserted into the bladder and connected to a drainage bag.

A midline abdominal incision was made from just below the xiphoid to the pubic symphysis. The subcutaneous tissue was incised with electrocautery, exposing the underlying rectus abdominis aponeurosis. This was incised at the linea alba and the rectus abdominis muscles were separated at the midline and retracted laterally, exposing the peritoneal cavity, which was entered sharply, taking care not the injure the underlying bowel. The falciform ligament was divided, allowing cranial displacement of the liver. A self-retaining retractor (e.g. Bookwalter, Omni-Tract) was positioned to optimize exposure, using padding on each retractor blade.

A thorough exploratory laparotomy was performed, confirming the absence of visible visceral metastases.

The transverse colon was moved cranially and the small bowel craniolaterally to expose the parietal peritoneum at the level of the aorta. The posterior peritoneum was incised medial to the inferior mesenteric vein over the aorta from the ligament of Treitz superiorly to the inferior mesenteric artery, inferiorly. The incision was extended superomedially to the duodenojejunal flexure, allowing mobilization of the terminal duodenum and pancreas, and laterally along the right paracolic gutter from the cecum to the hepatic flexure. The duodenum was Kocherized and the small bowel and right colon exteriorized onto the chest wall and placed in an intestinal (Lahey) bag.

***For right-sided tumors*:** Having carefully and thoroughly exposed the retroperitoneum, the right ureter was identified, surrounded with a vessel loop and gently retracted laterally. The lymphatic dissection was started by mobilizing the perivascular lymphatic tissue at the level of the left renal vein and taken laterally over the aorta and vena cava to the right renal vein. The right gonadal vein was identified, ligated with 3-0 silk ties, divided, and dissected distally.

Using a "split and roll" technique and delicate blunt and sharp dissection, the lymphatic tissues over the major vessels were gently mobilized. Multiple lumbar vessels were doubly ligated and divided allowing identification and preservation of the postganglionic sympathetic fibers. Posteriorly the lymphatic tissue was separated from the psoas fascia and anterior spinous ligament. Inferiorly the dissection was continued to the level of the right common iliac bifurcation, avoiding aortic dissection below the inferior mesenteric artery to prevent injury to the hypogastric plexus.

Meticulous hemo- and lymphostasis were achieved throughout the dissection using a combination of surgical clips and electrocautery. The nodal packet, consisting of the anterior aortocaval, interaortocaval, right paracaval, and right common iliac nodes, was removed in toto, along with the remnant of the right spermatic cord, and sent to pathology for evaluation.

***For left-sided tumors*:** Having carefully and thoroughly exposed the retroperitoneum, the left ureter was identified, surrounded with a vessel loop and gently retracted laterally. The lymphatic dissection was started at the level of the left renal vein by mobilizing the perivascular lymphatic tissue. The left adrenal and lumbar branches were identified and carefully dissected, ligated with 3-0 silk ties and divided. The left gonadal vein was similarly divided and dissected distally.

Using a "split and roll" technique and delicate blunt and sharp dissection, the pre- and para-aortic lymphatic tissues were gently mobilized. Multiple lumbar vessels were doubly ligated and divided, allowing identification and preservation of the postganglionic sympathetic fibers. Posteriorly, the lymphatic tissue was separated from the psoas fascia and anterior spinous ligament. Inferiorly the dissection was continued to the level of the left common iliac bifurcation, avoiding aortic dissection below the inferior mesenteric artery to prevent injury to the hypogastric plexus.

Meticulous hemo- and lymphostasis were achieved throughout the dissection using a combination of surgical clips and electrocautery. The nodal packet, consisting of the anterior aortic, paraaortic, and left common iliac nodes, was removed in toto, along with the remnant of the left spermatic cord, and sent to pathology for evaluation.

***Bilateral lymphadenectomy*:** Having carefully and thoroughly exposed the retroperitoneum, both ureters were identified, surrounded with a vessel loop and gently retracted laterally. The lymphatic dissection was started by mobilizing the perivascular lymphatic tissue at the level of the left renal vein and taken laterally over the aorta and vena cava to the right renal vein. The left adrenal and bilateral lumbar branches were identified, carefully dissected, ligated with 3-0 silk ties, and divided. The right and left gonadal veins were similarly divided and dissected distally.

Using a combination "split and roll" technique and delicate blunt and sharp dissection, the pre- and para-aortic, vena caval and interaortocaval lymphatic tissues were gently mobilized laterally to the corresponding ureters. Multiple lumbar vessels were doubly ligated and divided, allowing identification and preservation of the postganglionic sympathetic fibers. Posteriorly, the lymphatic tissue was separated from the psoas fascia and anterior spinous ligament. Inferiorly, the dissection was continued to the level of the common iliac bifurcation bilaterally. Limited anterior aortic dissection was performed below the inferior mesenteric artery to limit injury to the hypogastric plexus.

Meticulous hemo- and lymphostasis were achieved throughout the dissection using a combination of surgical clips and electrocautery. The nodal packet, consisting of the anterior aortic, paraaortic, interaortocaval, anterior caval, paracaval, and bilateral common iliac nodes, was removed in toto, along with the remnant of the spermatic cord ipsilaterally, and sent to pathology for evaluation.

Upon completion of the lymphadenectomy, the abdomen was irrigated with warm sterile water and carefully evaluated for bleeding. The contents of the bowel bag were placed back into the abdomen. Prior to closure, the abdominal vessels and visceral organs were inspected and found to be intact without any evidence of devascularization or injury.

The self-retaining retractor was removed and the abdominal incision was closed using a running 2-0 chromic to approximate the rectus muscles and 1-0 polydioxanone (PDS) for the rectus aponeurosis. 3-0 chromic sutures were used on Scarpa's fascia and the skin approximated with a subcuticular 4-0 poliglecaprone (Monocryl) suture. A sterile dressing was applied.

At the end of the procedure, all counts were correct.

The patient tolerated the procedure well and was taken to the recovery room in satisfactory condition.

Estimated blood loss: Approximately _____ml

Penis

23

Circumcision

Indications

- Phimosis
- Extensive preputial condylomata
- Patient preference (e.g. hygienic, aesthetic or religious reasons)

Essential Steps

1) Mark the foreskin over corona with a marking pen and incise this circumferentially.
2) Retract the foreskin proximally, free all preputial adhesions and make a second circumferential incision 1 cm below the coronal sulcus.
3) Remove the correct amount of preputial tissue to avoid chordee.
4) Ensure meticulous hemostasis with judicious electrocautery use to avoid inadvertent tissue necrosis.
5) Reapproximate the penile skin to the subcoronal cuff, using fine absorbable interrupted sutures.

Note These Variations

- A dorsal and ventral slit technique may be necessary in cases of severe phimosis where the foreskin cannot be retracted. A straight clamp is carefully placed below the foreskin ventrally and dorsally, and the foreskin is incised to the level of the corona, taking care not to injure the glans. The lateral foreskin flaps are then circumferentially excised just proximal to the corona. Skin closure is identical to the sleeve-technique procedure.

Complications

- Bleeding
- Infection

Operative Dictations in Urologic Surgery, First Edition. Noel A. Armenakas, John A. Fracchia, and Ron Golan.
© 2019 John Wiley & Sons Ltd. Published 2019 by John Wiley & Sons Ltd.

- Wound dehiscence
- Chordee
- Penile/urethral injury
- Meatal stenosis

Template Operative Dictation

Preoperative diagnosis: Phimosis
Postoperative diagnosis: Same
Procedure: Circumcision
Indications: The patient is a _____ -year-old male with *phimosis/extensive preputial condylomata* presenting for a circumcision.
Description of Procedure: The indications, alternatives, benefits, and risks were discussed with the *patient/patient's family* and informed consent was obtained.

The patient was brought onto the operating room table, positioned supine, and secured with a safety strap. All pressure points were carefully padded and pneumatic compression devices placed on the lower extremities.

After the administration of intravenous antibiotics and *general/regional/local* anesthesia, the genitalia were prepped and draped in the standard sterile manner.

A time-out was completed, verifying the correct patient, surgical procedure, and positioning, prior to beginning the procedure.

With the foreskin covering the glans in the normal anatomic position, the corona was marked with a marking pen. A circumferential incision was made at the level of the corona and taken down to the dartos fascia. The foreskin was retracted proximal to the glans and all preputial adhesions were freed. A second circumferential incision was made 1 cm below the coronal sulcus. Special care was taken not to disrupt the urethra on the ventral surface. All bleeding was carefully controlled with electrocautery.

The dorsal preputial skin was dissected superficially off the dartos fascia and divided longitudinally at the midline. The incision was carried out circumferentially removing a circular sleeve of foreskin, which was sent to pathology for evaluation. Meticulous hemostasis was achieved using electrocautery.

The skin edges were approximated with four-quadrant *3-0/4-0* chromic sutures. Similar interrupted sutures were placed between these in a circumferential manner, approximating the remainder of the incision.

A penile block was performed using _____cc of 0.25% bupivacaine HCL injected circumferentially in the proximal penile shaft for postoperative pain control.

Antibiotic ointment and a Vaseline gauze were placed on the suture line and the penis was wrapped loosely with a self-adherent (Coban) dressing.

At the end of the procedure, all counts were correct.

The patient tolerated the procedure well and was taken to the recovery room in satisfactory condition.

Estimated blood loss: Approximately _____ml

24

Inflatable Penile Prosthesis

Indications

- Erectile dysfunction

Essential Steps

1) Make a penoscrotal incision and expose the tunica albuginea of each corpus cavernosum.
2) Dilate each corpus cavernosum through a small corporotomy taking care not to perforate the tunica albuginea.
3) Measure the entire length of each corpus cavernosum using the Furlow insertion tool and choose the appropriate cylinders and rear tip extenders.
4) Place each cylinder through the corresponding corporotomy and confirm its correct position. Perform a watertight corporotomy closure.
5) Create a pocket in the paravesical space through the inguinal ring by perforating the transversalis fascia and position the reservoir within this.
6) Make a scrotal dartos pouch and situate the pump in a dependent position within this. (Usually, this is placed in the patient's dominant side to facilitate manual operation.)
7) Test the device to confirm its proper function and ensure proper placement and sizing of the cylinders.
8) Close the penoscrotal incision in two layers.

Note These Variations

- A "No-touch" technique can be used, eliminating any contact between the prosthesis and the skin, potentially minimizing the incidence of peri-prosthetic infection.
- There are several available options regarding the choice of manufacturer and the type of cylinders to use. The ultimate decision is dependent on the etiology of the erectile dysfunction, the specific penile characteristics, the surgeon's preference, and product availability.

Operative Dictations in Urologic Surgery, First Edition. Noel A. Armenakas, John A. Fracchia, and Ron Golan.
© 2019 John Wiley & Sons Ltd. Published 2019 by John Wiley & Sons Ltd.

- Alternatively, a transverse scrotal or infrapubic approach can be used for prosthesis placement.
- The Dilamezinsert can be used to aid in corporal dilation.
- The reservoir can be placed in the paravesical space through a separate small inguinal incision.
- Ectopic (submuscular) reservoir placement is preferable in cases of prior pelvic or inguinal surgery and in morbidly obese patients. The reservoir is placed in the abdominal wall anterior to the tranversalis fascia, avoiding the paravesical space.
- In patients with Peyronie's disease, penile modeling using a long-handled scalpel and nasal speculum or (Uramix) cavernotome may be required to incise and disrupt the fibrosis.

Complications

- Bleeding
- Infection
- Corpus cavernosal perforation
- Injuries to the urethra, bowel, vasculature
- SST glans deformity
- Chronic pain
- Erosion
- Mechanical failure
- Patient dissatisfaction

Template Operative Dictation

Preoperative diagnosis: Erectile dysfunction
Postoperative diagnosis: Same
Procedure: Insertion of a *(state type)*__ inflatable penile prosthesis
Indications: The patient is a _____-year-old male with erectile dysfunction presenting for insertion of an inflatable penile prosthesis.
Description of Procedure: The indications, alternatives, benefits, and risks were discussed with the patient and informed consent was obtained.

The patient was brought onto the operating room table, positioned supine with the hips abducted (frog leg) and secured with a safety strap. All pressure points were carefully padded and pneumatic compression devices were placed on the lower extremities.

After the administration of intravenous antibiotics and *general/regional* anesthesia, the genitalia perineum and lower abdomen were thoroughly prepped with *chlorhexidine-alcohol/povidone/iodine* and draped in the standard sterile manner.

A time-out was completed, verifying the correct patient, surgical procedure, and positioning, prior to beginning the procedure.

A 14 Fr urethral catheter was advanced into the bladder and connected to a drainage bag.

A 4 cm vertical penoscrotal incision was made at the median raphe and carried down through the dartos and superficial Buck's fascias. A self-retaining retractor (e.g. Lone Star) was appropriately positioned to optimize exposure.

The corpus spongiosum was retracted laterally and the *right/left* corpus cavernosum was identified. The deep layer of Buck's fascia was dissected off this, exposing the underlying tunica albuginea. Two, 2-0 polyglactin (Vicryl) stay sutures were placed laterally in the tunica albuginea and a 1.5 cm corporotomy was made between these. Using Metzenbaum scissors with the tips pointed laterally, the *right/left* corpora cavernosum was tunneled proximally and distally to the ischial tuberosities and mid glans, respectively. The entire corpus cavernosum was carefully dilated with sequentially placed #9-*13/14* Hegar dilators, without perforating the tunica albuginea. A catheter-tip syringe with sterile *normal saline/antibiotic solution* was used to irrigate intracor-porally. With the penis on stretch, the Furlow insertion tool was used to measure the length of the corpus cavernosum distally and proximally. The sum of the two measurements was _____cm.

The identical procedure was performed on the *left/right* corpus cavernosum, which was measured at _____cm.

Based on the measurements, a ____cm cylinder (with a ___ cm rear tip extender) was chosen for the right and a ____cm cylinder (with a ___cm rear tip extender) for the left corporal body.

The appropriate prosthesis components were opened, primed to the manufacturer's specifications and soaked in sterile *normal saline/antibiotic solution*. Rubber-shod hemostats were utilized on the tubing to avoid inadvertent injury to the device.

Using the Furlow insertion tool loaded with the Keith needle and traction suture, the *right/left* cylinder was positioned distally to the level of the mid glans with the penis on stretch. The needle was removed and the traction suture tagged with a rubber-shod hemostat. The cylinder was partially folded on itself, allowing the proximal end to be positioned in the ipsilateral crus. Once the cylinder was correctly situated proximally, the distal portion was repositioned by gently pulling on the traction suture. The entire cylinder lay flat within the corporotomy with the distal tip in the mid glans.

The contralateral cylinder was placed in the identical manner, and its correct position confirmed.

Each cylinder was inflated and deflated using a 60 cc syringe with 55 ml sterile normal saline, confirming proper placement without buckling, kinking, or leakage.

Attention was then directed to the *right/left* inguinal ring for placement of the reservoir. The dissection was carried out medial to the spermatic cord, and the transversalis fascia sharply incised at the level of the pubic tubercle. Using blunt and sharp dissection, a pocket was created to allow placement of the reservoir. The *65/100* ml reservoir was positioned over the index finger and placed through the defect into the paravesical space. The tubing was flushed, the reservoir was filled with *65/100* ml sterile normal saline, and the tubing clamped with a rubber-shod hemostat.

A dartos pouch was created in the dependent portion of the *right/left* hemiscrotum away from the testis, using blunt finger dissection. The pump was inserted into the dartos pouch and a Babcock clamp used to hold it in place. The pump and reservoir tubing were trimmed and flushed with sterile normal saline. The ends were connected using the quick-connectors, and the rubber-shod hemostats removed. *(When using a nonconnected system, connect the cylinder tubing to the pump tubing using quick-connectors, as well.)*

The corporotomy closure was completed bilaterally, tying the previously placed 2-0 Vicryl sutures, making sure not to puncture the underlying cylinders. The device was cycled through the activation and deactivation phases, ensuring proper function. With

the prosthesis inflated, the penis was straight and the cylinders were parallel to each other with the distal tips positioned symmetrically in the mid glans. The cylinders were left partially deflated and both traction sutures removed.

The wound was irrigated, meticulous hemostasis was obtained using electrocautery and the self-retaining retractor was removed.

The dartos fascia was approximated with a running 3-0 chromic suture and the peno-scrotal incision closed with a running subcuticular 4-0 poliglecaprone (Monocryl) suture. Sterile adhesive strips and a gauze dressing were used to secure the incision. The penis was wrapped loosely with a self-adherent (Coban) dressing and taped to the abdomen to limit postoperative swelling.

At the end of the procedure, all counts were correct.

The patient tolerated the procedure well and was taken to the recovery room in satisfactory condition.

Estimated blood loss: Approximately _____ml

25

Malleable Penile Prosthesis

Indications

- Erectile dysfunction

Essential Steps

1) Make a penoscrotal incision and expose the tunica albuginea of each corpus cavernosum.
2) Dilate each corpus cavernosum through a small corporotomy, taking care not to perforate the tunica albuginea. Determine the corporal diameter.
3) Use the Furlow insertion tool to measure the proximal and distal length of each corpus cavernosum and choose the appropriate cylinders and rear tip extenders.
4) Place each cylinder through the corresponding corporotomy and confirm its correct position. Perform a watertight corporotomy closure.
5) Close the penoscrotal incision in two layers.

Note These Variations

- A "No-touch" technique can be used, eliminating any contact between the prosthesis and the skin, possibly minimizing the incidence of peri-prosthetic infection.
- The choice of which single component device to use is based on the specific penile characteristics, the surgeon's preference, and product availability.
- An infrapubic, transverse scrotal or subcoronal approach can be used for prosthesis placement.
- The Dilamezinsert can be used to aid in corporal dilation.

Complications

- Bleeding
- Infection

Operative Dictations in Urologic Surgery, First Edition. Noel A. Armenakas, John A. Fracchia, and Ron Golan.
© 2019 John Wiley & Sons Ltd. Published 2019 by John Wiley & Sons Ltd.

- Urethral injury
- Corpus cavernosal perforation
- "SST" glans deformity
- Erosion
- Chronic pain
- Patient dissatisfaction

Template Operative Dictation

Preoperative diagnosis: Erectile dysfunction
Postoperative diagnosis: Same
Procedure: Insertion of a ___*(state type)*___ malleable penile prosthesis
Indications: The patient is a _____-year-old male with erectile dysfunction presenting for insertion of a malleable penile prosthesis.
Description of Procedure: The indications, alternatives, benefits, and risks were discussed with the patient and informed consent was obtained.

The patient was brought onto the operating room table, positioned supine, and secured with a safety strap. All pressure points were carefully padded and pneumatic compression devices were placed on the lower extremities.

After the administration of intravenous antibiotics and *general/regional* anesthesia, the genitalia perineum and lower abdomen were prepped and draped in the standard sterile manner.

A time-out was completed, verifying the correct patient, surgical procedure, and positioning, prior to beginning the procedure.

A 14 Fr urethral catheter was advanced into the bladder.

A 4 cm vertical penoscrotal incision was made at the median raphe and carried down through the dartos and superficial Buck's fascias. A self-retaining retractor (e.g. Lone Star) was appropriately positioned to optimize exposure.

The corpus spongiosum was retracted laterally and the *right/left* corpus cavernosum was identified. The deep layer of Buck's fascia was dissected off this, exposing the underlying tunica albuginea. Two, 2-0 polyglactin (Vicryl) stay sutures were placed laterally in the tunica albuginea, and a 2.5 cm corporotomy was made between these. Using Metzenbaum scissors with the tips pointed laterally, the corpora cavernosum was tunneled proximally and distally to the ischial tuberosities and mid glans, respectively. The entire corpus cavernosum was carefully dilated with sequentially placed #9-*13/14* Hegar dilators, without perforating the tunica albuginea. A catheter-tip syringe with sterile *normal saline/antibiotic solution* was used to irrigate intracorporally. With the penis on stretch, the Furlow insertion tool was used to measure the length of the corpus cavernosum distally and proximally. The sum of the two measurements was _____ cm.

The identical procedure was performed on the *left/right* corpus cavernosum, which was measured at _____ cm.

Based on the measurements, *9.5/11/13* mm diameter, _____ cm length rods were chosen and soaked in sterile *normal saline/antibiotic solution*. The ends were trimmed appropriately and a rear tip extender added to each.

With the penis on stretch, the *right/left* cylinder was positioned distally to the level of the mid glans. The cylinder was partially folded on itself, allowing the proximal end to

be positioned in the ipsilateral crus. The entire cylinder lay straight within the corporotomy with the distal tip in the mid glans.

The second cylinder was placed in the identical manner, and its correct position confirmed.

The corporotomy closure was completed bilaterally, tying the previously placed 2-0 Vicryl sutures, making sure not to injure the underlying cylinders.

The wound was irrigated, meticulous hemostasis was obtained using electrocautery, and the self-retaining retractor was removed.

The dartos fascia was approximated with a running 3-0 chromic suture and the peno-scrotal incision closed with a running subcuticular 4-0 poliglecaprone (Monocryl) suture. Sterile adhesive strips and a gauze dressing were used to secure the incision. The penis was wrapped loosely with a self-adherent (Coban) dressing.

The urethral catheter was connected to a drainage bag and the penis was taped to the abdomen to limit postoperative swelling.

At the end of the procedure, all counts were correct.

The patient tolerated the procedure well and was taken to the recovery room in satisfactory condition.

Estimated blood loss: Approximately _____ml

26

Partial Penectomy

Indications

- Penile cancer involving the glans and/or coronal sulcus (distal penis)

Essential Steps

1) Completely cover the entire tumor with a condom to avoid inadvertent spillage.
2) Remove at least a 1.0 cm cuff of healthy penile tissue proximal to the tumor.
3) Perform a hemostatic closure of each corpus cavernosum.
4) Create a spatulated urethral neomeatus.
5) Place a urethral catheter.

Note These Variations

- Select tumors which are limited to the glans can be managed with a glansectomy, achieving a satisfactory cosmetic and functional result.
- Alternatively, the penile skin can be closed using a "buttonhole" technique by fashioning a ventral flap of penile skin and advancing it dorsally.

Complications

- Bleeding
- Infection
- Neomeatal stenosis
- Penile skin necrosis

Operative Dictations in Urologic Surgery, First Edition. Noel A. Armenakas, John A. Fracchia, and Ron Golan.
© 2019 John Wiley & Sons Ltd. Published 2019 by John Wiley & Sons Ltd.

Template Operative Dictation

Preoperative diagnosis: Penile cancer
Postoperative diagnosis: Same
Procedure: Partial penectomy
Indications: The patient is a _____-year-old male with biopsy proven penile cancer on the *glans/corona/distal shaft* presenting for a partial penectomy.
Description of Procedure: The indications, alternatives, benefits, and risks were discussed with the patient and informed consent was obtained.

The patient was brought onto the operating room table, positioned supine, and secured with a safety strap. All pressure points were carefully padded and pneumatic compression devices placed on the lower extremities.

After the administration of intravenous antibiotics and *general endotracheal/regional* anesthesia, the genitalia were prepped and draped in the standard sterile manner.

A time-out was completed, verifying the correct patient, surgical procedure, and positioning, prior to beginning the procedure.

The penile tumor was completely isolated using a condom catheter, and an area approximately *1.0/1.5* cm proximal to the tumor was circumferentially outlined with a marking pen. A 0.25 in. Penrose drain was placed at the base of the penis and tightened as a tourniquet.

A circumferential skin incision was made following the markings and taken down through the dartos and Buck's fascial layers to the level of the tunica albuginea. The superficial penile vessels and deep dorsal neurovascular bundle were isolated and ligated with 2-0 silk ties. Additional hemostasis was achieved using electrocautery.

Both corpora cavernosa were transected symmetrically and the urethra dissected distally and transected, leaving a 1 cm urethral cuff to facilitate reconstruction of the corpus spongiosum. The amputated segment was sent to pathology for evaluation.

Each corpus cavernosum was closed by approximating the corresponding tunica albuginea with interrupted absorbable 2-0 polyglactin (Vicryl) sutures. The tourniquet was removed and cavernosal hemostasis was ensured.

The urethra was spatulated dorsally and an elliptical neomeatus fashioned by carefully suturing the dorsal corpus spongiosum to the previously approximated tunica albuginea, using interrupted 4-0 undyed Vicryl sutures. The penile skin was reapproximated with 3-0 chromic sutures. Additional interrupted 4-0 chromic sutures were used to circumferentially secure the urethra to the penile skin. A 16 Fr urethral catheter was used for bladder drainage.

Antibiotic ointment and a Vaseline gauze were placed on the suture line, and the penis was wrapped loosely with a self-adherent (Coban) dressing.

At the end of the procedure, all counts were correct.

The patient tolerated the procedure well and was taken to the recovery room in satisfactory condition.

Estimated blood loss: Approximately _____ml

27

Penile Arterial Revascularization

Indications

- Healthy individuals with erectile dysfunction secondary to isolated occlusion of the internal pudendal artery (e.g. after pelvic trauma)

Essential Steps

- Perform a preoperative iliac arteriogram to ensure patency of the inferior epigastric artery and identify the site of obstruction of the inferior pudendal/penile artery.
- Make an abdominal incision and harvest the inferior epigastric artery from its origin to the level of the umbilicus, and divide it superiorly.
- Expose the deep dorsal penile artery, through a separate incision at the base of the penis.
- Tunnel the inferior epigastric artery through the ipsilateral inguinal ring, and place it within the penile incision.
- Anastomose the inferior epigastric artery to the dorsal penile artery using the operating microscope. Use topical papaverine to prevent vasospasm.
- Confirm the patency of the anastomosis.

Note These Variations

- There are numerous techniques described for penile revascularization, which include anastomosing the inferior epigastric artery to the cavernosal tunica albuginea (Michel I); anastomosing the inferior epigastric artery to the dorsal vein (Virag 5); using a venous autograft to divert blood flow from the femoral to the dorsal artery (Crespo); anastomosing the inferior epigastric artery to both the deep dorsal vein and dorsal artery (Hauri); anastomosing the dorsal artery to the cavernosal artery (Goldstein).
- Alternatively, the inferior epigastric artery can be accessed through a paramedian vertical or transverse abdominal incision, and the dorsal penile artery through a penoscrotal approach.
- An end-to-end inferior epigastric to dorsal penile artery anastomosis may be fashioned.
- Doppler ultrasound can be used to further confirm the patency of the arterial anastomosis.

Operative Dictations in Urologic Surgery, First Edition. Noel A. Armenakas, John A. Fracchia, and Ron Golan.
© 2019 John Wiley & Sons Ltd. Published 2019 by John Wiley & Sons Ltd.

Complications

- Bleeding
- Infection
- Penile edema/ecchymosis
- Penile pain
- Decreased penile sensation
- Glans hyperemia
- Penile shortening
- Priapism
- Persistent erectile dysfunction

Template Operative Dictation

Preoperative diagnosis: Erectile dysfunction from secondary isolated occlusion of the internal pudendal/penile artery
Postoperative diagnosis: Same
Procedure: Penile arterial revascularization
Indications: The patient is a _____ -year-old male with erectile dysfunction from secondary isolated occlusion of the internal pudendal artery presenting for penile revascularization.
Description of Procedure: The indications, alternatives, benefits, and risks were discussed with the patient and informed consent was obtained.

The patient was brought onto the operating room table, positioned supine, and secured with a safety strap. All pressure points were carefully padded and pneumatic compression devices placed on the lower extremities.

After the administration of intravenous antibiotics and *general/regional* anesthesia, the entire abdomen and genitalia were prepped and draped in the standard sterile manner.

A time-out was completed, verifying the correct patient, surgical procedure, and positioning, prior to beginning the procedure.

A 16 Fr urethral catheter was inserted into the bladder and connected to a drainage bag.

A midline abdominal incision was made from just below the umbilicus to the pubic symphysis. The subcutaneous tissue was incised with electrocautery, exposing the underlying rectus abdominis aponeurosis. This was incised at the linea alba and the rectus abdominis muscles were separated at the midline.

The *left/right* rectus abdominis muscle was retracted superolaterally, using two padded Richardson retractors, exposing the inferior epigastric neurovascular bundle. Using optical magnification with surgical loupes, the inferior epigastric artery was dissected from its origin at the external iliac artery to the level of the umbilicus. All branches of the artery were ligated with *vascular titanium clips/4-0 silk ties* and divided. 3000 units of heparin were administered intravenously. The distal end of the inferior epigastric artery was secured with a microvascular clamp and divided at the level of the umbilicus.

A 5 cm dorsal incision was made at the base of the penis and carried down through the dartos and Buck's fascias, preserving the fundiform and suspensory penile ligaments. A self-retaining retractor (e.g. Weitlaner, Lone Star) was appropriately positioned to optimize exposure.

The operating microscope was draped and brought into the field for the vascular anastomosis.

The deep dorsal penile neurovascular bundle was identified and the *left/right* deep dorsal penile artery was carefully isolated and circumferentially mobilized for a distance of approximately 3 cm, avoiding injury to the adjacent dorsal penile vein and nerves.

The harvested inferior epigastric artery was tunneled through the floor of the ipsilateral inguinal canal, medial to the spermatic cord, and brought out through a subcutaneous tunnel into the penile incision using a curved Adson (Tonsil) clamp. Meticulous hemostasis was achieved using bipolar electrocautery throughout the procedure.

Two microvascular clamps were placed on the deep dorsal penile artery and a 3 mm anterior arteriotomy made between these. Topical papaverine was applied to the inferior epigastric and deep dorsal arteries, confirming excellent blood flow.

An end-to-side microsurgical vascular anastomosis was performed between the inferior epigastric and deep dorsal artery, using *interrupted/two running* 10-0 *polypropylene (Prolene)/nylon (Ethilon)* sutures. All three microvascular clamps were removed, confirming a good pulsatile flow with Doppler sonography and the absence of any bleeding.

Both incisions were irrigated with sterile *normal saline/antibiotic solution* and meticulous hemostasis was again confirmed prior to removing the self-retaining retractors.

The dartos fascia was approximated with a 3-0 polyglactin (Vicryl) suture and the penile skin incision closed with a running subcuticular 4-0 poliglecaprone (Monocryl) suture.

The abdominal incision was closed using a running 2-0 chromic suture to approximate the rectus muscles and a 1-0 polydioxanone (PDS) suture for the rectus aponeurosis. 3-0 chromic sutures were used on Scarpa's fascia and the skin approximated with a subcuticular 4-0 poliglecaprone (Monocryl) suture.

Sterile adhesive strips and a gauze dressing were applied to secure both incisions.

At the end of the procedure, all counts were correct.

The patient tolerated the procedure well and was taken to the recovery room in satisfactory condition.

Estimated blood loss: Approximately _____ ml

28

Penile Reimplantation

Indications

- Penile amputation

Essential Steps

- Preserve the amputed segment by wrapping it in a sterile gauze soaked with normal saline and placing it in a dry bag. Immerse the bag in an ice slush.
- Irrigate the distal penile stump with antibiotic solution, and perform minimal debridement confirming its viability.
- Place a urethral catheter to stabilize the penile stump, and approximate the tunica albuginea of the each corpus cavernosum.
- Perform a spatulated anastomotic urethroplasty.
- Identify and isolate the deep dorsal neurovascular bundle.
- Using the operating microscope, reanastomose the deep dorsal vein and, at least, one dorsal artery and nerve.
- Confirm the patency of the anastomosis and the viability of the reimplanted penile segment.
- Close the incision in two layers.

Note These Variations

- If both deep dorsal arteries and nerves are identified and appear viable, bilateral neurovascular anastomoses can be performed.
- A percutaneous suprapubic tube can be placed at the end of the procedure.

Complications

- Bleeding
- Infection
- Skin/penile necrosis

Operative Dictations in Urologic Surgery, First Edition. Noel A. Armenakas, John A. Fracchia, and Ron Golan.
© 2019 John Wiley & Sons Ltd. Published 2019 by John Wiley & Sons Ltd.

- Decreased penile sensation
- Erectile dysfunction
- Urethral stricture
- Urethrocutaneous fistula

Template Operative Dictation

Preoperative diagnosis: Penile amputation
Postoperative diagnosis: Same
Procedure: Microsurgical penile reimplantation
Indications: The patient is a ____-year-old male with a *self-inflicted/accidental* penile amputation presenting for penile reimplantation.
Description of Procedure: The indications, alternatives, benefits, and risks were discussed with the patient and informed consent was obtained.

The patient was brought onto the operating room table, positioned supine, and secured with a safety strap. All pressure points were carefully padded and pneumatic compression devices placed on the lower extremities.

After the administration of intravenous antibiotics and *general/regional* anesthesia, the genitalia and lower abdomen were prepped and draped in the standard sterile manner.

A time-out was completed, verifying the correct patient, surgical procedure, and positioning, prior to beginning the procedure.

Using optical magnification with surgical loupes, the amputated penile segment, which had been preserved using cold ischemia, was examined and thoroughly irrigated with warm sterile normal saline and an antibiotic solution. Minimal debridement was performed, confirming its viability.

A tourniquet was applied on the penile stump using a 0.25 in. Penrose drain. The penile skin and dartos fascia were dissected proximally for a distance of 1–2 cm, exposing the dorsal neurovascular bundle and corpora. The tourniquet was released intermittently throughout the procedure, and meticulous hemostasis achieved using electrocautery and 4-0 chromic ties.

The amputated segment was placed in its normal position adjacent to the penile stump, and stabilized using a 16 Fr urethral catheter inserted through the meatus into the bladder.

The corpora cavernosa were properly aligned and their corresponding tunica albuginea approximated circumferentially with interrupted 3-0 polydioxanone (PDS) sutures.

The proximal and distal penile urethral ends were minimally debrided and spatulated on opposite ends. A one-layer urethro-urethral anastomosis was completed with interrupted 5-0 PDS sutures.

The operating microscope was draped and brought into the field for the microneurovascular anastomoses.

The deep dorsal penile vein was identified and freed proximally and distally. The ends were spatulated on opposite sides, and a venovenous anastomosis completed using *interrupted/two running* 10-0 *polypropylene (Prolene)/nylon (Ethilon)* sutures.

The *left/right* deep dorsal penile artery was then identified and similarly dissected. An arterio-arterial anastomosis was performed in the identical manner. The tourniquet

was removed and the microvascular anastomoses inspected confirming a good pulsatile flow without bleeding. Finally, the dorsal nerve was reapproximated using interrupted 9-0 *Prolene/Ethilon* sutures placed in the epineurium.

The wound was irrigated with sterile *normal saline/antibiotic solution* and meticulous hemostasis again confirmed.

The dartos fascia and penile skin were individually approximated with interrupted 3-0 polyglactin (Vicryl) sutures.

Antibiotic ointment and a sterile gauze dressing were placed on the suture line, and the penis wrapped very loosely with a self-adherent (Coban) dressing. The urethral catheter was connected to a drainage bag and the penis was taped to the abdomen to limit postoperative swelling.

At the end of the procedure, all counts were correct.

The patient tolerated the procedure well and was taken to the recovery room in satisfactory condition.

Estimated blood loss: Approximately _____ml

29

Plication for Penile Curvature (Lue "16-Dot" Technique)

Indications

- Penile curvature ≤60°

Essential Steps

1) Induce an intraoperative simulated saline artificial erection to establish the point of maximal curvature.
2) Expose the tunica albuginea at that level.
3) In cases of ventral and dorsal curvature, avoid injury to the neurovascular bundle and urethra, respectively.
4) Place the plication sutures through the tunica albugineal layers, avoiding the underlying cavernosal tissue.
5) Repeat the simulated erection to confirm adequate penile straightening.

Note These Variations

- Alternatively, a Nesbit or Yacchia procedure can be performed. The former involves the elliptical excision of small segments of tunica albuginea, whereas the latter incorporates longitudinal incisions in the tunica albuginea, which are closed transversely (using the Heineke-Mikulicz principle).
- A penoscrotal or direct penile incision can be used instead of a subcoronal circumferential incision.
- More than two pairs of parallelly placed sutures may be needed to correct curvatures >30°.
- A urethral catheter may be used intraoperatively to avoid urethral injury.

Complications

- Bleeding
- Infection

Operative Dictations in Urologic Surgery, First Edition. Noel A. Armenakas, John A. Fracchia, and Ron Golan.
© 2019 John Wiley & Sons Ltd. Published 2019 by John Wiley & Sons Ltd.

- Persistent curvature
- Penile or urethral injury
- Penile shortening

Template Operative Dictation

Preoperative diagnosis: Penile curvature
Postoperative diagnosis: Same
Procedure: Penile plication
Indications: The patient is a _____-year-old male with a _____ degree *dorsal/lateral/ventral* penile curvature presenting for reconstruction.
Description of Procedure: The indications, alternatives, benefits, and risks were discussed with the patient and informed consent was obtained.

The patient was brought onto the operating room table, positioned supine, and secured with a safety strap. All pressure points were carefully padded and pneumatic compression devices placed on the lower extremities.

After the administration of intravenous antibiotics and *general/regional* anesthesia, the genitalia were prepped and draped in the standard sterile manner.

A time-out was completed, verifying the correct patient, surgical procedure, and positioning, prior to beginning the procedure.

A 2-0 polypropylene (Prolene) stay suture was placed through the anterior mid glans for traction. A circumferential penile skin incision was made 1 cm below the coronal sulcus and carried down through the dartos and superficial Buck's fascias. The penile shaft was degloved proximally within this avascular plane. Meticulous hemostasis was achieved with electrocautery. An artificial saline erection was induced using sterile normal saline injected through a 21-gauge butterfly needle. The area of maximal curvature was outlined using a marking pen. A self-retaining retractor (e.g. Lone Star) was appropriately positioned to optimize exposure.

Buck's fascia was elevated at the level of maximal curvature on the *ventral/right lateral/left lateral/dorsal surface*, over the previously made marking.

A 16-dot repair was performed placing two lateral sets of 2-0 nonabsorbable polyester sutures (Ethibond) in parallel, just proximal and distal to the maximal point of curvature. Each of the four sutures had two entry and two exit points, incorporating approximately a 1 cm full-thickness segment of tunica albuginea.

The sutures were carefully tied and an artificial saline erection was again induced, ensuring satisfactory penile straightening.

Meticulous hemostasis was achieved using bipolar electrocautery. Prior to closure, the penis was inspected, confirming the absence of injury to the urethra or neurovascular bundle.

The dartos fascia and penile skin were reapproximated using 4-0 interrupted chromic sutures. The mid glans traction suture and self-retaining retractor were removed.

Antibiotic ointment and a Vaseline gauze were placed on the suture line, and the penis wrapped loosely with a self-adherent (Coban) dressing.

At the end of the procedure, all counts were correct.

The patient tolerated the procedure well and was taken to the recovery room in satisfactory condition.

Estimated blood loss: Approximately _____ml

30

Priapism Reduction (Al-Ghorab Open Distal Shunt)

Indications

- Ischemic (low-flow) priapism refractory to corporal aspiration and irrigation, intracorporal injection of sympathomimetic agents, and percutaneous corpoglanular shunts

Essential Steps

1) Make a transverse dorsal incision in glans and expose both distal corpora cavernosa.
2) Excise a wedge of tunica albuginea bilaterally and drain the intracorporal stagnant blood and clots.
3) Once adequate detumescence is confirmed, close the glans incision.

Note These Variations

- There are several distal shunting options available. The percutaneous techniques include puncturing the corpora cavernosa through the glans using a large biopsy needle (Winter), or advancing a #11 blade from the glans into the corpora cavernosa (Ebbehoj, T-shunt).
- Hegar dilators can be introduced through each corporotomy to facilitate removal of the stagnant intracorporal blood (Burnett modification).
- A urethral catheter can be placed to avoid injury to the urethra.

Complications

- Bleeding
- Infection
- Persistent priapism
- Erectile dysfunction

Operative Dictations in Urologic Surgery, First Edition. Noel A. Armenakas, John A. Fracchia, and Ron Golan.
© 2019 John Wiley & Sons Ltd. Published 2019 by John Wiley & Sons Ltd.

Template Operative Dictation

Preoperative diagnosis: Priapism
Postoperative diagnosis: Same
Procedure: Open corpoglanular penile shunt
Indications: The patient is a _____-year-old male with priapism of _____ hours duration, who failed conservative management, presenting for an open corpoglanular penile shunt.
Description of Procedure: The indications, alternatives, benefits, and risks were discussed with the patient and informed consent was obtained.

The patient was brought onto the operating room table, positioned supine, and secured with a safety strap. All pressure points were carefully padded and pneumatic compression devices were placed on the lower extremities.

After the administration of intravenous antibiotics and *general/regional* anesthesia, the genitalia were prepped and draped in the standard sterile manner.

A time-out was completed, verifying the correct patient, surgical procedure, and positioning, prior to beginning the procedure.

A tourniquet was applied at the base of the penis using a 0.25 in. Penrose drain.

A 2 cm transverse incision was made in the dorsum of the glans, 1 cm distal to the corona. This was taken down sharply through the dartos and Buck's fascias to the tunica albuginea of the corpora cavernosa. The dorsal tunica albuginea of each corpora cavernosum was grasped with an *Allis/Kocher* clamp, and a wedge of tissue excised bilaterally. Using external pressure on the corpora, the stagnant dark intracorporal blood was removed, confirming restoration of arterial blood flow and adequate detumescence.

The glans incision was closed with interrupted 3-0 chromic sutures. The tourniquet was removed and meticulous hemostasis was confirmed.

A gauze dressing was used to secure the incision and the penis was wrapped loosely with a self-adherent (Coban) dressing. The penis was taped to the abdomen to limit postoperative swelling.

At the end of the procedure, all counts were correct.

The patient tolerated the procedure well and was taken to the recovery room in satisfactory condition.

Estimated blood loss: Approximately _____ml

31

Repair of Penile Fracture

Indications

- Rupture of the tunica albuginea of the corpus cavernosum

Essential Steps

1) Patients presenting with hematuria or blood at the meatus, or who are unable to urinate, should be evaluated with either retrograde urethrography or cystoscopy to identify a concomitant urethral injury.
2) Deglove the penis and expose the corpora cavernosa and spongiosum.
3) Identify the tear(s) in the tunica albuginea (unilateral or bilateral) and close it in one layer.
4) Repair a concomitant urethral injury.
5) Reapproximate the penile skin to the subcoronal cuff.

Note These Variations

- The penile fracture can be accessed through various incisions, including a midline penoscrotal, a longitudinal ventral penile, or at the level of the presumed rupture site.
- For dorsal lacerations, the neurovascular bundle should be carefully dissected to expose the entire involved tunica albugineal segment.
- A concomitant urethral injury should be identified and repaired. Small tears in the corpora spongiosum can be simply sutured; large tears or complete urethral transections should be reconstructed using an anastomotic approach.
- At the completion of the tunica albugineal repair, an artificial saline erection can be induced to assess penile orientation and the integrity of the tunical closure.

Complications

- Bleeding
- Infection

Operative Dictations in Urologic Surgery, First Edition. Noel A. Armenakas, John A. Fracchia, and Ron Golan.
© 2019 John Wiley & Sons Ltd. Published 2019 by John Wiley & Sons Ltd.

- Penile curvature
- Painful erections
- Urethral stricture
- Erectile dysfunction
- Fistula (urethrocutaneous)

Template Operative Dictation

Preoperative diagnosis: Penile fracture
Postoperative diagnosis: Same
Procedure: Surgical exploration and repair of penile fracture
Indications: The patient is a _____-year-old male with a clinical diagnosis of a penile fracture presenting for penile exploration and repair.
Description of Procedure: The indications, alternatives, benefits, and risks were discussed with the patient and informed consent was obtained.

The patient was brought onto the operating room table, positioned supine, and secured with a safety strap. All pressure points were carefully padded and pneumatic compression devices were placed on the lower extremities.

After the administration of intravenous antibiotics and *general/regional* anesthesia, the genitalia were prepped and draped in the standard sterile manner.

A time-out was completed, verifying the correct patient, surgical procedure, and positioning, prior to beginning the procedure.

A 16 Fr urethral catheter was placed for urethral identification and bladder drainage.

A circumferential penile skin incision was made 1 cm below the coronal sulcus and carried down through the dartos and superficial Buck's fascias. The penis was carefully degloved, using sharp and blunt dissection, exposing both corpora cavernosa and the corpora spongiosum. Meticulous hemostasis was achieved with electrocautery. A self-retaining retractor (e.g. Lone Star) was appropriately positioned to optimize exposure.

The wound was irrigated with sterile normal saline and the clot evacuated. Buck's fascia was further dissected at this level, exposing the underlying ____cm tunica albugineal disruption on the *ventral/dorsal* surface of the *right/left* corpus cavernosum. The edges of the tunica albuginea were minimally debrided, avoiding injury to the cavernosal tissue. The tunica albuginea was closed, in the same axis as the laceration, with a running 2-0 *polydioxanone (PDS)/polyglactin (Vicryl)/polyester (Ethibond)* suture.

The urethral catheter was removed, sterile normal saline was instilled through the meatus, and the urethra was inspected, confirming its patency.

Hemostasis was again confirmed and the penis examined for any additional injuries. The dartos fascia and penile skin were reapproximated separately using interrupted 3-0 chromic sutures, and the self-retaining retractor removed.

Antibiotic ointment and a Vaseline gauze were placed on the suture line, and the penis was wrapped loosely with a self-adherent (Coban) dressing.

At the end of the procedure, all counts were correct.

The patient tolerated the procedure well and was taken to the recovery room in satisfactory condition.

Estimated blood loss: Approximately _____ml

32

Total Penectomy

Indications

- Penile cancer, where its location precludes salvage of a functional remnant

Essential Steps

1) Completely cover the entire tumor with a condom to avoid inadvertent spillage.
2) Remove at least a 2 cm cuff of healthy penile tissue proximal to the tumor.
3) Perform a hemostatic closure of each corpus cavernosum, individually.
4) Avoid angulation of the urethra during scrotal tunneling.
5) Create a patulous perineal urethrostomy to avoid meatal stenosis.
6) Place a urethral catheter.

Note These Variations

- Alternatively, a perineal approach using an inverted-Y incision can be used.

Complications

- Bleeding
- Infection
- Neomeatal stenosis
- Penile skin necrosis

Template Operative Dictation

Preoperative diagnosis: Penile cancer
Postoperative diagnosis: Same
Procedure: Total penectomy
Indications: The patient is a _____-year-old male with biopsy-proven penile cancer on the *mid/distal/proximal* shaft presenting for a total penectomy.

Operative Dictations in Urologic Surgery, First Edition. Noel A. Armenakas, John A. Fracchia, and Ron Golan.
© 2019 John Wiley & Sons Ltd. Published 2019 by John Wiley & Sons Ltd.

Description of Procedure: The indications, alternatives, benefits, and risks were discussed with the patient and informed consent was obtained.

The patient was brought onto the operating room table, positioned supine, and secured with a safety strap. All pressure points were carefully padded and pneumatic compression devices were placed on the lower extremities.

After the administration of intravenous antibiotics and *general endotracheal/regional* anesthesia, the patient was repositioned in dorsal lithotomy and the genitalia were prepped and draped in the standard sterile manner.

A time-out was completed, verifying the correct patient, surgical procedure, and positioning, prior to beginning the procedure.

The penile tumor was completely isolated using a condom catheter. A diamond-shaped area was marked at the base of the penis extending superiorly to the infrapubic region and inferiorly to the anterior scrotal wall, leaving a 2 cm margin of healthy tissue. A skin incision was made following the markings and taken down through the dartos fascia. Superiorly, the dissection was carried down to the suspensory ligament, which was divided to facilitate exposure and penile mobility. The superficial penile vessels and the deep dorsal neurovascular bundle were isolated and ligated with 2-0 silk ties. Additional hemostasis was achieved using electrocautery.

The penis was reflected cephalad and the scrotum retracted caudally, exposing the ventral surface of the urethra. Buck's fascia was sharply incised, exposing the corpus spongiosum, which was carefully separated from the corpora cavernosa using sharp and blunt dissection. The urethra was transected at this level and its proximal portion was placed within the scrotum.

The corpora cavernosa were individually isolated circumferentially at the level of the ischiopubic rami. They were then transected symmetrically, again ensuring a 2 cm margin proximal to the tumor. The amputated segment was sent to pathology for evaluation. Each corpus cavernosum was individually closed by approximating the corresponding tunica albuginea with interrupted 2-0 polydioxanone (PDS) sutures, ensuring adequate hemostasis.

Having completed the penectomy, attention was turned to the creation of a perineal urethrostomy. A 1.5 cm mid-perineal elliptical skin incision was made over the median raphe and carried down through Colles' fascia and the subcutaneous fat. Using a right-angle clamp, the distal urethral end was tunneled caudally beneath the scrotum and brought out through the perineal incision, avoiding any angulation.

The urethra was spatulated dorsally and an elliptical neomeatus fashioned by carefully suturing the urethra to the perineal skin, using interrupted 4-0 polyglactin (Vicryl) sutures. A 16 Fr urethral catheter was placed for bladder drainage.

Meticulous hemostasis was again achieved using electrocautery.

The dartos fascia and scrotal skin were approximated transversally in two layers using interrupted 3-0 Vicryl sutures.

Antibiotic ointment and a Vaseline gauze were placed on the suture line, and a pressure dressing and scrotal supporter was applied. The patient was repositioned supine.

At the end of the procedure, all counts were correct.

The patient tolerated the procedure well and was taken to the recovery room in satisfactory condition.

Estimated blood loss: Approximately _____ml

Prostate

33

Radical Perineal Prostatectomy

Indications

- Clinically organ-confined prostate cancer

Essential Steps

1) Place a Lowsley retractor in the bladder, transurethrally.
2) Make a semicircular incision anteriorly between the ischial tuberosities.
3) Expose the prostate by retracting the external anal sphincter anteriorly and dividing the rectourethralis muscles.
4) Incise Denonvilliers' fascia vertically in the midline, from the vesicoprostatic junction to the prostatic apex, taking care not to injure the neurovascular bundles.
5) Divide the urethra.
6) Inject intravenous indigo carmine/methylene blue to assist in identifying the ureteral orifices.
7) Incise the bladder neck and place a red rubber catheter through the prostatic urethra for traction.
8) Remove the entire specimen (prostate, ampullae, seminal vesicles) and complete the bladder neck closure and vesicourethral anastomosis.
9) Inspect for inadvertent rectal injury prior to closing the incision.

Note These Variations

- The more commonly performed Belt procedure is described (i.e. a subsphincteric approach beneath the anal sphincter), which is a modification of the classic Young perineal prostatectomy.

Complications

- Bleeding
- Infection

Operative Dictations in Urologic Surgery, First Edition. Noel A. Armenakas, John A. Fracchia, and Ron Golan.
© 2019 John Wiley & Sons Ltd. Published 2019 by John Wiley & Sons Ltd.

- Rectal/ureteral injury
- Urine leak/urinoma
- Erectile dysfunction
- Bladder neck stenosis/urethral stricture
- Urinary incontinence

Template Operative Dictation

Preoperative diagnosis: Prostate cancer
Postoperative diagnosis: Same
Procedure: Radical perineal prostatectomy
Indications: The patient is a ____-year-old male with clinical stage T____, Gleason score _____ prostate cancer presenting for radical perineal prostatectomy.
Description of Procedure: The indications, alternatives, benefits, and risks were discussed with the patient and informed consent was obtained.

The patient was brought onto the operating room table, positioned supine, and secured with a safety strap. Pneumatic compression devices were placed on the lower extremities.

After the administration of intravenous antibiotics and *general endotracheal/regional* anesthesia, the patient was repositioned in high dorsal lithotomy, using (Allen) universal stirrups, with care taken not to hyperextend either hip or place traction on the hamstrings. The perineum was slightly elevated with an under-buttock gel pad, and the table was placed in the Trendelenburg position. All pressure points were carefully padded. The abdomen, genitalia, perineum, and upper thighs were prepped and draped in the standard sterile manner. A sterile towel was placed around the anus from the 9 o'clock to the 3 o'clock position. *(Alternatively, an adhesive finger cot drape can be used.)*

A time-out was completed, verifying the correct patient, surgical procedure, and positioning, prior to beginning the procedure.

An 18 Fr urethral catheter was inserted to empty the bladder and subsequently removed.

A curved Lowsley retractor was passed transurethrally into the bladder and secured by opening its wings. The right and left ischial tuberosities were palpated and a semicircular incision was made between these, anterior to the anus. Entrance into the space between the superficial and deep layers of the external anal sphincter was accomplished using blunt and sharp dissection. Hemostasis was obtained with electrocautery.

The fibers of the external anal sphincter were retracted anteriorly, and with gentle continuous dorsal traction on the rectum, the posterior layer of Denonvilliers' fascia was identified anterior to the rectum. The levator ani muscles were retracted laterally and anteriorly, leading to the rectourethralis muscle, which was sharply divided, taking care not to injure the rectum or urethra.

Gentle traction on the Lowsley retractor toward the anterior abdominal wall exposed the prostate into the field. The prostate was carefully dissected inferiorly off the rectum using blunt dissection. Denonvilliers' fascia was incised transversely in the midline, several centimeters proximal to the prostatic apex, taking care not to injure the neurovascular bundles between the layers of Denonvilliers' and the posterolateral prostate.

The distal posterior layer of Denonvilliers' was then incised vertically in the midline. Additional adhesions near the prostatic apex were sharply divided. The dissection continued laterally and posteriorly to the level of the seminal vesicles.

The posterior aspect of the urethra was identified at the prostatic apex with the aid of the Lowsley retractor, and incised transversely. The curved Lowsley retractor was removed and replaced with a straight Lowsley retractor entering through the apex of the prostate and passed into the bladder. The wings were opened to secure the retractor within the bladder. Using traction on the Lowsley retractor, the remaining anterior aspect of the urethra was incised.

The anesthesiologist was asked to inject 10 cc of intravenous *indigo carmine/methylene blue* to facilitate visualization of the ureteral orifices.

A self-retaining retractor (e.g. Lone Star, Bookwalter) was appropriately positioned to optimize exposure. The anterior prostate was bluntly dissected from the prostatic apex to the bladder neck, with dorsal traction placed on the Lowsley retractor, taking care not to injure the dorsal venous complex.

Once at the bladder neck, the Lowsley retractor was removed. A right-angle clamp was placed through the prostatic urethra at the apex and brought into the bladder neck. A small rent was made in the anterior bladder neck with the right-angle clamp, and a red rubber catheter was brought through this and out the apical prostatic urethra. The two ends of the red rubber catheter were secured with a heavy clamp and used to apply traction to the prostate.

The anterior bladder neck was incised and any areas of bleeding were cauterized. Blue efflux was noted from both ureteral orifices.

The bladder neck was circumferentially divided from the base of the prostate exposing the seminal vesicles and ampullae of the vasa. The lateral pedicles were identified bilaterally, sequentially divided close to the prostate, and ligated with 2-0 polyglactin (Vicryl) sutures and surgical clips. Electrocautery was not used in this area to avoid inadvertent injury to the neurovascular bundles.

A vein retractor was placed under the trigone exposing the vas deferens and seminal vesicles. Each of these were individually dissected, clamped and divided between 3-0 Vicryl suture ligatures. The entire specimen, consisting of the prostate, ampullae, and seminal vesicles was removed *en bloc* and sent to pathology for evaluation.

The bladder neck was closed in a "tennis racquet" configuration around the diameter of the small finger, with a 3-0 Vicryl suture. A 20 Fr red rubber catheter was passed from the urethral meatus to the proximal urethra and into the newly constructed bladder neck.

The vesicourethral anastomosis was performed with 2-0 poliglecaprone (Monocryl) sutures placed full-thickness, beginning at the 2 o'clock and 10 o'clock positions, circumferentially, approximating the proximal urethra and bladder neck. The red rubber catheter was removed and a 20 Fr urethral catheter was advanced transurethrally into the bladder and irrigated with sterile normal saline, ensuring a watertight anastomosis.

The perineal wound was irrigated with warm sterile water and inspected thoroughly confirming meticulous hemostasis and the absence of a rectal injury. A surgical drain (e.g. Jackson-Pratt, 0.25 in. Penrose) was positioned near the anastomosis and brought through the lateral aspect of the incision where it was secured at the skin with a 2-0 silk suture.

The levator ani, central tendon and Colles' fascia were individually approximated with 2-0 Vicryl sutures. The skin was closed with interrupted 3-0 chromic sutures and a sterile dressing applied.

The urethral catheter was connected to a drainage bag and the patient was repositioned supine.

At the end of the procedure, all counts were correct.

The patient tolerated the procedure well and was taken to the recovery room in satisfactory condition.

Estimated blood loss: Approximately _____ml

34

Radical Retropubic Prostatectomy with Bilateral Pelvic Lymph Node Dissection

Indications

- Prostate cancer

Essential Steps

1) Expose the right and left pelvic paravesical and paraprostatic areas via a retroperitoneal approach.
2) Perform bilateral pelvic lymph node dissections and incise the endopelvic fascia.
3) Ligate the dorsal vein complex, avoiding damage to the striated sphincter, and obtain meticulous hemostasis.
4) Transect the urethra at the prostatic apex and incise the prostatic fascia anteriorly to avoid the neurovascular bundles bilaterally.
5) Dissect and remove the prostate and seminal vesicles *en bloc*.
6) Fashion a new bladder neck that will accommodate the tip of the surgeon's index finger.
7) Perform a watertight urethrovesical anastomosis.

Note These Variations

- In patients with a low likelihood of pelvic node metastasis, a limited lymphadenectomy can be performed, or the procedure may be eliminated altogether.
- The dorsal vein can be accessed without transecting the puboprostatic ligaments.
- The vesicourethral anastomotic sutures may be placed once the specimen is removed, rather than after dividing the anterior urethral wall.
- Excision of one or both neurovascular bundles may be required, depending on the preoperative clinical and imaging findings.
- Intravenous methylene blue or indigo carmine can be given to assist in identifying the ureteral orifices. Alternatively, the ureteral orifices can be cannulated with infant feeding tubes.
- In addition to conventional bladder neck reconstruction, the bladder neck can be intussuscepted, which may improve postoperative urinary continence.

Operative Dictations in Urologic Surgery, First Edition. Noel A. Armenakas, John A. Fracchia, and Ron Golan.
© 2019 John Wiley & Sons Ltd. Published 2019 by John Wiley & Sons Ltd.

Complications

- Bleeding
- Infection
- Rectal/ureteral injury
- Obturator nerve injury
- Urine leak/urinoma
- Lymphocele
- Erectile dysfunction
- Bladder neck stenosis/urethral stricture
- Urinary incontinence

Template Operative Dictation

Preoperative diagnosis: Prostate cancer
Postoperative diagnosis: Same
Procedure: Radical retropubic prostatectomy, bilateral pelvic lymph node dissection
Indications: The patient is a ___-year-old male with a clinical stage T___, Gleason score ____ prostate cancer presenting for radical retropubic prostatectomy and bilateral pelvic lymph node dissection.
Description of Procedure: The indications, alternatives, benefits, and risks were discussed with the patient and informed consent was obtained.

The patient was brought onto the operating room table, positioned supine, with the break just above the anterosuperior iliac spine and secured with a safety strap. All pressure points were carefully padded and pneumatic compression devices were placed on the lower extremities.

After the administration of intravenous antibiotics and *general endotracheal/regional* anesthesia, the entire abdomen and external genitalia were prepped and draped in the standard sterile manner. The table was flexed 15° and adjusted in mild Trendelenburg.

A time-out was completed, verifying the correct patient, surgical procedure, and positioning, prior to beginning the procedure.

A 20 Fr urethral catheter with a 30 cc balloon was advanced into the bladder and the balloon inflated with 30 ml sterile water.

A 10 cm midline abdominal incision was made between the umbilicus and the symphysis pubis, and carried down through the subcutaneous tissue using electrocautery. The underlying rectus abdominis aponeurosis was identified and incised at the linea alba. The rectus abdominis muscles were separated at the midline and retracted laterally, taking care not to injure the underlying inferior epigastric vessels.

The space of Retzius was developed by sweeping the infrapubic space posterolaterally and mobilizing the peritoneum cranially on both sides of the pelvic sidewall. The vasa deferentia were ligated and divided to facilitate mobilization of the peritoneal sac. Care was taken to avoid entry into the peritoneal cavity. A self-retaining retractor (e.g. Bookwalter, Omni-Tract, Balfour) was appropriately positioned to optimize exposure, using padding on each retractor blade.

The iliac vessels were exposed from just above the common iliac bifurcation to the femoral canal. The ureters were identified anteriorly at the bifurcation of the external

and internal iliac vessels, and protected. The lymph nodes appeared *unremarkable/enlarged/matted* on palpation.

The nodal dissection was started at the medial aspect of the *left/right* external iliac artery by incising the perivascular fibroareolar sheath. Using gentle medial traction, the obturator neurovascular bundle was identified posteriorly and preserved. The dissection was carried laterally to the genitofemoral nerve and medially to the ipsilateral ureter. The cranial and caudal limits of dissection were the common iliac bifurcation and femoral canal (node of Cloquet), respectively. Small vessels and lymphatic branches were fulgurated or ligated with surgical clips to maintain meticulous hemo- and lymphostasis. A large surgical clip was used to individually secure the distal and proximal extents of the lymph node packet. The nodal packet was removed and sent to pathology for evaluation.

The identical lymph node dissection was performed on the contralateral side.

The superficial branch of the dorsal vein was coagulated and divided. The endopelvic fascia was incised bilaterally from the lateral edge of the puboprostatic ligament to the medial prostatic fascia, using gentle lateral traction on the bladder and prostate. The puboprostatic ligaments were sharply divided superficially at the inferior border of the pubic symphysis and a plane developed below the dorsal vein complex staying above the urethra. A right-angle clamp was passed anterior to the urethra through the opening in the endopelvic fascia, encompassing the dorsal vein complex distal to the prostatic apex. The dorsal vein complex was ligated at this level using two 2-0 *polyglactin (Vicryl)/poliglecaprone (Monocryl)* sutures and divided between these, exposing the urethra. Residual bleeding was controlled with a similar *running/figure-of-eight Vicryl/Monocryl* suture.

The right-angle clamp was then passed beneath the smooth musculature of the urethra just beyond the prostatic apex. The anterior two-thirds of the urethral wall were sharply divided, exposing the urethral catheter, which was clamped and cut distally. Its severed end was removed transurethrally.

The prostate was gently displaced posteriorly and six anastomotic 3-0 Monocryl sutures on UR-5 needles were placed into the distal urethral segment at the 12, 2, 5, 6, 7 and 10 o'clock positions. The residual posterior urethral lip of tissue was divided and the anastomotic sutures were clamped and covered with towels, avoiding inadvertent displacement.

The posterior striated urethral sphincter was divided midway between the apex of the prostate and the urethra while displacing the neurovascular bundles posteriorly. The superficial layers of the levator fascia were carefully dissected from the bladder neck to the apex, releasing the neurovascular bundles laterally. The dissection was extended caudally and residual layers of the striated sphincter were divided at the midline, exposing the anterior rectal wall.

Using blunt dissection, a plane was developed between the anterior rectum and Denonvillier's fascia, separating the prostate at the midline. The lateral aspects of the prostate were dissected parallel to the neurovascular bundles to the junction of the seminal vesicles and bladder, carefully dividing the lateral pedicles in layers using clips.

Having completely mobilized the lateral pedicles bilaterally, the anterior bladder neck was incised at its junction with the prostate. The balloon was deflated and the two ends of the catheter were clamped and placed on gentle upward traction. Both ureteral orifices were visualized with clear efflux. The posterior bladder wall was divided and the

dissection continued posterolaterally, developing a plane between the anterior surface of the seminal vesicles and the posterior bladder wall. The ampullae of the vasa were identified, isolated, and transected. The seminal vesicles were individually dissected off Denonvillier's fascia and their corresponding vessels ligated with surgical clips. The prostate, ampullae, and seminal vesicles were removed *en bloc* and sent to pathology for evaluation. The pelvis was irrigated with warm sterile water and minor bleeding sites were coagulated, avoiding the neurovascular bundles.

The bladder neck was reconstructed using interrupted 2-0 chromic sutures to approximate full-thickness muscularis and mucosa forming a "tennis racquet" closure. Additional interrupted 4-0 chromic sutures were used to evert the mucosa to allow a mucosa-mucosal anastomosis. The caliber of the newly constructed bladder neck was approximately the size of the tip of the index finger.

A new 20 Fr urethral catheter was inserted through the urethral meatus and retrieved in the true pelvis. The six Monocryl sutures previously inserted in the distal urethra were placed inside-out in their corresponding positions on the bladder neck using a french-eye needle. The catheter was advanced into the bladder and its balloon inflated with 15 ml sterile water. Using gentle manual caudal bladder compression, each suture was securely tied, completing the vesicourethral anastomosis.

The urethral catheter was irrigated with normal saline confirming a watertight anastomosis. Prior to closure, the pelvis was inspected and found to be without any evidence of bleeding or injury to any structures.

A surgical drain (e.g. Jackson-Pratt, 0.25 in. Penrose) was placed into the space of Retzius, brought out through a separate lateral skin incision and secured at the skin with a 2-0 silk suture.

The self-retaining retractor was removed and the abdominal incision was closed using a running 2-0 chromic suture to approximate the rectus muscles and 1-0 polydioxanone (PDS) suture for the rectus aponeurosis. Chromic sutures were used on Scarpa's fascia and the skin approximated with a subcuticular 4-0 Monocryl suture. The incision was reinforced with sterile adhesive strips and a sterile dressing was applied.

The urethral catheter was secured to the patient's anterior thigh.

At the end of the procedure, all counts were correct.

The patient tolerated the procedure without difficulty and was taken to the recovery room in satisfactory condition.

Estimated blood loss: Approximately _____ml

35

Retropubic Simple Prostatectomy

Indications

- Bladder outlet obstruction with prostate volume >100 g

Essential Steps

1) Gently dissect the preprostatic fat to identify and ligate the superficial dorsal venous branches.
2) Make a transverse mid-anterior capsulotomy to expose the prostate.
3) Enucleate the prostate, staying in the plane between the prostatic capsule and the adenoma.
4) Excise a wedge of posterior bladder neck ("trigonization") to limit the likelihood of a bladder neck contracture.
5) Pass a three-way urethral catheter into the bladder and close the prostatic capsulotomy.
6) Place a retroperitoneal drain.
7) Begin continuous bladder irrigation.

Note These Variations

- Alternatively, a suprapubic longitudinal incision (modified Pfannenstiel) may be used.
- Intravenous methylene blue or indigo carmine can be given to assist in identifying the ureteral orifices. Additionally, the ureteral orifices can be cannulated with infant feeding tubes.
- Hemostasis may be enhanced by incising the endopelvic fascia and obtaining control of the lateral pedicles at the bladder neck (similar to what is done during a radical retropubic prostatectomy).
- Persistent fossa bleeding, after prostatic enucleation, can be managed with figure-of-eight sutures placed at the 5 o'clock and 7 o'clock positions at the prostatovesical junction.

Complications

- Bleeding
- Infection
- Urine leak/urinoma
- Ureteral injury
- Urinary incontinence
- Bladder neck contracture/urethral stricture

Template Operative Dictation

Preoperative diagnosis: Obstructive, clinically benign prostatic enlargement
Postoperative diagnosis: Same
Procedure: Retropubic simple prostatectomy
Indications: The patient is a ___-year-old male with bladder outlet obstruction *and/or urinary retention* with a large prostate presenting for retropubic prostatectomy.
Description of Procedure: The indications, alternatives, benefits, and risks were discussed with the patient and informed consent was obtained.

The patient was brought onto the operating room table, positioned supine, and secured with a safety strap. All pressure points were carefully padded and pneumatic compression devices were placed on the lower extremities.

After the administration of intravenous antibiotics and *general endotracheal/regional* anesthesia, the entire abdomen and external genitalia were prepped and draped in the standard sterile manner. The operating table was flexed and positioned in mild Trendelenburg.

A time-out was completed, verifying the correct patient, surgical procedure, and positioning, prior to beginning the procedure.

A 20 Fr urethral catheter was inserted into the bladder and clamped.

A 10 cm midline abdominal incision was made between the umbilicus and the symphysis pubis, and carried down through the subcutaneous tissue using electrocautery. The underlying rectus abdominis aponeurosis was identified and incised at the linea alba. The rectus abdominis muscles were separated at the midline and retracted laterally, taking care not to injure the underlying inferior epigastric vessels. A self-retaining retractor (e.g. Balfour, Bookwalter, Omni-Tract) was appropriately positioned to optimize exposure, using padding on each retractor blade. A malleable blade was used to displace the bladder superiorly and posteriorly.

The peritoneum was swept cranially, after incising the perivesical fat just below the peritoneal reflection, and the anterior surface of the bladder and prostate were exposed. Care was taken to avoid entry into the peritoneal cavity. The preprostatic fat was gently dissected, exposing the superficial dorsal vein, which was ligated with 2-0 chromic sutures.

A full-thickness transverse prostatic capsulotomy was made approximately 2 cm caudal to the bladder neck and sufficiently extended in each direction. A 2-0 polyglactin (Vicryl) figure-of-eight suture was placed on each lateral margin of the capsulotomy to avoid inadvertent tearing. The urethral catheter was removed. The anterior prostatic commissure was sharply divided from the bladder neck to the apex, separating the

lateral prostatic lobes, anteriorly. Prostatic enucleation was begun anteriorly and continued circumferentially with the index finger, staying in a plane between the adenoma and the capsule. The apical dissection was performed, taking care not to avulse the urethra or injure the external sphincter.

Having completed the enucleation, the adenoma was removed and sent to pathology for evaluation. The prostatic fossa was inspected confirming the absence of residual adenoma. A sterile rolled gauze packing was placed deep into the prostatic fossa to tamponade any bleeding. After several minutes, the packing was removed and additional hemostasis achieved with electrocautery.

A small wedge resection of the posterior bladder neck was performed and the mucosa advanced into the prostatic fossa where it was sutured with interrupted 2-0 chromics. Both ureteral orifices were visualized with clear efflux, confirming their integrity.

A *22/24* Fr three-way urethral catheter with a 30 cc balloon was advanced transurethrally into the bladder and the balloon inflated with _____ ml sterile water. The catheter was placed on gentle traction and connected to a drainage bag.

The prostatic capsulotomy was closed using a single running 2-0 polyglactin (Vicryl) suture. The urethral catheter was irrigated with sterile normal saline, confirming a watertight capsular closure and satisfactory hemostasis.

A surgical drain (e.g. Jackson Pratt, 0.25 in. Penrose) was placed into the space of Retzius, brought out through a separate lateral skin incision and secured at the skin with a 2-0 silk suture.

The self-retaining retractor was removed and the pelvis was irrigated with sterile normal saline and inspected, confirming the absence of any bleeding or injury. The abdominal incision was closed using a running 2-0 chromic suture to approximate the rectus muscles and a 1-0 polydioxanone (PDS) suture for the rectus aponeurosis. 3-0 chromic sutures were used on Scarpa's fascia and the skin approximated with a subcuticular 4-0 poliglecaprone (Monocryl) suture. The incision was reinforced with sterile adhesive strips and a sterile dressing was applied.

Continuous bladder irrigation was started and the urethral catheter was secured to the patient's anterior thigh.

At the end of the procedure, all counts were correct.

The patient tolerated the procedure without difficulty and was taken to the recovery room in satisfactory condition.

Estimated blood loss: Approximately _____ ml

36

Suprapubic Prostatectomy

Indications

- Bladder outlet obstruction with prostate volume >100 g

Essential Steps

1) Distend the bladder with sterile saline through a urethral catheter.
2) Make a vertical midline cystotomy.
3) Identify and protect the ureteral orifices.
4) Enucleate the gland, staying in the plane between the prostatic capsule and the adenoma.
5) Place hemostatic sutures at the prostatovesical junction at the 5 o'clock and 7 o'clock positions.
6) Insert a suprapubic and transurethral catheter.
7) Place a retroperitoneal drain.
8) Begin continuous bladder irrigation.

Note These Variations

- Alternatively, a suprapubic longitudinal incision (modified Pfannenstiel) may be used.
- The ureteral orifices can be cannulated with infant feeding tubes to assist in their identification.
- Persistent fossa bleeding after prostatic enucleation can be managed with capsular plication sutures and/or distal traction on the bladder neck.
- In the presence of a large poorly draining bladder diverticulum, a diverticulectomy may be performed concomitantly.

Complications

- Bleeding
- Infection

Operative Dictations in Urologic Surgery, First Edition. Noel A. Armenakas, John A. Fracchia, and Ron Golan.
© 2019 John Wiley & Sons Ltd. Published 2019 by John Wiley & Sons Ltd.

- Urine leak/urinoma
- Ureteral injury
- Urinary incontinence
- Bladder neck contracture/urethral stricture

Template Operative Dictation

Preoperative diagnosis: Obstructive, clinically benign prostatic enlargement
Postoperative diagnosis: Same
Procedure: Suprapubic prostatectomy
Indications: The patient is a ___ -year-old male with bladder outlet obstruction *and/ or urinary retention* with a large prostate presenting for suprapubic prostatectomy.
Description of Procedure: The indications, alternatives, benefits, and risks were discussed with the patient and informed consent was obtained.

The patient was brought onto the operating room table, positioned supine, and secured with a safety strap. All pressure points were carefully padded and pneumatic compression devices placed on the lower extremities.

After the administration of intravenous antibiotics and *general endotracheal/regional* anesthesia, the entire abdomen and external genitalia were prepped and draped in the standard sterile manner.

A time-out was completed, verifying the correct patient, surgical procedure, and positioning, prior to beginning the procedure.

A 20 Fr urethral catheter was used to fill the bladder with sterile normal saline.

The anesthesiologist was asked to inject 10 cc *indigo carmine/methylene blue* intravenously to facilitate visualization of the ureteral orifices.

A 10 cm midline abdominal incision was made between the umbilicus and the symphysis pubis and carried down through the subcutaneous tissue using electrocautery. The underlying rectus abdominis aponeurosis was identified and incised at the linea alba. The rectus abdominis muscles were separated at the midline and retracted laterally, taking care not to injure the underlying inferior epigastric vessels. A self-retaining retractor (e.g. Balfour, Bookwalter, Omni-Tract) was appropriately positioned to optimize exposure, using padding on each retractor blade.

The peritoneum was swept superiorly with a sponge stick after transversely incising the transversalis fascia just below the peritoneal reflection. Care was taken to avoid entry into the peritoneal cavity. Two 2-0 polyglactin (Vicryl) sutures were placed into the mid-anterior bladder wall and a full-thickness vertical stab incision made between these. The incised bladder wall was grasped with Allis clamps and the cystotomy extended cephalad and caudally to within 1 cm of the bladder neck. Additional pairs of 2-0 Vicryl stay sutures were placed on each side of the cystotomy, and a figure-of-eight suture placed caudally to prevent tearing of the anterior commissure during enucleation of the adenoma. A well-padded malleable blade was positioned cephalad into the bladder and connected to the self-retaining retractor. The bladder was thoroughly inspected and blue dye was seen effluxing from both ureteral orifices. There were no bladder stones or tumors noted.

The intravesical prostatic mucosa at the bladder neck was identified and incised with electrocautery in a circular fashion, proceeding from posterior to anterior. Care

was taken to avoid injury to the ureteral orifices. Hemostasis was achieved with electrocautery.

Prostatic enucleation was begun anteriorly and continued circumferentially with the index finger, staying in a plane between the adenoma and the capsule. The apical dissection was performed carefully using a gentle pinching action, taking care not to avulse the urethra or injure the external sphincter. Having completed the enucleation, the adenoma was removed and sent to pathology for evaluation. The prostatic fossa was inspected confirming the absence of residual adenoma.

A sterile rolled gauze packing was placed deep into the prostatic fossa to tamponade any bleeding. After several minutes, the packing was removed and the posterior bladder neck was grasped at the 5 o'clock and 7 o'clock positions with long Allis clamps. Two, 1-0 chromic figure-of-eight sutures were placed to ensure hemostasis.

A 22 Fr urethral catheter with a 30 cc balloon was advanced transurethrally into the bladder. Sterile water was used to inflate the balloon to ____ml and the catheter was placed on gentle traction. Additionally, a 24 Fr Malecot suprapubic tube was placed into the bladder dome, secured with a 2-0 chromic purse-string suture and brought out cephalad through a separate skin incision.

The cystotomy was closed in two layers using running 3-0 and 2-0 Vicryl sutures on the mucosal and muscularis/adventitial layers, respectively. Through-and-through catheter irrigation with sterile normal saline ensured patency of both the transurethral and suprapubic catheters, and a watertight bladder closure.

A surgical drain (e.g. Jackson Pratt, 0.25 in. Penrose) was placed into the space of Retzius and brought out through a separate lateral skin incision. The drain and suprapubic catheter were secured at the skin with 2-0 silk sutures.

The self-retaining retractor was removed and the pelvis was irrigated with warm normal saline and inspected confirming the absence of any bleeding or injury. The abdominal incision was closed using a running 2-0 chromic to approximate the rectus muscles and 1-0 polydioxanone (PDS) for the rectus aponeurosis. 3-0 chromic sutures were used on Scarpa's fascia and the skin approximated with a subcuticular 4-0 poliglecaprone (Monocryl) suture. The incision was reinforced with sterile adhesive strips and a sterile dressing applied.

Continuous bladder irrigation was started through the transurethral catheter and a four-liter drainage bag was attached to the suprapubic tube. The output was noted to be *clear/light pink tinged* with the urethral catheter on gentle traction. Both tubes were appropriately secured to the skin.

At the end of the procedure, all counts were correct.

The patient tolerated the procedure without difficulty and was taken to the recovery room in satisfactory condition.

Estimated blood loss: Approximately _____ml

Testis and Scrotum

37

Epididymal Cyst Excision (Spermatocelectomy)

Indications

- Scrotal discomfort secondary to epididymal cyst
- Cosmetic concern secondary to epididymal cyst
- Chronic epididymal pain (*Note:* Pain may not be relieved by excision.)

Essential Steps

1) Make an incision in the ipsilateral anterior scrotal wall.
2) Spread the dartos muscle, incise the tunica vaginalis, and deliver the testis and epididymis.
3) Carefully dissect the epididymal cyst from the epididymis.
4) Ligate the single tubule or vasa efferentia leading from the epididymis to the cyst.
5) Replace the testis and epididymis in their normal anatomic position within the scrotum.

Note These Variations

- During the wound closure, a drain may be placed at the discretion of the surgeon.

Complications

- Bleeding
- Scrotal swelling
- Infection
- Scrotal abscess
- Persistent scrotal pain
- Loss of sperm transport from the ipsilateral epididymis

Operative Dictations in Urologic Surgery, First Edition. Noel A. Armenakas, John A. Fracchia, and Ron Golan.
© 2019 John Wiley & Sons Ltd. Published 2019 by John Wiley & Sons Ltd.

Template Operative Dictation

Preoperative diagnosis: *Right/left* epididymal cyst (Spermatocele)
Postoperative diagnosis: Same
Procedure: *Right/left* epididymal cyst excision (Spermatocelectomy)
Indications: The patient is a _____-year-old male with a *right/left* epididymal cyst presenting for excision.
Description of Procedure: The indications, alternatives, benefits, and risks were discussed with the patient and informed consent was obtained.

The patient was brought onto the operating room table, positioned supine, and secured with a safety strap. All pressure points were carefully padded and pneumatic compression devices were placed on the lower extremities.

After the administration of intravenous antibiotics and *general/regional* anesthesia, the patient's scrotum was examined and the *right/left* epididymal cyst palpated. The lower abdomen and external genitalia were prepped and draped in the standard sterile manner.

A time-out was completed, verifying the correct patient, surgical procedure, site, and positioning, prior to beginning the procedure.

A skin incision was made over the *right/left* anterior hemiscrotum. The dartos fascia and tunica vaginalis were divided and the testicle and epididymis delivered. The cyst was identified at the epididymal *caput/cauda/body* and carefully dissected from the remaining epididymis. The attachment at its epididymal origin was ligated with a 4-0 chromic suture and divided, freeing the cyst, which was sent to pathology for evaluation. The surgical base was lightly cauterized, maintaining meticulous hemostasis.

After excising the cyst, the epididymis, testis, and spermatic cord were inspected and found to be intact without any evidence of injury. They were then carefully placed back into the scrotum in their normal anatomic position, making sure that the spermatic cord was not twisted.

The dartos fascia and scrotal skin were closed with running and interrupted 3-0 chromic sutures, respectively. The incision was covered with a sterile dressing and gauze fluffs, and an athletic supporter was applied to help minimize swelling.

At the end of the procedure, all counts were correct.

The patient tolerated the procedure well and was taken to the recovery room in satisfactory condition.

Estimated blood loss: Approximately _____ml

38

Epididymectomy

Indications

- Chronic infection refractory to antibiotics and/or antitubercular therapy; epididymal abscess formation
- Suggestion of neoplasm
- Chronic epididymal pain (*Note:* Pain may not be relieved by epididymectomy.)

Essential Steps

1) Make an incision in the ipsilateral anterior scrotal wall.
2) Spread the dartos muscle, incise the tunica vaginalis, and deliver the testis and epididymis.
3) Transect the ipsilateral vas deferens proximal to the epididymis.
4) Resect the epididymis and lightly cauterize the residual base.
5) Replace the testis and epididymis in their normal anatomic position within the scrotum.
6) Place a drain if an underlying infection is suspected.

Note These Variations

- An inguinal approach can be utilized in selected cases.
- The use of a scrotal drain is optional.

Complications

- Bleeding
- Scrotal swelling
- Infection
- Scrotal abscess
- Persistent scrotal pain

Operative Dictations in Urologic Surgery, First Edition. Noel A. Armenakas, John A. Fracchia, and Ron Golan.
© 2019 John Wiley & Sons Ltd. Published 2019 by John Wiley & Sons Ltd.

Template Operative Dictation

Preoperative diagnosis: *Right/left chronic epididymitis/epididymal tumor/epididymal abscess*

Postoperative diagnosis: Same

Procedure: *Right/left* epididymectomy

Indications: The patient is a _____-year-old male with *chronic epididymitis/an epididymal tumor* presenting for *right/left* epididymectomy.

Description of Procedure: The indications, alternatives, benefits, and risks were discussed with the patient and informed consent was obtained.

The patient was brought onto the operating room table, positioned supine, and secured with a safety strap. All pressure points were carefully padded and pneumatic compression devices were placed on the lower extremities.

After the administration of intravenous antibiotics and *general/regional* anesthesia, the patient's scrotum was examined and the *right/left indurated epididymis/epididymal mass* palpated. The lower abdomen and external genitalia were prepped and draped in the standard sterile manner.

A time-out was completed, verifying the correct patient, surgical procedure, site, and positioning, prior to beginning the procedure.

A skin incision was made over the *right/left* anterior hemiscrotum. The dartos fascia and tunica vaginalis were divided and the testicle and epididymis were delivered. The vas deferens proximal to the epididymis was isolated, ligated with 2-0 chromic sutures, and divided. The tail of the epididymis was lifted off the testis, exposing the artery of the epididymis near the junction of the upper and middle third of the testis. This was ligated with 3-0 chromic sutures, taking care not to injure the testicular artery. The remainder of the epididymis was carefully dissected off the testicular tunica albuginea and the entire vasoepididiymal complex was removed and sent to pathology for evaluation. The surgical base was lightly cauterized, maintaining meticulous hemostasis.

The testis and spermatic cord were inspected and found to be intact without any evidence of injury. They were then carefully placed into the scrotum in their normal anatomic position, making sure that the spermatic cord was not twisted.

A 0.25 in. Penrose drain was placed through a separate scrotal stab incision, and a sterile safety pin was inserted through this to prevent its migration into the wound.

The dartos fascia and scrotal skin were closed with running and interrupted 3-0 chromic sutures, respectively. The incision was covered with a sterile dressing and gauze fluffs, and an athletic supporter was applied to help minimize swelling.

At the end of the procedure, all counts were correct.

The patient tolerated the procedure well and was taken to the recovery room in satisfactory condition.

Estimated blood loss: Approximately _____ml

39

Hydrocelectomy

Indications

- Scrotal discomfort
- Cosmetic concerns

Essential Steps

1) Make an incision in the ipsilateral anterior scrotal wall.
2) Dissect the hydrocele sac in an inferior to superior direction to the origin of the sac from the spermatic cord.
3) Incise the sac and suction off the contents.
4) Excise the redundant sac and surgically evert the edges with a running absorbable suture loosely around the spermatic cord.
5) Replace the testis and epididymis in their normal anatomic position within the scrotum.
6) Consider leaving a drain to minimize postoperative swelling.

Note These Variations

- A hydrocele plication (Lord technique) can be performed by placing 6–12 plicating sutures into the incised edge of the tunica and gathering the inverted sac to the edge of the testis.
- The tunica vaginalis may be excised close to the testicle and epididymis, and simply oversewn with interlocking running sutures placed circumferentially for hemostasis.
- The use of a scrotal drain is optional.

Complications

- Bleeding
- Scrotal swelling

Operative Dictations in Urologic Surgery, First Edition. Noel A. Armenakas, John A. Fracchia, and Ron Golan.
© 2019 John Wiley & Sons Ltd. Published 2019 by John Wiley & Sons Ltd.

- Infection
- Scrotal abscess
- Testicular/epididymal injury
- Persistent scrotal pain
- Recurrent hydrocele

Template Operative Dictation

Preoperative diagnosis: *Right/left* hydrocele
Postoperative diagnosis: Same
Procedure: *Right/left* hydrocelectomy
Indications: The patient is a ___-year-old male with a *right/left* hydrocele presenting for hydrocelectomy.
Description of Procedure: The indications, alternatives, benefits, and risks were discussed with the patient and informed consent was obtained.

The patient was brought onto the operating room table, positioned supine, and secured with a safety strap. All pressure points were carefully padded and pneumatic compression devices were placed on the lower extremities.

After the administration of intravenous antibiotics and *general/regional* anesthesia, the patient's scrotum was examined and the *right/left* hydrocele palpated. The lower abdomen and external genitalia were prepped and draped in the standard sterile manner.

A time-out was completed, verifying the correct patient, surgical procedure, site, and positioning, prior to beginning the procedure.

A skin incision was made over the *right/left* anterior hemiscrotum. The dartos fascia was incised, exposing the hydrocele. The sac was separated from the scrotal wall with sharp and blunt dissection. Using manual pressure, the hydrocele and testicle were delivered through the incision and dissected from the spermatic cord in an inferior to superior direction. The hydrocele sac was carefully freed from the surrounding tissue with a moist sponge, cleanly exposing the parietal layer of the tunica vaginalis. The hydrocele was incised and approximately ___ml straw-colored fluid aspirated. The redundant hydrocele sac was excised and sent to pathology for evaluation. The edges of the sac were everted loosely behind the testis and sutured to each other using a running 3-0 *polyglycolic (Vicryl)/chromic* suture. All bleeding points were cauterized, maintaining meticulous hemostasis.

The testis, epididymis and spermatic cord were inspected and found to be intact without any evidence of injury. They were carefully placed back into the scrotum, in their normal anatomic position, making sure that the spermatic cord was not twisted.

A 0.25 in. Penrose drain was placed through a separate scrotal stab incision and a sterile safety pin inserted through this to prevent its migration into the wound.

The dartos fascia and scrotal skin were closed with running and interrupted 3-0 chromic sutures, respectively. The incision was covered with a sterile dressing and gauze fluffs, and an athletic supporter was applied to help minimize swelling.

At the end of the procedure, all counts were correct.

The patient tolerated the procedure well and was taken to the recovery room in satisfactory condition.

Estimated blood loss: Approximately ____ ml

40

Microsurgical Testicular Sperm Extraction (MicroTESE)

Indications

- Nonobstructive azoospermia (after assessment of Y chromosomal microdeletions)
- Failure to find sperm in the epididymis in the presence of spermatogenesis, or complete absence of the vas deferens

Essential Steps

1) Make an incision in the anterior scrotum and deliver the testis into the wound.
2) Under magnification, find an avascular area to incise on the tunica albuginea.
3) Identify sperm-containing seminiferous tubules, dissect them from the adjacent tissue and excise them.
4) Examine the fluid under the microscope to determine if sperm are present. If no sperm are identified, repeat the procedure at another location.

Note These Variations

- Percutaneous testicular or epididymal sperm aspiration may be sufficient in retrieving sperm in some patients.
- Bilateral testicular exploration may be required if sperm is not found in the initial testis.

Complications

- Bleeding
- Infection
- Inability to identify any sperm-laden seminiferous tubules
- Epididymal/testicular injury
- Testicular atrophy
- Hypogonadism

Operative Dictations in Urologic Surgery, First Edition. Noel A. Armenakas, John A. Fracchia, and Ron Golan.
© 2019 John Wiley & Sons Ltd. Published 2019 by John Wiley & Sons Ltd.

Template Operative Dictation

Preoperative diagnosis: Infertility
Postoperative diagnosis: Same
Procedure: Microsurgical testicular sperm extraction
Indications: The patient is a _____-year-old male with azoospermia presenting for microsurgical testicular sperm extraction.
Description of Procedure: The indications, alternatives, benefits, and risks were discussed with the patient and informed consent was obtained.

The patient was brought onto the operating room table, positioned supine, and secured with a safety strap. All pressure points were carefully padded and pneumatic compression devices were placed on the lower extremities.

After the administration of intravenous antibiotics and *local anesthesia with a spermatic cord block/regional anesthesia/general anesthesia*, the external genitalia were prepped and draped in the standard sterile manner.

A time-out was completed, verifying the correct patient, surgical procedure, and positioning, prior to beginning the procedure.

A 5 cm transverse scrotal skin incision was made through the *right/left anterior scrotal wall/median raphe* and carried down through the dartos fascia with electrocautery. The tunica vaginalis was opened and the *right/left* testis delivered through the incision.

The operating microscope was draped and brought into the field.

A 15° microknife was used to make a transverse incision in a relatively avascular area of the tunica albuginea at the midportion of the testis.

Under 15–25x magnification, sperm-containing tubules were identified by their relatively larger size and opaque color. These were carefully dissected from the surrounding parenchyma with a microneedle holder. A sharp curved iris scissor was used to excise the tubules and the specimen placed in human tubal fluid media, microdissected and immediately examined under 200x power using phase contrast microscopy. The presence of sperm was confirmed and the microdissection completed. The specimen was placed in human tubal fluid media and sent for cryopreservation.

Meticulous hemostasis was obtained with microbipolar cautery. The tunica albuginea was closed with a 6-0 nylon (Ethilon). The testis was correctly repositioned into the scrotum within the tunica vaginalis, which was closed with a running 5-0 polyglactin (Vicryl) suture. The dartos fascia was approximated with a running 4-0 Vicryl and the skin with a subcuticular 5-0 poliglecaprone (Monocryl) suture. The incision was reinforced with sterile adhesive strips and a sterile dressing was applied. Gauze fluffs and an athletic supporter were used to help minimize swelling.

At the end of the procedure, all counts were correct.

The patient tolerated the procedure without difficulty and was taken to the recovery room in satisfactory condition.

Estimated blood loss: Approximately _____ml

41

Microsurgical Varicocelectomy

Indications

- Male infertility with impaired semen analysis that is potentially correctable with a varicocele repair
- Impaired testicular growth in an adolescent associated with a varicocele
- Disfiguring varicocele
- Chronic intrascrotal pain attributed to a large varicocele

Essential Steps

1) Make a 2–3 cm subinguinal incision over the external ring.
2) Gently grasp the spermatic cord and open the external and internal spermatic fascias.
3) Identify and isolate the testicular artery using papaverine and a micro-Doppler probe.
4) Doubly clip or ligate all nonvasal veins within the spermatic cord as well as any perforating and gubernacular veins, while preserving the lymphatics.

Note These Variations

- Alternatively, an inguinal microsurgical approach can be used. This is preferred in children or prepubertal adolescents because of the smaller vessels encountered with the subinguinal approach. Similarly, it is should be used when an ipsilateral herniorrhaphy is simultaneously performed.

Complications

- Bleeding
- Infection
- Injury to the epididymis, testicle, or vas deferens
- Testicular atrophy

Operative Dictations in Urologic Surgery, First Edition. Noel A. Armenakas, John A. Fracchia, and Ron Golan.
© 2019 John Wiley & Sons Ltd. Published 2019 by John Wiley & Sons Ltd.

- Lack of improvement in semen analysis
- Hydrocele
- Recurrent varicocele

Template Operative Dictation

Preoperative diagnosis: *Right/left/bilateral* varicocele(s)
Postoperative diagnosis: Same
Procedure: Microsurgical varicocelectom*y(ies)*
Indications: The patient is a _____-year-old male with *infertility/impaired testicular growth/chronic intrascrotal pain/a disfiguring varicocele* presenting for *right/left/bilateral* varicocelectom*y(ies)*.
Description of Procedure: The indications, alternatives, benefits, and risks were discussed with the patient/guardian and informed consent was obtained.

The patient was brought onto the operating room table, positioned supine, and secured with a safety strap. All pressure points were carefully padded and pneumatic compression devices were placed on the lower extremities.

After the administration of intravenous antibiotics and *general/regional* anesthesia, the patient's scrotum was examined. The lower abdomen and external genitalia were prepped and draped in the standard sterile manner.

A time-out was completed, verifying the correct patient, surgical procedure, site, and positioning, prior to beginning the procedure.

A 3 cm *right/left* subinguinal incision was made through the skin overlying the ipsilateral pubic tubercle. Camper's and Scarpa's fascia were divided with electrocautery. The spermatic cord was gently grasped with a Babcock clamp, delivered into the field, and placed over a 0.25 in. Penrose drain for support.

The operating microscope was draped and brought into the field.

The external and internal spermatic fascias were incised vertically and extended superiorly exposing the dilated internal spermatic veins. Care was taken to preserve the genital and ilioinguinal branches of the genitofemoral nerve, the cremasteric vessels and all lymphatics.

The spermatic cord was irrigated with 1 ml papaverine. Under 25x magnification and with the aid of a micro-Doppler probe, *one/two* testicular artery*(ies) was/were* identified and microdissected, separating *it/them* from the adjacent network of veins. A vessel loop was placed loosely around *the/each* testicular artery.

Microsurgical dissection of the cord was performed in an orderly linear fashion, transversely. All nonvasal veins in the spermatic cord were identified and *doubly clipped/suture ligated with 4-0 silk*, transected and sent to pathology. The spermatic cord was thoroughly examined confirming the absence of any remaining patent external or internal spermatic veins. The Penrose drain and arterial vessel loop were removed.

The testis was delivered into the field, using light traction on the cord and gentle pressure on the testis from below. The gubernaculum was inspected for veins entering from the tunica vaginalis. Small veins were fulgurated with a microbipolar cautery, and large veins clipped and divided. The testis was carefully placed back into the scrotum in its normal anatomic position, and the spermatic cord was again examined, confirming meticulous hemostasis.

Prior to closure, the testicular artery, vas deferens, deferential vessels, and testicle were noted to be intact. Camper's and Scarpa's fascia were approximated with running 3-0 chromic sutures and the wound was infiltrated with 0.25% bupivacaine. The skin was closed with a subcuticular 5-0 poliglecaprone (Monocryl) suture and the incision reinforced with sterile adhesive strips.

> *For bilateral varicocelectomies*: The identical procedure was performed on the contralateral side.

The incision(s) *was/were* covered with a sterile dressing and gauze fluffs, and an athletic supporter was applied to help minimize swelling.

At the end of the procedure, all counts were correct.

The patient tolerated the procedure without difficulty and was taken to the recovery room in satisfactory condition.

Estimated blood loss: Approximately _____ml

42

Radical Orchiectomy

Indication

- Suspected testis neoplasm

Essential Steps

1) Make an inguinal incision.
2) Dissect the spermatic cord circumferentially and occlude it at the level of the internal ring before manipulating the testis.
3) Free all attachments of the spermatic cord and testis from the internal ring to the gubernaculum.
4) Separately ligate the spermatic cord vessels and vas deferens, and then remove the specimen. (Use silk ties and leave a long tail for subsequent identification, should a retroperitoneal lymphadenectomy be performed.)

Note These Variations

- A testicular prosthesis may be inserted at the time of orchiectomy, at the patient's discretion.

Complications

- Inguinal/retroperitoneal bleeding
- Infection
- Postoperative swelling
- Inguinal neuralgia
- Prosthesis infection/erosion (if inserted)

Operative Dictations in Urologic Surgery, First Edition. Noel A. Armenakas, John A. Fracchia, and Ron Golan.
© 2019 John Wiley & Sons Ltd. Published 2019 by John Wiley & Sons Ltd.

Template Operative Dictation

Preoperative diagnosis: Suspected testis neoplasm
Postoperative diagnosis: Same
Procedure: *Right/left* radical orchiectomy
Indications: The patient is a ___-year-old male with a suspected *right/left* testicular neoplasm presenting for radical orchiectomy.
Description of Procedure: The indications, alternatives, benefits, and risks were discussed with the patient and informed consent was obtained.

The patient was brought onto the operating room table, positioned supine, and secured with a safety strap. All pressure points were carefully padded and pneumatic compression devices were placed on the lower extremities.

After the administration of intravenous antibiotics and *general/regional* anesthesia, the lower abdomen and external genitalia were prepped and draped in the standard sterile manner.

A time-out was completed, verifying the correct patient, surgical procedure, site, and positioning, prior to beginning the procedure.

A *right/left* inguinal skin incision was made between the ipsilateral pubic tubercle and the anterosuperior iliac spine. Scarpa's fascia was divided with electrocautery and the aponeurosis of the external oblique was incised in the direction of its fibers. The ilioinguinal nerve was identified, isolated and carefully retracted out of the operative field. The spermatic cord was dissected circumferentially and occluded with a 0.25 in. Penrose drain encircled twice at the level of the internal ring. The dissection proceeded inferiorly from the internal ring toward the testicle, freeing the cord of all attachments. The scrotum was then grasped and inverted, bringing the testicle into the operative field, where it was isolated with a towel. The gubernaculum was clamped and cut, completely freeing the testicle inferiorly. Palpation of the testicle confirmed the presence of an irregular hard mass, consistent with a neoplasm.

The spermatic cord vessels and vas deferens were individually doubly ligated with 2-0 silk sutures leaving long "tails" to facilitate easy identification should a retroperitoneal node dissection be indicated. The spermatic cord was transected at the level of the internal ring. The specimen was removed and sent to pathology for evaluation.

The inguinal canal and inner scrotum were irrigated with warm sterile water and thoroughly examined for bleeding. Meticulous hemostasis was achieved with electrocautery. The ilioinguinal nerve was inspected, noted to be intact, and replaced in its normal anatomic position below the external oblique aponeurosis.

The inguinal incision was closed using a running 3-0 polyglactin (Vicryl) suture on the external oblique aponeurosis and a 3-0 chromic on Scarpa's fascia. The skin was approximated with a 4-0 subcuticular polyglecaprone (Monocryl) suture. The incision was reinforced with sterile adhesive strips and a sterile dressing was applied. Gauze fluffs and an athletic supporter were used to help minimize swelling.

At the end of the procedure, all counts were correct.

The patient tolerated the procedure without difficulty and was taken to the recovery room in satisfactory condition.

Estimated blood loss: Approximately _____ml

43

Simple Orchiectomy (Unilateral or Bilateral)

Indications

- Inflammatory, ischemic or necrotic testicular disease, not amenable to testicular preservation
- Endocrine ablation for prostate cancer

Essential Steps

1) Make an incision in the ipsilateral anterior scrotal wall.
2) Dissect the spermatic cord circumferentially superior to the testis.
3) Free all intrascrotal attachments of the spermatic cord and testis.
4) Ligate the spermatic cord and remove the testis.

Note These Variations

- If both testes are to be removed, a median raphe incision can be used.
- A drain should be placed if bacterial contamination is suspected.

Complications

- Bleeding
- Infection
- Postoperative swelling

Template Operative Dictation

Preoperative diagnosis: *Right/left testicular inflammation/ischemia/necrosis// prostate cancer*
Postoperative diagnosis: Same
Procedure: *Right/left/bilateral* orchiectomy*(ies)*

Operative Dictations in Urologic Surgery, First Edition. Noel A. Armenakas, John A. Fracchia, and Ron Golan.
© 2019 John Wiley & Sons Ltd. Published 2019 by John Wiley & Sons Ltd.

Indications: The patient is a _____-year-old male with ____ *an ischemic/infected testicle//prostate cancer* presenting for *right/left/bilateral* scrotal orchiectomy*(ies)*.

Description of Procedure: The indications, alternatives, benefits, and risks were discussed with the patient and informed consent was obtained.

The patient was brought onto the operating room table, positioned supine, and secured with a safety strap. All pressure points were carefully padded and pneumatic compression devices were placed on the lower extremities.

After the administration of intravenous antibiotics and *general/regional* anesthesia, the patient's scrotum was examined. The external genitalia were prepped and draped in the standard sterile manner.

A time-out was completed, verifying the correct patient, surgical procedure, site, and positioning, prior to beginning the procedure.

A 5 cm *transverse/longitudinal* skin incision was made through the *right/left anterior scrotal wall/median raphe* and the dartos fascia divided using electrocautery. The *right/left* testicle was delivered and the ipsilateral spermatic cord was identified and isolated superior to the testicle. The spermatic cord and vas deferens were clamped individually within the scrotum, doubly ligated with 2-0 polyglactin (Vicryl) ties, and divided. The specimen was removed and sent to pathology for evaluation.

> ***For bilateral orchiectomies:*** The identical procedure was completed on the contralateral side.

The wound was irrigated with sterile normal saline and thoroughly inspected for bleeding. Meticulous hemostasis was achieved with electrocautery.

The dartos fascia and scrotal skin were closed with running and interrupted 3-0 chromic sutures, respectively. The incision was covered with a sterile dressing and gauze fluffs, and an athletic supporter was applied to help minimize swelling.

At the end of the procedure, all counts were correct.

The patient tolerated the procedure without difficulty and was taken to the recovery room in satisfactory condition.

Estimated blood loss: Approximately _____ml

44

Testicular Prosthesis Insertion

Indications

- Psychologic/cosmetic choice in a patient with an absent testicle

Essential Steps

1) Make an incision in the anterior scrotal wall superior to the proposed placement of the testicular prosthesis.
2) Choose the appropriate-sized prosthesis to match the contralateral testis.
3) Secure the prosthesis by placing a suture through the plastic loop on the prosthesis to the dartos muscle in order to prevent its cranial migration.

Note These Variations

- Alternatively, a low inguinal incision can be used.
- Prior to insertion, the prosthesis may be bathed in antibiotic solution.
- The neck of the scrotum can be closed using a 3-0 polyglactin (Vicryl) purse-string suture, to prevent cranial migration of the prosthesis.

Complications

- Bleeding
- Postoperative swelling
- Prosthesis infection/erosion

Template Operative Dictation

Preoperative diagnosis: Absent *right/left* testis
Postoperative diagnosis: Same
Procedure: Insertion of *right/left* testicular prosthesis

Operative Dictations in Urologic Surgery, First Edition. Noel A. Armenakas, John A. Fracchia, and Ron Golan.
© 2019 John Wiley & Sons Ltd. Published 2019 by John Wiley & Sons Ltd.

Indications: The patient is a _____-year-old male with an absent *right/left* testis presenting for insertion of a testicular prosthesis.

Description of Procedure: The indications, alternatives, benefits, and risks were discussed with the patient and informed consent obtained.

The patient was brought onto the operating room table, positioned supine, and secured with a safety strap. All pressure points were carefully padded and pneumatic compression devices were placed on the lower extremities.

After the administration of intravenous antibiotics and *general/regional* anesthesia, the lower abdomen and external genitalia were prepped and draped in the standard sterile manner.

A time-out was completed, verifying the correct patient, surgical procedure, site, and positioning, prior to beginning the procedure.

A _____size saline testicular prosthesis was chosen based on the approximate volume of the contralateral testis.

A skin incision was made through the *right/left* superior anterior scrotal wall and the dartos muscle divided with electrocautery. A scrotal pouch was bluntly created with two fingers. The inferior base of the scrotum was inverted with an Allis clamp, and a 3-0 polyglactin (Vicryl) suture was placed in the inner scrotal wall and through the plastic dependent loop on the prosthesis. The prosthesis was then maneuvered to fit comfortably in the scrotum. Care was taken not to damage the prosthesis.

The wound was irrigated with sterile *normal saline/antibiotic solution* and thoroughly inspected for bleeding. Meticulous hemostasis was achieved using electrocautery. The dartos muscle was approximated with a running 3-0 chromic suture. The scrotal skin closure was completed using a subcuticular 4-0 poliglecaprone (Monocryl) and reinforced with sterile adhesive strips. The incision was covered with a sterile dressing and gauze fluffs, and an athletic supporter was applied to help minimize swelling.

At the end of the procedure, all counts were correct.

The patient tolerated the procedure without difficulty and was taken to the recovery room in satisfactory condition.

Estimated blood loss: Approximately _____ ml

45

Testis Biopsy

Indications

- Azoospermia with testis of normal consistency and size, palpable vasa deferentia, a normal serum follicle-stimulating hormone, and a normal chromosome analysis

Essential Steps

1) Make an incision in the anterior scrotal wall, with an assistant orienting the testis anteriorly and the epididymis posteriorly.
2) Incise the tunica albuginea and squeeze the testes to extrude spermatic tubules for biopsy; avoid distorting the testis tissue by limiting excessive handling of biopsy material.
3) Gently handle the biopsy specimen and place it in Bouin's solution. Perform a touch-prep cytological examination.
4) If no sperm are found on the touch prep or wet squash prep, perform another biopsy from another site within the testicle.
5) Place any retrieved sperm in the appropriate medium for cryopreservation.

Note These Variations

- An operating microscope can be used to enhance visualization.
- Alternatively, a testis biopsy can be performed percutaneously by fine-needle aspiration or a biopsy gun.

Complications

- Bleeding
- Infection
- Inability to identify any sperm-laden seminiferous tubules

Operative Dictations in Urologic Surgery, First Edition. Noel A. Armenakas, John A. Fracchia, and Ron Golan.
© 2019 John Wiley & Sons Ltd. Published 2019 by John Wiley & Sons Ltd.

- Postoperative swelling
- Epididymal/testicular injury
- Testicular atrophy

Template Operative Dictation

Preoperative diagnosis: Infertility
Postoperative diagnosis: Same
Procedure: Testis biopsy
Indications: The patient is a _____-year-old male with azoospermia presenting for testis biopsy.
Description of Procedure: The indications, alternatives, benefits, and risks were discussed with the patient and informed consent was obtained.

The patient was brought onto the operating room table, positioned supine, and secured with a safety strap. All pressure points were carefully padded and pneumatic compression devices were placed on the lower extremities.

After the administration of intravenous antibiotics and *local anesthesia with a spermatic cord block/regional anesthesia/general anesthesia*, the external genitalia were prepped and draped in the standard sterile manner.

A time-out was completed, verifying the correct patient, surgical procedure, site, and positioning, prior to beginning the procedure.

Using optical magnification with surgical loupes, a 2 cm transverse skin incision was made through the *right/left anteromedial/anterolateral* scrotal wall and carried down through the dartos fascia with electrocautery. With the assistant applying manual pressure to orient the testis anteriorly and the epididymis posteriorly, a small window was created in the tunica vaginalis, exposing the underlying testis. A 5 mm incision was made in an avascular area of the tunica albuginea, and using gentle testicular compression the underlying seminiferous tubules were extruded and carefully excised with sharp iris scissors. The specimen was placed in *Bouin's solution/human tubule fluid medium*.

A touch-prep cytologic examination was performed by blotting the cut surface of the testis several times with a glass slide. The specimen was examined under a microscope, confirming the presence of motile spermatids.

(If no sperm are seen, excise another specimen for a wet squash prep by placing it on a slide and adding a drop of saline. If sperm are retrieved, remove additional tissue and place it in the appropriate medium for cryopreservation.)

The tunica albuginea was closed with 6-0 nylon (Ethilon) to aid in identifying a site for future sperm retrieval if necessary.

The wound was thoroughly inspected for bleeding and hemostasis was meticulously obtained with bipolar electrocautery. The tunica vaginalis was closed with a running 5-0 polyglactin (Vicryl), the dartos fascia with a running 4-0 Vicryl, and the skin with a subcuticular 5-0 poliglecaprone (Monocryl) suture. The incision was reinforced with sterile adhesive strips and covered with a sterile dressing. Gauze fluffs and an athletic supporter were applied to help minimize swelling.

At the end of the procedure, all counts were correct.

The patient tolerated the procedure without difficulty and was taken to the recovery room in satisfactory condition.

Estimated blood loss: Approximately _____ml

46

Vasectomy

Indications

- Elective male sterilization

Essential Steps

1) Make two incisions in the (left and right) anterolateral scrotal wall or one incision in the superior scrotal median raphe.
2) Palpate each vas deferens and deliver it into the wound.
3) Open the vassal sheath, resect a small segment of the vas deferens, and ligate (clip, cauterize, suture) each end of each vas deferens.
4) Send the specimens for pathologic confirmation.

Note These Variations

- A "no-scalpel" technique can be used to enter the scrotum by piercing the scrotal wall with a sharpened-tip curved hemostat.
- The vasal sheath can be closed over the vassal remnant, which may decrease the risk of recanalization.

Complications

- Bleeding
- Infection
- Postoperative swelling
- Ligation of a vessel mistaken for the vas
- Post-vasectomy pain
- Recanalization with persistent fertility

Operative Dictations in Urologic Surgery, First Edition. Noel A. Armenakas, John A. Fracchia, and Ron Golan.
© 2019 John Wiley & Sons Ltd. Published 2019 by John Wiley & Sons Ltd.

Template Operative Dictation

Preoperative diagnosis: Elective sterilization
Postoperative diagnosis: Same
Procedure: Bilateral vasectomy
Indications: The patient is a _____-year-old male presenting for elective bilateral vasectomy.
Description of Procedure: The indications, contraceptive alternatives to male vasectomy as well as the benefits and risks were discussed with the patient and informed consent was obtained.

The patient was brought onto the operating room table, positioned supine, and secured with a safety strap. All pressure points were carefully padded and pneumatic compression devices were placed on the lower extremities.

The external genitalia were prepped and draped in the standard sterile manner.

A time-out was completed, verifying the correct patient, surgical procedure, and positioning, prior to beginning the procedure.

The vasa deferentia were palpated bilaterally and 2% xylocaine anesthesia administered intrascrotally.

> *Using two incisions*: An anterolateral scrotal skin incision was made over the *left/right* vas deferens.

> *Using one incision*: A skin incision was made in the superoanterior scrotal median raphe.

The *left/right* vas deferens was grasped with a ring-tipped fixation clamp and brought into the wound. The fascia of the vas deferens was then sharply incised and a 1 cm segment of the underlying vas deferens was isolated. Small titanium hemoclips were placed on each end of the vas, and the isolated segment between these was transected and sent to pathology for evaluation. Both ends of the vas deferens and their lumens were cauterized. Meticulous hemostasis was achieved throughout the procedure with electrocautery.

An identical procedure was performed on the contralateral side.

The skin incision(s) *was/were* closed with a 4-0 chromic suture. A sterile dressing and athletic supporter were applied.

At the end of the procedure, all counts were correct.

The patient tolerated the procedure without difficulty and was sent home in satisfactory condition.

Estimated blood loss: Approximately _____ml

47

Vasoepididymostomy

Indications

- Absence of sperm in the vasal lumen with no vasal obstruction in the setting of spermatogenesis on testis biopsy or history of prior vasectomy

Essential Steps

1) Make a high scrotal incision to expose the testicle.
2) Confirm the presence of sperm in the epididymal tubule distal to the proposed anastomosis.
3) Perform a saline vasogram to establish testicular vasal patency.
4) Complete a two-layer microsurgical vasoepididymostomy.

Note These Variations

- Alternate techniques include end-to-end or triangulated end-to-side anastomoses and intussusception.
- A one-layer modified anastomosis can be performed with full-thickness inside-out 9-0 nylon sutures buttressed with similar muscularis sutures.

Complications

- Bleeding
- Infection
- Testicular atrophy
- Persistent azoospermia
- Persistent infertility

Operative Dictations in Urologic Surgery, First Edition. Noel A. Armenakas, John A. Fracchia, and Ron Golan.
© 2019 John Wiley & Sons Ltd. Published 2019 by John Wiley & Sons Ltd.

Template Operative Dictation

Preoperative diagnosis: Infertility
Postoperative diagnosis: Same
Procedure: Vasoepididymostomy
Indications: The patient is a _____-year-old male with epididymal obstruction presenting for a vasoepididymostomy.
Description of Procedure: The indications, alternatives, benefits, and risks were discussed with the patient and informed consent was obtained.

The patient was brought onto the operating room table, positioned supine, and secured with a safety strap. All pressure points were carefully padded and pneumatic compression devices were placed on the lower extremities.

After the administration of intravenous antibiotics and *general endotracheal/regional* anesthesia, the patient's scrotum was examined. The lower abdomen and external genitalia were prepped and draped in the standard sterile manner.

A time-out was completed, verifying the correct patient, surgical procedure and positioning, prior to beginning the procedure.

A 3–4 cm high vertical skin incision was made through the *right/left anterior scrotal wall//median raphe* and taken down through the dartos fascia, exposing the tunica vaginalis. The testis was delivered with the tunica vaginalis intact. Babcock clamps were placed on the vas deferens and an avascular plane was identified within the periadventitial sheath and punctured, allowing passage of a 0.25 in. Penrose drain for traction.

The operating microscope was draped and brought into the field for the reconstructive portion of the procedure.

The vas was carefully dissected free from the surrounding scar, preserving the vasal artery. The abdominal and testicular vasal segments were mobilized to the external inguinal ring and vasoepididymal junction, respectively. The vas was secured with a slotted nerve clamp and an ultra-sharp knife was used to provide a clean 90° cut across it.

The testicular fluid was placed on a slide with Lactated Ringer's solution and examined using a microscope in the operating room, confirming the absence of sperm.

The lumen of the abdominal vas was gently dilated with a microvessel dilator, cannulated with a 23-gauge angiocatheter sheath, and irrigated with sterile normal saline solution, ensuring its patency. The vasal vessels were ligated with 6-0 nylon (Ethilon) and the abdominal vas recut to obtain a fresh surface. All three vasal layers were identified and bleeding was seen from the cut edge of the mucosa and muscularis. Using microbipolar cautery, small bleeders on the vasal edge were carefully coagulated, taking care not to injure the mucosa.

The epididymis was exposed by opening its tunical covering and carefully inspected, starting at the cauda and advancing toward the caput. A dilated epididymal tubule was identified and punctured with a 70-μm diameter tapered needle. Again, the fluid was examined using microscopy, this time confirming the presence of motile sperm.

The abdominal vas was brought through a small window in the tunica vaginalis, positioned adjacent to the dilated epididymal tubule. Its adventitia was secured to the anastomotic site with 9-0 Ethilon sutures.

A 3 mm incision was made in the longitudinal axis of the dilated epididymal tubule using a microknife. The posterior edge of the epididymal tubule was approximated to the vasal mucosa in an end-to-side fashion with 10-0 Ethilon sutures placed inside-out.

The lumen was irrigated with heparinized Lactated Ringer's solution before each suture placement to ensure its patency. Six 9-0 Ethilon sutures were used to secure the adventitia of the vas to the tunica. Additional sutures were placed approximating the vasal sheath to the epididymal tunica. The completed vasoepididymostomy was inspected, confirming a tension-free repair. The wound was irrigated with sterile normal saline. Meticulous hemostasis was obtained throughout the procedure with the microbipolar electrocautery.

The tunica vaginalis was closed over the testis using a running 5-0 polyglactin (Vicryl) suture, and the testis was repositioned anatomically within the *right/left* hemiscrotum. The dartos fascia was approximated with a running 4-0 Vicryl and the skin with a subcuticular 5-0 poliglecaprone (Monocryl) suture.

The identical procedure was carried out on the contralateral side.

Each incision was reinforced with sterile adhesive strips and covered with a sterile dressing.

Gauze fluffs and an athletic supporter were applied to help minimize swelling.

At the end of the procedure, all counts were correct.

The patient tolerated the procedures without difficulty and was taken to the recovery room in satisfactory condition.

Estimated blood loss: Approximately _____ml

48

Vasovasostomy

Indications

- Obstructive azoospermia in men with testis of normal consistency and size. (These patients usually have a prior history of fertility or vasectomy and often have had a testis biopsy documenting spermatogenesis.)

Essential Steps

1) Make a superior scrotal or inguinal incision. The choice depends on the etiology of obstruction (e.g. history of scrotal vasectomy, inguinal hernia repair, etc.).
2) Secure each end of the vas deferens above and below the obstructed area and transect the vas sharply at 90°.
3) Confirm the presence of sperm and vasal patency from the testicular and abdominal vasal segments, respectively.
4) Perform a two- to four-layer microsurgical vasovasostomy bilaterally.

Note These Variations

- Magnification loupes can be used if a microscope is not available.
- The testicular portion of the vas can be barbotoged to assess for seminal fluid if none is seen upon initial transection.
- If the vasal gap is long, additional length can be obtained by dissecting the testicular end of the vas distally to the vasoepididymal junction.
- In cases of unilateral atrophic testes, a crossed vasovasostomy can be performed.

Complications

- Bleeding
- Infection
- Testicular atrophy (from injury to the testicular artery)
- Persistent azoospermia/infertility

Operative Dictations in Urologic Surgery, First Edition. Noel A. Armenakas, John A. Fracchia, and Ron Golan.
© 2019 John Wiley & Sons Ltd. Published 2019 by John Wiley & Sons Ltd.

Template Operative Dictation

Preoperative diagnosis: Infertility
Postoperative diagnosis: Same
Procedure: Vasovasostomy
Indications: The patient is a _____-year-old male with obstructive azoospermia presenting for a vasovasostomy.
Description of Procedure: The indications, alternatives, benefits, and risks were discussed with the patient and informed consent was obtained.

The patient was brought onto the operating room table, positioned supine, and secured with a safety strap. All pressure points were carefully padded and pneumatic compression devices were placed on the lower extremities.

After the administration of intravenous antibiotics and *general endotracheal/regional* anesthesia, the patient's scrotum was examined. The lower abdomen and external genitalia were prepped and draped in the standard sterile manner.

A time-out was completed, verifying the correct patient, surgical procedure, and positioning, prior to beginning the procedure.

A 3–4 cm high vertical skin incision was made through the *right/left anterior scrotal wall//median raphe* and taken down through the dartos fascia, exposing the tunica vaginalis. The *right/left* testis was delivered with the tunica vaginalis intact. Babcock clamps were placed on the vas deferens above and below the obstructed segments. An avascular plane was identified within the periadventitial sheath and punctured, allowing passage of a 0.25 in. Penrose drain for traction.

The operating microscope was draped and brought into the field for the reconstructive portion of the procedure.

The vas was carefully dissected free from the surrounding scar and its abdominal end was mobilized to the external inguinal ring. The vas was secured with a slotted nerve clamp and an ultra-sharp knife was used to cut it cleanly at 90°, proximal and distal to the defect.

The testicular end of the vas was inspected, and the *thin cloudy/copious clear/creamy yellow* fluid placed on a slide was mixed with a drop of Lactated Ringer's solution and examined using a microscope in the operating room, confirming the presence of *motile/immotile* sperm.

The vasal vessels were ligated with 6-0 nylon (Ethilon) and the abdominal vas recut, obtaining a fresh surface. All three vasal layers were identified and healthy bleeding was seen from the cut edge of the mucosa and muscularis. Using a microbipolar cautery, small bleeders on the vasal edge were carefully coagulated, taking care not to injure the mucosa. The lumen of the abdominal vas was gently dilated with a microvessel dilator, cannulated with a 23-gauge angiocatheter sheath, and irrigated with sterile normal saline, ensuring its patency.

An approximating clamp (Microspike approximator) was used to stabilize the abdominal and testicular ends of the vas deferens in preparation for the anastomosis. A rubber damn was placed to isolate the surgical field.

A microdot technique was utilized by marking both cut ends of the vas for each of the six mucosal suture sites. Three 10-0 double-armed Ethilon sutures were placed inside-out on the anterior vas incorporating the mucosa and superficial muscularis. Next, three 9-0 Ethilon sutures were used to approximate the deep muscularis. The vas was

rotated 180° and its lumen irrigated with heparinized Lactated Ringer's solution. The posterior anastomosis was completed using a similar two-layer suturing technique. The anastomosis was further secured by approximating the vasal sheath with six 8-0 Ethilon sutures. The completed vasovasostomy was inspected, confirming a tension-free repair, and the wound was irrigated with sterile normal saline. Meticulous hemostasis was obtained throughout the procedure with the microbipolar electrocautery.

The tunica vaginalis was closed over the testis using a running 5-0 polyglactin (Vicryl) suture, and the testis was repositioned anatomically within the *right/left* hemiscrotum. The dartos fascia was closed with a running 4-0 Vicryl and the skin with a subcuticular 5-0 poliglecaprone (Monocryl) suture.

The identical procedure was carried out on the contralateral side.

Each incision was reinforced with sterile adhesive strips and covered with a sterile dressing. Gauze fluffs and an athletic supporter were applied to help minimize swelling.

At the end of the procedure, all counts were correct.

The patient tolerated the procedures without difficulty and was taken to the recovery room in satisfactory condition.

Estimated blood loss: Approximately _____ ml

Ureter

49

Bladder Flap (Boari-Ockerblad)

Indications

• Mid-distal ureteral reconstruction not amenable to a psoas hitch alone

Essential Steps

1) Ensure preoperatively that the bladder capacity is adequate.
2) Expose the bladder and sweep the peritoneum cephalad.
3) Dissect the ureter extraperitoneally, preserving its vascular adventitia.
4) Divide the contralateral superior bladder pedicle to aid in bladder mobilization.
5) Create an appropriate size anterior bladder flap with at least a 4 cm base and a 3 cm apex.
6) Through the cystotomy, manually advance the posterior bladder to the ipsilateral psoas tendon and perform a psoas hitch.
7) Spatulate the ureter and anastomose it to the flap.
8) Tubularize the flap and close it in two layers.

Note These Variations

• Alternatively, a suprapubic longitudinal incision (modified Pfannenstiel) may be used.
• For additional mobilization, the ipsilateral superior bladder pedicle can be divided.
• In cases of significant ureteral fibrosis, an intraperitoneal approach may be required.
• Longer defects can be bridged using an "L-shaped" flap configuration.
• If there is any question of tension on the repair, a downward nephropexy can be performed by mobilizing the ipsilateral kidney and fixing the renal capsule caudally to the underlying retroperitoneal muscles; an additional 3–4 cm of proximal ureteral length can be obtained with this technique.
• The contralateral ureteral orifice can be intubated temporarily to avoid injury during bladder closure.

Operative Dictations in Urologic Surgery, First Edition. Noel A. Armenakas, John A. Fracchia, and Ron Golan.
© 2019 John Wiley & Sons Ltd. Published 2019 by John Wiley & Sons Ltd.

Complications

- Bleeding
- Infection
- Urine leak/urinoma
- Ileus/bowel obstruction
- Ureteral obstruction/stricture
- Neuropraxia

Template: Operative Dictation

Preoperative diagnosis: *Right/left mid/distal* ureteral *obstruction/stricture/injury/malignancy*

Postoperative diagnosis: Same

Procedure: Creation of a bladder flap and psoas hitch

Indications: The patient is a _____-year-old *male/female* with a *right/left* ureteral *obstruction/stricture/injury/malignancy* presenting for a bladder flap and psoas hitch.

Description of Procedure: The indications, alternatives, benefits, and risks were discussed with the patient and informed consent was obtained.

The patient was brought onto the operating room table, placed supine, and secured with a safety strap. All pressure points were carefully padded and pneumatic compression devices were placed on the lower extremities.

After the administration of intravenous antibiotics and general endotracheal anesthesia, the patient's entire abdomen was prepped and draped in the standard sterile manner.

The radiographic images were in the room.

A time-out was completed, verifying the correct patient, surgical procedure, site, and positioning, prior to beginning the procedure.

An 18 Fr urethral catheter was inserted to drain the bladder.

A midline abdominal incision was made starting just below the umbilicus and carried down to the pubic symphysis. The subcutaneous tissue was incised with electrocautery, exposing the underlying rectus abdominis aponeurosis. This was incised at the linea alba and the rectus abdominis muscles were separated at the midline and retracted laterally, taking care not to injure the underlying inferior epigastric vessels. The anterior bladder wall was exposed and the peritoneum was swept cephalad. A self-retaining retractor (e.g. Bookwalter, Omni-Tract, Balfour) was appropriately positioned to optimize exposure, using padding on each retractor blade.

The colon was reflected medially and the *right/left* ureter was identified above the iliac artery bifurcation, circumferentially mobilized, and encircled with a vessel loop. Ureteral dissection was continued distally to the area of *narrowing/obliteration*. The ureter was transected proximal to the diseased portion and the distal end tagged with a long 4-0 chromic suture. Urinary efflux was noted. Cephalad ureteral dissection was completed, leaving the medial periureteral tissue intact to avoid vascular compromise. Hemostasis was obtained throughout the dissection.

The contralateral superior vesical pedicle was divided using the electrothermal bipolar tissue sealing device (LigaSure), facilitating bladder mobilization. The distance from

the transected ureter to the bladder was measured at _____cm. The bladder was filled with 300 ml sterile normal saline and the catheter clamped.

A U-shaped anterior bladder flap was marked beginning posteriorly on the ipsilateral side and extending anteriorly to the contralateral bladder wall. The width of the base and apex of the flap was 4 and 3 cm, respectively. Four 2-0 chromic stay sutures were placed on the corners of the flap and the bladder wall was incised along the markings using cutting current. The contralateral ureteral orifice was identified with clear efflux. Using manual manipulation, the ipsilateral posterior bladder wall was elevated toward the psoas tendon, where it was secured with three interrupted 2-0 polyglactin (Vicryl) sutures. Care was taken not to injure the underlying genitofemoral nerve.

A 2 cm submucosal tunnel was created in the apex of the flap, using sharp dissection. The distal ureter was spatulated for 1 cm on its lateral border and placed submucosally within the tunnel. A tension free ureterovesical anastomosis was performed using interrupted 4-0 chromic sutures. Two additional chromic sutures were placed extravesically to anchor the ureteral adventitia to the bladder flap. A ___Fr ____cm double-J stent was advanced over a guidewire with its proximal and distal ends positioned within the renal pelvis and bladder, respectively, and the guidewire was withdrawn.

The bladder wall was closed in continuity with the flap in two layers, using running 2-0 Vicryl sutures. The patency of the repair was confirmed by irrigating the urethral catheter with sterile normal saline. Meticulous hemostasis was obtained throughout the procedure with electrocautery.

A surgical drain (e.g. Jackson-Pratt) was placed in the pelvis away from the cystotomy and brought out at the skin through a separate stab incision, where it was secured with a 2-0 silk suture. Prior to closure, the operative field was irrigated with warm sterile saline and inspected, confirming the absence of bleeding or any injury.

The self-retaining retractor was removed, and the abdominal incision was closed using a running 2-0 chromic suture to approximate the rectus muscles and a 1-0 polydioxanone (PDS) suture for the rectus aponeurosis. The subcutaneous tissue was approximated with 3-0 chromic sutures and the skin closed with a running 4-0 poliglecaprone (Monocryl) suture.

A sterile dressing was applied.

At the end of the procedure, all counts were correct.

The patient tolerated the procedure without difficulty and was taken to the recovery room in satisfactory condition.

Estimated blood loss: Approximately _____ml

50

Ileal Ureter

Indications

- Replacement of extensive ureteral defects (caused by injury, stricture, fistula, retroperitoneal fibrosis, tuberculosis, etc.), when other less invasive procedures are not feasible

Essential Steps

1) Isolate and divide a 25–35 cm segment of distal ileum approximately 15–20 cm from the ileocecal valve. Use transillumination to identify the vascular arcades.
2) Perform a functional end-to-end ileoileal anastomosis, restoring bowel continuity.
3) Orient the ileal segment in an isoperistaltic direction and place it in the lateral retroperitoneum adjacent to the renal pelvis.
4) Incise the renal pelvis obliquely and complete a one-layer ileopyelostomy.
5) Open the bladder at the midline and create a full-thickness posterior bladder window through which the distal ileal segment is advanced and anastomosed to the bladder wall.
6) Prior to closing the cystotomy, irrigate the ileal ureter to ensure a watertight repair; similarly, ensure that the cystotomy is watertight.
7) Place a drain.

Note These Variations

- The ileoileal anastomosis may be hand-sewn, using a two-layer technique.
- In the presence of a scarred or intrarenal pelvis, the proximal ileal segment can be anastomosed to the lower pole calyx, after excising the inferior renal parenchyma (ileocalicostomy).
- For short ureteral defects, segmental (rather than total) ureteral replacement can be performed utilizing a shorter piece of ileum and anastomosing the native ureter to the ileal segment.

Operative Dictations in Urologic Surgery, First Edition. Noel A. Armenakas, John A. Fracchia, and Ron Golan.
© 2019 John Wiley & Sons Ltd. Published 2019 by John Wiley & Sons Ltd.

- In cases of bilateral ureteral replacement, a longer segment of ileum can be isolated and placed in a reverse L-configuration. The ileopyelostomies are completed using end-to-end and end-to-side anastomoses.
- A nephrostomy tube can be used for temporary urinary diversion.

Complications

- Bleeding
- Infection
- Ileus/bowel obstruction
- Bowel injury/leak
- Urinary leak/stricture (ileopyelo and ileovesical anastomoses)
- Pyelonephritis
- Stone formation
- Metabolic abnormalities (hypokalemic, hyperchloremic metabolic acidosis)
- Renal failure

Template Operative Dictation

Preoperative diagnosis: Need for *right/left* ureteral replacement, following _____.

Postoperative diagnosis: Same

Procedure: *Right/left* ileal ureter

Indications: The patient is a _____-year-old *male/female* presenting for an ileal ureter as management of a _____.

Description of Procedure: The indications, alternatives, benefits, and risks were discussed with the patient and informed consent was obtained.

The patient was brought onto the operating room table, positioned supine, and secured with a safety strap. All pressure points were carefully padded and pneumatic compression devices were placed on the lower extremities.

After the administration of intravenous antibiotics and general endotracheal anesthesia, the patient's entire abdomen was prepped and draped in the standard sterile manner.

A time-out was completed, verifying the correct patient, surgical procedure, site, and positioning prior to beginning the procedure.

An 18 Fr urethral catheter was inserted into the bladder and connected to a drainage bag.

A midline abdominal incision was made starting just above the umbilicus and carried down to the pubic symphysis. The subcutaneous tissue was incised with electrocautery, exposing the underlying rectus abdominis aponeurosis. This was incised at the linea alba and the rectus abdominis muscles separated at the midline and retracted laterally, taking care not to injure the underlying inferior epigastric vessels.

The peritoneal cavity was entered sharply, avoiding any injury to the bowel. A self-retaining retractor (e.g. Bookwalter, Omni-Tract, Balfour) was appropriately positioned to optimize exposure, using padding on each retractor blade. The bowel was carefully examined, confirming the absence of any inflammatory disease *(or radiation enteritis)*.

On the right: The parietal peritoneum was incised on the white line of Toldt, and the cecum and entire ascending colon were mobilized and reflected medially. A small window was created in the mesentery of the descending colon to permit the ileal segment to reach the bladder with ease.

On the left: The parietal peritoneum was incised on the white line of Toldt and the entire descending and sigmoid colon were mobilized and reflected superomedially to facilitate subsequent placement of the ileal segment.

The *right/left* ureter was identified and inspected, confirming extensive scarring.

Attention was turned to the distal ileum, which was carefully inspected. With the aid of transillumination, the watershed area between the ileocolic and right colic artery was identified. A 30 cm segment of distal ileum was selected approximately 15–20 cm from the ileocecal valve. An avascular mesenteric window was opened on each side of the desired ileal segment using an electrothermal bipolar tissue sealing device (LigaSure) to incise and ligate the mesentery on both sides, avoiding injury to the main intestinal vasculature. *(Alternatively, the mesentery can be incised and its blood vessels individually clamped, divided, and doubly ligated with chromic or silk ties)*. Additional hemostasis was achieved using 3-0 *chromic/silk* ties. The isolated ileal segment was transected at its proximal and distal antimesenteric borders, using a GIA60 stapler. The isolated ileal segment was placed caudal to the small bowel mesenteric defect.

The continuity of the ileum was restored using a stapled technique as follows: The antimesenteric corners of the proximal and distal ileal segments were identified and a small segment of tissue was resected off each end of the stapled suture lines. One limb of the GIA60 stapler was inserted into the proximal and the other into the distal ileal segment with care taken not to injure the bowel mesentery. The ileal segments were rotated ensuring that the antimesenteric bowel walls faced each other prior to firing the stapler. Four small clamps were then placed on the ends of the transected bowel. The two clamps on the lines of the original bowel transection were held together, while the others were spread apart, creating a wide opening. A TA55 stapler was used to complete the functional end-to-end ileoileal anastomosis. The staple line was checked to confirm its integrity and was additionally reinforced with interrupted 3-0 silk sutures. The mesenteric window was closed with a running 4-0 chromic suture to avoid internal herniation.

The ileal segment's proximal and distal staple lines were resected and its lumen copiously irrigated with sterile normal saline. Once free of mucous and enteric material, the isolated ileal segment was oriented in an isoperistaltic direction and positioned high in the *right/left* retroperitoneum, taking care not to injure its mesenteric vasculature.

Using sharp dissection, Gerota's fascia was opened and the underlying *right/left* kidney and renal pelvis were identified. The renal pelvis was carefully dissected and thoroughly mobilized, preserving its vasculature. 4-0 chromic stay sutures were placed superiorly and inferiorly, and the renal pelvis incised obliquely at a 45° angle, for a distance equal to the proximal ileal opening. The ileopyelo anastomosis was completed using interrupted 3-0 polyglactin (Vicryl) sutures.

Attention was then directed to the bladder. Two 2-0 chromic stay sutures were placed into the mid-anterior bladder wall and a 1 cm full-thickness vertical stab incision was made between these using electrocautery. The partially filled bladder was drained using suction. Allis clamps were placed on both edges of the cystotomy and the incision

extended cranially and caudally for a total distance of 8 cm. The urethral catheter was removed, optimizing visualization, and the bladder was thoroughly inspected confirming the absence of any tumors, stones, foreign bodies or diverticula. The bladder wall was *minimally/moderately/significantly/not* trabeculated, with a normal appearing mucosa. Both ureteral orifices were in the normal anatomic position.

A full-thickness segment of the posterolateral *right/left* bladder wall was excised. A Babcock clamp was passed through this window and the distal ileal segment grasped and advanced into the bladder. The ileovesical anastomosis was completed using interrupted 3-0 and 4-0 Vicryl sutures for the outer seromuscular and inner mucosal layers, respectively.

Having completed the ileal interposition, the ileal ureter was irrigated with sterile normal saline, confirming a watertight repair. The midline cystotomy was closed in two layers with 2-0 Vicryl sutures. A new 20 Fr urethral catheter was inserted into the bladder, irrigated with sterile normal saline ensuring a patent bladder closure, and connected to a drainage bag.

The abdomen and pelvis were examined for any bleeding sites and meticulous hemostasis was achieved with electrocautery. A surgical drain (e.g. Jackson-Pratt) was placed in the retroperitoneum and brought out at the skin through a separate stab incision, where it was secured with a 2-0 silk suture. Prior to closure, the operative field was irrigated with warm sterile normal saline and thoroughly inspected confirming the absence of bleeding or injury.

The self-retaining retractor was removed and the abdominal incision was closed using a running 2-0 chromic suture to approximate the rectus muscles and a 1-0 polydioxanone (PDS) suture for the rectus aponeurosis. The subcutaneous tissue was approximated with 3-0 chromic sutures and the skin was closed with staples. A sterile dressing was applied.

At the end of the procedure, all counts were correct.

The patient tolerated the procedure without difficulty and was taken to the recovery room in satisfactory condition.

Estimated blood loss: Approximately _____ml

51

Psoas Hitch

Indications

- Pelvic ureteral reconstruction not amenable to a ureteroneocystostomy alone

Essential Steps

1) Ensure preoperatively that the bladder capacity is adequate.
2) Expose the bladder and sweep the peritoneum cephalad.
3) Dissect the ureter extraperitoneally, preserving its vascular adventitia.
4) Divide the contralateral superior bladder pedicle to aid in bladder mobilization.
5) Make an oblique anterior cystotomy perpendicular to the ipsilateral ureter and, through this, manually manipulate the bladder to the ipsilateral psoas.
6) Suture the posterior bladder wall to the psoas tendon, taking care not to injure the underlying genitofemoral nerve.
7) Spatulate the ureter and anastomose it to the bladder wall.
8) Close the cystotomy transversely, in two layers.

Note This Variation

- Alternatively, a suprapubic longitudinal incision (modified Pfannenstiel) may be used.
- For additional mobilization, the ipsilateral superior bladder pedicle can be divided.
- In cases of significant ureteral fibrosis, an intraperitoneal approach may be required.
- A direct (refluxing), rather than an antifluxing ureterovesical anastomosis can be performed.

Complications

- Bleeding
- Infection
- Urine leak/urinoma

Operative Dictations in Urologic Surgery, First Edition. Noel A. Armenakas, John A. Fracchia, and Ron Golan.
© 2019 John Wiley & Sons Ltd. Published 2019 by John Wiley & Sons Ltd.

- Ileus/bowel obstruction
- Ureteral obstruction/stricture
- Neuropraxia

Template: Operative Dictation

Preoperative diagnosis: *Right/left* distal ureteral *stricture/injury/malignancy*
Postoperative diagnosis: Same
Procedure: Creation of a psoas hitch
Indications: The patient is a _____-year-old *male/female* with a *right/left* ureteral *stricture/injury/malignancy* presenting for a psoas hitch.
Description of Procedure: The indications, alternatives, benefits, and risks were discussed with the patient and informed consent was obtained.

The patient was brought onto the operating room table, placed supine, and secured with a safety strap. All pressure points were carefully padded and pneumatic compression devices were placed on the lower extremities.

After the administration of intravenous antibiotics and general endotracheal anesthesia, the patient's entire abdomen was prepped and draped in the standard sterile manner.

The radiographic images were in the room.

A time-out was completed, verifying the correct patient, surgical procedure, site, and positioning, prior to beginning the procedure.

An 18 Fr urethral catheter was inserted to drain the bladder.

A midline abdominal incision was made, starting just below the umbilicus and carried down to the pubic symphysis. The subcutaneous tissue was incised with electrocautery, exposing the underlying rectus abdominis aponeurosis. This was incised at the linea alba and the rectus abdominis muscles separated at the midline and retracted laterally, taking care not to injure the underlying inferior epigastric vessels. The anterior bladder wall was exposed and the peritoneum was swept cephalad. A self-retaining retractor (e.g. Bookwalter, Omni-Tract, Balfour) was appropriately positioned to optimize exposure, using padding on each retractor blade.

The colon was reflected medially and the *right/left* ureter was identified below the iliac artery bifurcation, circumferentially mobilized, and encircled with a vessel loop. Ureteral dissection was continued distally to the area of *narrowing/obliteration*. The ureter was transected proximal to the diseased portion and the distal end was tagged with a long 4-0 chromic suture. Urinary efflux was noted. Cephalad ureteral dissection was completed, leaving the periureteral tissue intact to avoid vascular compromise.

The contralateral superior vesical pedicle was divided using the electrothermal bipolar tissue sealing device (LigaSure), facilitating bladder mobilization. The bladder was filled with 300 ml sterile normal saline and the catheter clamped.

A 6 cm oblique incision was made in the *right/left* anterior bladder wall, perpendicular to the ipsilateral ureter. Using manual manipulation, the posterior bladder wall was elevated toward the ipsilateral psoas tendon, where it was secured with three interrupted 2-0 polyglactin (Vicryl) sutures. Care was taken not to injure the underlying genitofemoral nerve.

A 2 cm submucosal tunnel was created posteriorly at the apex of the bladder using sharp dissection. The distal ureter was spatulated for 1 cm on its lateral border and

placed submucosally within the tunnel. A tension-free ureterovesical anastomosis was performed using interrupted 4-0 chromic sutures. Two additional chromic sutures were placed extravesically to anchor the ureteral adventitia to the bladder flap. A ___Fr ____cm double-J stent was advanced over a guidewire, with its proximal and distal ends positioned within the renal pelvis and bladder, respectively, and the guidewire was withdrawn.

The bladder wall was closed transversely in two layers using running 2-0 Vicryl sutures. The patency of the repair was confirmed by irrigating the urethral catheter with sterile normal saline. Meticulous hemostasis was obtained throughout the procedure.

A surgical drain (e.g. Jackson-Pratt) was placed in the pelvis, away from the cystotomy, and brought out at the skin through a separate stab incision, where it was secured with a 2-0 silk suture. Prior to closure, the operative field was irrigated with warm sterile saline and inspected, confirming the absence of bleeding or any injury.

The self-retaining retractor was removed and the abdominal incision was closed using a running 2-0 chromic suture to approximate the rectus muscles and 1-0 polydioxanone (PDS) suture for the rectus aponeurosis. The subcutaneous tissue was approximated with 3-0 chromic sutures and the skin was closed with a running 4-0 poliglecaprone (Monocryl) suture.

A sterile dressing was applied.

At the end of the procedure, all counts were correct.

The patient tolerated the procedure without difficulty and was taken to the recovery room in satisfactory condition.

Estimated blood loss: Approximately _____ml

52

Transureteroureterostomy

Indications

- Mid-ureteral injuries precluding adequate bladder mobilization
- Bilateral ureteral injuries managed with a contralateral Boari flap and/or a psoas hitch
- Ureteral reconstruction during urinary undiversion

Essential Steps

1) Expose both ureters at the level of the common iliac bifurcation.
2) Dissect the donor ureter, preserving its vascular adventitia.
3) Transect the donor ureter above the diseased portion, mobilize it cephalad, and advance it to the recipient ureter above the inferior mesenteric artery through a posterior peritoneal window. Avoid ureteral kinking or angulation.
4) Make a 1.5 cm incision in the anteromedial wall of the recipient ureter.
5) Spatulate the donor ureter and anastomose it in an end-to-side fashion to the recipient ureter.

Note These Variations

- Select distal transureteroureterostomies can be performed exclusively through a retroperitoneal approach.
- If the recipient distal ureter requires tapering or reimplantation, this should be done prior to performing the ureteroureteral anastomosis.
- An omental or peritoneal flap can be used to protect the anastomosis.
- A ureteral stent can be placed in the recipient ureter intraoperatively and removed after completion of the ureteroureteral anastomosis or maintained postoperatively.

Complications

- Bleeding
- Infection

Operative Dictations in Urologic Surgery, First Edition. Noel A. Armenakas, John A. Fracchia, and Ron Golan.
© 2019 John Wiley & Sons Ltd. Published 2019 by John Wiley & Sons Ltd.

- Urine leak/urinoma
- Pyelonephritis
- Ileus/bowel obstruction
- Ureteral obstruction/stricture (unilateral or bilateral)

Template: Operative Dictation

Preoperative diagnosis: *Right/left* mid-ureteral *obstruction/stricture/injury*
Postoperative diagnosis: Same
Procedure: *Right/left* transureteroureterostomy
Indications: The patient is a _____-year-old *male/female* with a *right/left* mid ureteral *obstruction/stricture/injury* presenting for a transureteroureterostomy.
Description of Procedure: The indications, alternatives, benefits, and risks were discussed with the patient and informed consent was obtained.

The patient was brought onto the operating room table, placed supine, and secured with a safety strap. All pressure points were carefully padded and pneumatic compression devices were placed on the lower extremities.

After the administration of intravenous antibiotics and general endotracheal anesthesia, the patient's entire abdomen was prepped and draped in the standard sterile manner.

The radiographic images were in the room.

A time-out was completed, verifying the correct patient, surgical procedure, site, and positioning, prior to beginning the procedure.

A 16 Fr urethral catheter was advanced into the bladder and connected to a drainage bag.

A midline abdominal incision was made starting just above the umbilicus and carried down to the pubic symphysis. The subcutaneous tissue was incised with electrocautery, exposing the underlying rectus abdominis aponeurosis. This was incised at the linea alba and the rectus abdominis muscles separated at the midline and retracted laterally, taking care not to injure the underlying inferior epigastric vessels.

The peritoneal cavity was entered and the ascending and descending colon mobilized along the white line of Toldt. The bowel was thoroughly packed and a self-retaining retractor (e.g. Bookwalter, Omni-Tract, Balfour) was appropriately positioned to optimize exposure, using padding on each retractor blade.

The ureters were identified and exposed at the level of the common iliac bifurcation. The *right/left* (donor) ureter was dissected proximal to the diseased portion, transected, and its distal end and tagged with a long 4-0 chromic suture. Urinary efflux was noted. Cephalad ureteral dissection was completed for a distance of approximately 10 cm, leaving the medial periureteral tissue intact to avoid vascular compromise.

The inferior mesenteric artery was identified and a posterior peritoneal window created superior to this and anterior to the great vessels. The sufficiently mobilized donor ureter was brought gently through this opening above the inferior mesenteric artery, without kinking or angulation. The donor ureter was positioned adjacent to the recipient ureter without tension, and was spatulated distally for 1 cm.

Two 4-0 chromic stay sutures were placed on the recipient ureteral adventitia superiorly and inferiorly to the intended site of anastomosis. A 1.5 cm vertical ureterotomy was made between these on the anteromedial surface, preserving the ureteral blood supply.

An end-to-side, tension-free ureteroureteral anastomosis was fashioned using *interrupted/running* 4-0 chromic sutures, beginning with the superior and inferior apices and continuing with the posterior and anterior ureteral walls.

The previously made posterior peritoneal window was loosely approximated, using running 3-0 chromic sutures bilaterally. Meticulous hemostasis was obtained throughout the procedure.

A surgical drain (e.g. Jackson-Pratt) was placed away from the ureteroureteral anastomosis and brought out at the skin through a separate stab incision, where it was secured with a 2-0 silk suture. Prior to closure, the operative field was irrigated with warm sterile saline and inspected, confirming the absence of bleeding or any injury.

The self-retaining retractor was removed and the abdominal incision was closed using a running 2-0 chromic suture to approximate the rectus muscles and 1-0 polydioxanone (PDS) suture for the rectus aponeurosis. The subcutaneous tissue was approximated with 3-0 chromic sutures and the skin was closed with a running 4-0 poliglecaprone (Monocryl) suture.

A sterile dressing was applied.

At the end of the procedure, all counts were correct.

The patient tolerated the procedure without difficulty and was taken to the recovery room in satisfactory condition.

Estimated blood loss: Approximately _____ml

53

Ureterocalicostomy

Indications

- Salvage of a failed prior pyeloplasty or endopyelotomy
- Primary repair for a ureteropelvic junction obstruction where there is a small intra-renal pelvis, significant lower pole caliectasis, and overlying thin renal parenchyma
- Traumatic ureteropelvic junction avulsion

Essential Steps

1) Identify the area of obstruction and transect the ureter distal to this.
2) Mobilize the healthy ureter and advance it cranially, preserving its vascular adventia.
3) Perform a lower pole heminephrectomy to expose the lower pole calyx. Obtain meticulous parenchymal hemostasis.
4) Generously spatulate the ureter and complete a tension-free ureterocalyceal anastomosis over a stent.
5) Approximate the renal capsule inferiorly.

Note These Variations

- Alternatively, a subcostal incision off the 12th rib can be used for exposure.
- The repair can be further stabilized with a nephropexy, fixing the renal capsule caudally to the underlying retroperitoneal muscles.

Complications

- Bleeding
- Infection
- Urine leak/urinoma
- Ileus/bowel obstruction
- Ureteral obstruction/stricture

Operative Dictations in Urologic Surgery, First Edition. Noel A. Armenakas, John A. Fracchia, and Ron Golan.
© 2019 John Wiley & Sons Ltd. Published 2019 by John Wiley & Sons Ltd.

Template: Operative Dictation

Preoperative diagnosis: *Right/left* ureteral pelvic junction *obstruction/avulsion*
Postoperative diagnosis: Same
Procedure: *Right/left* ureterocalicostomy
Indications: The patient is a _____-year-old *male/female* presenting for a *right/left* ureterocalicostomy.
Description of Procedure: The indications, alternatives, benefits, and risks were discussed with the *patient/patient's family* and informed consent was obtained.

The patient was brought onto the operating room table, placed supine, and secured with a safety strap. All pressure points were carefully padded and pneumatic compression devices were placed on the lower extremities.

After the administration of intravenous antibiotics and general endotracheal anesthesia, a 16 Fr urethral catheter was inserted into the bladder and connected to a drainage bag. The patient was placed in the lateral decubitus position at a 90° angle with the lower leg flexed 90° and the upper leg extended. An axillary roll was positioned to protect the brachial plexus and a gel pad placed to support the back. Multiple pillows were used to pad beneath and between both the upper and lower extremities to ensure adequate cushioning. The kidney rest was elevated and the table flexed and adjusted horizontally, obtaining optimal flank exposure. The patient was secured to the table with 3 in. surgical tape and safety straps and prepped and draped in the standard sterile manner.

The radiographic images were in the room.

A time-out was completed, verifying the correct patient, surgical procedure, site, and positioning, prior to beginning the procedure.

The space between the 11th and 12th ribs was palpated and an incision made at this level from the mid-axillary line and extended medially to the lateral border of the rectus abdominis muscle. Using electrocautery, the external oblique and latissimus dorsi muscles were incised, exposing the underlying ribs. The intercostal attachments were transected, taking care to avoid injury to the pleura and neurovascular bundle on the inferior surface of the 11th rib. The internal oblique muscle and lumbodorsal fascia were divided with cautery and the transversus abdominis carefully split in the direction of its fibers, avoiding entry into the peritoneum. A generous paranephric space was created by sweeping the peritoneum medially and the retroperitoneal connective tissue superiorly and inferiorly. A self-retaining retractor (e.g. Bookwalter, Omni-Tract, Finochietto) was appropriately positioned to optimize exposure, using padding on each retractor blade.

The parietal peritoneum was incised on the white line of Toldt and the colon reflected medially, exposing Gerota's fascia. Using sharp dissection, Gerota's fascia was incised posteriorly and the underlying kidney and renal pelvis were identified. The inferior pole of the *right/left* kidney, renal pelvis, and proximal ureter were carefully dissected and thoroughly mobilized. The site of *obstruction/avulsion* was identified and the ureter traced inferiorly and transected at its superior most viable segment, preserving the periureteral adventitial blood supply. The proximal end of the transected ureter was tagged with a 4-0 chromic suture.

The lower pole renal parenchyma was excised, exposing the lower pole calyx. Parenchymal bleeders were carefully ligated with figure-of-eight 4-0 chromic sutures, ensuring adequate hemostasis.

The end of the healthy transected ureter was spatulated on its lateral aspect for a distance of 2 cm. A tension-free mucosa-to-mucosal ureterocalyceal anastomosis was fashioned using interrupted 4-0 chromic sutures placed further apart on the calyx than on the ureter to achieve a widely patent repair. The anastomosis was began posteriorly and completed anteriorly over a _____Fr _____cm double-J stent. Meticulous hemostasis was obtained throughout the procedure.

An absorbable gelatin sponge (Gelfoam) bolster was placed in the parenchymal defect and the renal capsule loosely approximated over this using interrupted 2-0 polydioxanone (PDS) sutures. Available perirenal fat was secured over the defect and Gerota's fascia loosely approximated covering the repair.

A surgical drain (e.g. Jackson-Pratt, 0.25 in. Penrose) was placed in the infrarenal space, away from the repair, and brought out through a separate, more caudal-cutaneous incision where it was secured at the skin with a 2-0 silk suture.

Prior to closure, the operative field was irrigated with warm sterile saline and inspected confirming the absence of bleeding or any injury. The self-retaining retractor was removed, the kidney rest lowered, and the table taken out of flexion.

The incision was closed using running 1-0 PDS to approximate the three muscle layers, individually, taking care not to entrap the intercostal neurovascular bundle. 3-0 chromic sutures were used on Scarpa's fascia and the skin approximated with a subcuticular 4-0 poliglecaprone (Monocryl) suture. A sterile dressing was applied and the patient repositioned supine.

At the end of the procedure, all counts were correct.

The patient tolerated the procedure without difficulty and was taken to the recovery room in satisfactory condition.

Estimated blood loss: Approximately _____ml

54

Ureterolithotomy

Indications

- Ureteral stone removal where less-invasive approaches would have a very low likelihood of success, are not available, or have failed.

Essential Steps

1) Access the ureter extraperitoneally.
2) Carefully dissect the ureter, preserving its vascular adventitia, and avoid dislodging the stone.
3) Identify the stone using gentle palpation.
4) Isolate the ureter above and below the stone.
5) Make a longitudinal ureterotomy over the stone and carefully extract the stone.
6) Complete a watertight ureterotomy closure.

Note These Variations

- The surgical approach for open ureterolithotomy is dependent on the stone's location. Stones in the abdominal portion of the ureter are usually approached through a flank incision (and less commonly through a dorsal lumbotomy). Pelvic ureteral stones can be accessed through a Gibson, infrapubic midline, or Pfannenstiel incision. Stones impacted in the intramural ureter may require transvesical exposure.
- Once identified within the ureter, the stone can be immobilized using a variety of techniques, including Babcock clamps or vessel loops placed proximally and distally, or a Satinsky clamp placed longitudinally.

Complications

- Bleeding
- Infection

Operative Dictations in Urologic Surgery, First Edition. Noel A. Armenakas, John A. Fracchia, and Ron Golan.
© 2019 John Wiley & Sons Ltd. Published 2019 by John Wiley & Sons Ltd.

- Urine leak/urinoma
- Infection
- Ureteral obstruction/stricture

Template: Operative Dictation

Preoperative diagnosis: *Right/Left* ureteral obstruction secondary to a ___cm *proximal/mid/distal* ureteral calculus
Postoperative diagnosis: Same
Procedure: *Right/Left* ureterolithotomy
Indications: The patient is a ____-year-old *male/female* with a *right/left proximal/mid/distal* ureteral stone presenting for a ureterolithotomy.
Description of Procedure: The indications, alternatives, benefits, and risks were discussed with the patient and informed consent was obtained.

The patient was brought onto the operating room table, placed supine, and secured with a safety strap. All pressure points were carefully padded and pneumatic compression devices were placed on the lower extremities.

(The incision presented herein is for exposure of a proximal ureteral stone.)

After the administration of intravenous antibiotics and general endotracheal anesthesia, a 16 Fr urethral catheter was inserted into the bladder and connected to a drainage bag. The patient was placed in the lateral decubitus position at a 90° angle with the lower leg flexed 90° and the upper leg extended. An axillary roll was positioned to protect the brachial plexus and a gel pad placed to support the back. Multiple pillows were used to pad beneath and between both the upper and lower extremities to ensure adequate cushioning. The kidney rest was elevated and the table flexed and adjusted horizontally, obtaining optimal flank exposure. The patient was secured to the table with 3 in. surgical tape and safety straps, and prepped and draped in the standard sterile manner.

The radiographic images were in the room.

A time-out was completed, verifying the correct patient, surgical procedure, site, and positioning, prior to beginning the procedure.

A *right/left* flank incision was made off the tip of the 12th rib, starting at the mid-axillary line and extended medially to the lateral border of the rectus abdominis muscle. Using electrocautery, the external oblique and latissimus dorsi muscles were incised and the neurovascular bundle identified, dissected free and retracted out of the way. The internal oblique muscle and lumbodorsal fascia were divided with cautery and the transversus abdominis split in the direction of its fibers, avoiding entry into the peritoneum. A generous paranephric space was created by sweeping the peritoneum medially and the retroperitoneal connective tissue superiorly and inferiorly. A self-retaining retractor (e.g. Bookwalter, Omni-Tract, Finochietto) was appropriately positioned to optimize exposure, using padding on each retractor blade.

The parietal peritoneum was incised on the white line of Toldt and the colon reflected medially, exposing Gerota's fascia. Using sharp dissection, Gerota's fascia was incised posteriorly and the underlying kidney and renal pelvis identified. The *right/left* proximal ureter was carefully dissected and mobilized, preserving the periureteral tissues.

The stone was palpated in the proximal ureter, and two Babcock clamps positioned above and below it. A longitudinal ureterotomy was made over the stone and a 4-0 chromic stay suture was placed full-thickness through both the medial and lateral edges of the incised ureter. The stone was removed very gently using a Randall's forceps avoiding fragmentation or damage to the ureteral wall, and sent for chemical analysis. A 5Fr infant feeding tube was advanced proximally and distally through the ureterotomy and irrigated with sterile normal saline, confirming ureteral patency. A _____ Fr _____cm double-J stent was positioned intraureterally. The ureter was closed over the stent in a watertight fashion using interrupted 5-0 chromic sutures. Meticulous hemostasis was obtained throughout the procedure.

A surgical drain (e.g. Jackson-Pratt, 0.25 in. Penrose) was placed away from the ureteral repair and brought out at the skin through a separate stab incision, where it was secured with a 2-0 silk suture. Prior to closure, the operative field was irrigated with warm sterile saline and inspected confirming the absence of bleeding or any injury.

The self-retaining retractor was removed, the kidney rest lowered and the table taken out of flexion.

The incision was closed using running 1-0 polydioxanone (PDS) sutures to approximate the three muscle layers, individually, taking care not to entrap the neurovascular bundle. 3-0 chromic sutures were used on Scarpa's fascia and the skin approximated with a subcuticular 4-0 poliglecaprone (Monocryl) suture. A sterile dressing was applied and the patient was repositioned supine.

At the end of the procedure, all counts were correct.

The patient tolerated the procedure without difficulty and was taken to the recovery room in satisfactory condition.

Estimated blood loss: Approximately _____ml

55

Ureterolysis (with Omental Flaps)

Indications

- Ureteral obstruction secondary to retroperitoneal fibrosis

Essential Steps

1) Place bilateral ureteral stents or catheters to assist in identifying the ureters.
2) Expose the retroperitoneum through a midline transperitoneal approach.
3) Identify the dilated ureters proximally and trace them distally where they enter the fibrosis.
4) Biopsy the fibrotic tissue encasing the ureters.
5) Carefully mobilize and release each ureter.
6) Position the ureters laterally within the peritoneal cavity and close the peritoneal incision posteriorly.
7) Protect the ureters with bilateral omental flaps.
8) Place a drain.

Note These Variations

- The use of ureteral stents/catheters is at the discretion of the surgeon.
- Rather than placing the ureters intraperitoneally and covering them with omental flaps, they can be positioned retroperitoneally by securing the overlying peritoneum to the psoas muscle, medially.

Complications

- Bleeding
- Infection
- Ureteral injury
- Urine leak/urinoma

Operative Dictations in Urologic Surgery, First Edition. Noel A. Armenakas, John A. Fracchia, and Ron Golan.
© 2019 John Wiley & Sons Ltd. Published 2019 by John Wiley & Sons Ltd.

- Ileus/bowel obstruction
- Ureteral obstruction/stricture
- Intraabdominal organ injuries

Template: Operative Dictation

Preoperative diagnosis: Ureteral obstruction secondary to retroperitoneal fibrosis
Postoperative diagnosis: Same
Procedure: Bilateral ureterolysis
Indications: The patient is a _____-year-old *male/female* with retroperitoneal fibrosis presenting for bilateral ureterolysis.
Description of Procedure: The indications, alternatives, benefits, and risks were discussed with the patient and informed consent was obtained.

The patient was brought onto the operating room table, placed supine, and secured with a safety strap. All pressure points were carefully padded and pneumatic compression devices were placed on the lower extremities.

After the administration of intravenous antibiotics and initiation of general endotracheal anesthesia, the lower chest, abdomen, and genitalia were prepped and draped in the standard sterile manner.

The radiographic images were in the room.

A time-out was completed, verifying the correct patient, surgical procedure, and positioning, prior to beginning the procedure.

A 22 Fr rigid cystoscope with a 30° lens was inserted per meatus and advanced under direct vision into the urinary bladder. Urethroscopy revealed a normal urethra. *(In a male patient, comment on the prostate size, lobes and degree of obstruction.)* The bladder was evaluated with both the 30° and 70° lenses. The media was clear, the bladder capacity was normal, and the bladder wall was noted to expand symmetrically in all dimensions. There were no tumors, stones, foreign bodies, or diverticula present. The bladder wall was *minimally/moderately/significantly/not* trabeculated with a normal appearing mucosa. Both ureteral orifices were in the normal anatomic position.

_____ Fr _____ cm double-J ureteral stents/5 Fr open-ended ureteral catheters were placed bilaterally to facilitate ureteral identification. The cystoscope was removed and a 16 Fr urethral catheter advanced into the bladder and connected to a drainage bag.

A midline abdominal incision was made starting 5 cm above the umbilicus and carried down to the pubic symphysis. The subcutaneous tissue was incised with electrocautery, exposing the underlying rectus abdominis aponeurosis. This was incised at the linea alba and the rectus abdominis muscles separated at the midline and retracted laterally, taking care not to injure the underlying inferior epigastric vessels.

The peritoneal cavity was entered and the ascending and descending colon were mobilized along the white line of Toldt. A self-retaining retractor (e.g. Bookwalter, Omni-Tract, Balfour) was appropriately positioned to optimize exposure, using padding on each retractor blade.

An exploratory laparotomy was performed, confirming the absence of visible malignant disease. The bowel was then thoroughly packed using moist laparotomy pads.

The dilated proximal *right/left* ureter was identified. It was carefully dissected, taking care not to injure its vascular adventitia, and encircled with a vessel loop. With the indwelling ureteral stent as a guide, the ureter was traced distally to the area of dense scarring. A biopsy of the periureteral fibrotic tissue was sent for pathologic evaluation.

Using sharp and blunt dissection, the ureter was carefully released from the encasing retroperitoneal fibrosis, from a cranial to caudal direction. Once entirely freed, the ureter was noted to fill with urine maintaining a pink color, confirming its patency and viability. Meticulous hemostasis was obtained throughout the dissection with electrocautery.

The identical procedure was performed on the contralateral ureter.

The ureters were positioned laterally without tension, and the posterior peritoneum was closed beneath each ureter with a running 4-0 chromic suture.

Bilateral omental flaps were created by mobilizing the omentum off the stomach, preserving the left and right gastroepiploic arteries. The omentum was divided transversely at the approximate midline of the greater gastric curvature using *an electrothermal bipolar tissue sealing device (LigaSure)/surgical clips,* creating two well-vascularized flaps. Each ureter was wrapped circumferentially and the omental flaps individually secured with several interrupted 3-0 chromic sutures.

Upon completion of the reconstructive procedure, the abdomen was irrigated with warm sterile water and carefully evaluated for bleeding.

A surgical drain (e.g. Jackson-Pratt) was placed in the retroperitoneum and brought out at the skin through a separate stab incision, where it was secured with a 2-0 silk suture. Prior to closure, the abdominal vessels and visceral organs were inspected and found to be intact without any evidence of devascularization or injury.

The self-retaining retractor was removed and the abdominal incision was closed using a running 2-0 chromic to approximate the rectus muscles and 1-0 polydioxanone (PDS) for the rectus aponeurosis. Scarpa's fascia was closed with 3-0 chromic sutures and staples were used on the skin. A sterile dressing was applied.

At the end of the procedure, all counts were correct.

The patient tolerated the procedure well and was taken to the recovery room in satisfactory condition.

Estimated blood loss: Approximately _____ml

56

Ureteroureterostomy

Indications

- Short (≤2 cm) proximal and mid-ureteral defects

Essential Steps

1) Identify and transect the ureter proximal and distal to the diseased area.
2) Mobilize the ureter proximally, preserving its vascular adventitia.
3) Spatulate both ureteral ends on opposite sides and perform a tension-free end-to-end ureteroureteral anastomosis over a stent.

Note These Variations

- Alternatively, a Gibson incision can be used to access the mid-ureter.
- Ureteral injuries caused by high-velocity gunshot wounds require more extensive debridement.
- An omental or peritoneal flap can be used to protect the anastomosis.

Complications

- Bleeding
- Infection
- Ileus/bowel obstruction
- Urine leak/urinoma
- Ureteral obstruction/stricture

Operative Dictations in Urologic Surgery, First Edition. Noel A. Armenakas, John A. Fracchia, and Ron Golan.
© 2019 John Wiley & Sons Ltd. Published 2019 by John Wiley & Sons Ltd.

Template: Operative Dictation

Preoperative diagnosis: *Right/left proximal/mid*-ureteral *obstruction/stricture/injury*
Postoperative diagnosis: Same
Procedure: *Right/left* ureteroureterostomy
Indications: The patient is a _____-year-old *male/female* with a _____ cm *right/left proximal/mid* ureteral *obstruction/stricture/injury* presenting for a ureteroureterostomy.
Description of Procedure: The indications, alternatives, benefits, and risks were discussed with the patient and informed consent was obtained.

The patient was brought onto the operating room table, placed supine, and secured with a safety strap. All pressure points were carefully padded and pneumatic compression devices were placed on the lower extremities.

After the administration of intravenous antibiotics and general endotracheal anesthesia, a 16 Fr urethral catheter was inserted into the bladder and connected to a drainage bag. The patient was placed in the lateral decubitus position at a 90° angle with the lower leg flexed 90° and the upper leg extended. An axillary roll was positioned to protect the brachial plexus and a gel pad placed to support the back. Multiple pillows were used to pad beneath and between both the upper and lower extremities to ensure adequate cushioning. The kidney rest was elevated and the table flexed and adjusted horizontally, obtaining optimal flank exposure. The patient was secured to the table with 3 in. surgical tape and safety straps and prepped and draped in the standard sterile manner.

The radiographic images were in the room.

A time-out was completed, verifying the correct patient, surgical procedure, site, and positioning, prior to beginning the procedure.

A *right/left* flank incision was made off the tip of the 12th rib, starting at the mid-axillary line and extended medially to the lateral border of the rectus abdominis muscle. Using electrocautery, the external oblique and latissimus dorsi muscles were incised and the neurovascular bundle identified, dissected free, and retracted out of the way. The internal oblique muscle and lumbodorsal fascia were divided with cautery and the transversus abdominis carefully split in the direction of its fibers, avoiding entry into the peritoneum. A generous paranephric space was created by sweeping the peritoneum medially and the retroperitoneal connective tissue superiorly and inferiorly. A self-retaining retractor (e.g. Bookwalter, Omni-Tract, Finochietto) was appropriately positioned to optimize exposure, using padding on each retractor blade.

The parietal peritoneum was incised on the white line of Toldt and the colon reflected medially, exposing Gerota's fascia. Using sharp dissection, Gerota's fascia was incised posteriorly and the underlying kidney and renal pelvis were identified. The proximal ureter was carefully dissected and thoroughly mobilized, preserving the periureteral tissues.

The site of *obstruction/stricture/injury* was identified and a long 4-0 chromic traction suture was placed above and below this. The entire diseased ureteral segment was excised, leaving two healthy ends. Urinary efflux was noted from the proximal segment. The distal ureter was briefly intubated with a 5 Fr infant feeding tube, confirming its patency.

The ureteral ends were spatulated for a distance of 1 cm on opposite sides and an end-to-end tension free ureteroureteral anastomosis was fashioned using interrupted

4-0 chromic sutures, beginning posteriorly. A ____ Fr _____cm double-J stent was carefully positioned to bridge the repair prior to completing the anterior anastomosis. Meticulous hemostasis was obtained throughout the procedure.

A surgical drain (e.g. Jackson-Pratt) was placed away from the ureteroureteral anastomosis and brought out at the skin through a separate stab incision, where it was secured with a 2-0 silk suture. Prior to closure, the operative field was irrigated with warm sterile saline and inspected, confirming the absence of bleeding or any injury.

The self-retaining retractor was removed, the kidney rest lowered, and the table taken out of flexion. The incision was closed, using running 1-0 polydioxanone (PDS) sutures to approximate the three muscle layers individually, taking care not to entrap the intercostal neurovascular bundle. 3-0 chromic sutures were used on Scarpa's fascia and the skin was approximated with a subcuticular 4-0 poliglecaprone (Monocryl) suture. A sterile dressing was applied and the patient was repositioned supine.

At the end of the procedure, all counts were correct.

The patient tolerated the procedure without difficulty and was taken to the recovery room in satisfactory condition.

Estimated blood loss: Approximately _____ml

Urethra

57

Artificial Urinary Sphincter (Male)

Indications

- Moderate to severe stress urinary incontinence

Essential Steps

1) Prepare the three components of the artificial urinary sphincter according to the manufacturer's specifications.
2) Insert a small urethral catheter and keep the bladder decompressed.
3) Expose the bulbar urethra through a vertical midline perineal incision.
4) Dissect the proximal bulbar urethra circumferentially and create a 2 cm tunnel to allow unobstructed passage of the cuff.
5) Measure the urethral circumference on its bare surface. Choose a urethral cuff size smaller than the measured circumference.
6) Make an inguinal (or suprapubic) incision and create a small pocket in the ipsilateral prevesical space to insert the pressure-regulating balloon. Fill the balloon with sterile normal saline per the manufacturer's recommendations.
7) Create a scrotal dartos pouch on the same side and situate the pump in a dependent position. (Usually this is placed in the patient's dominant side to facilitate manual operation).
8) Bring the cuff tubing through the perineum and out the inguinal incision. Trim, flush, and connect the tubing.
9) Test the device to confirm its proper function.
10) Perform a cystoscopy and repeat the cycling process to ensure adequate urethral coaptation and the absence of an inadvertent urethral injury.

Note These Variations

- The procedure can be performed through a single transcrotal incision.
- Tandem urethral cuffs can be used in patients with severe stress urinary incontinence.
- The urethral cuff can be placed transcorporally (e.g. for revisions or post-radiation) or at the bladder neck (e.g. for neurogenic bladder disorders).

Operative Dictations in Urologic Surgery, First Edition. Noel A. Armenakas, John A. Fracchia, and Ron Golan.
© 2019 John Wiley & Sons Ltd. Published 2019 by John Wiley & Sons Ltd.

- The pressure-regulating balloon may be filled with a solution of sterile normal saline *with* contrast media. It can be inserted through the external inguinal ring or a suprapubic incision.
- The 71–80 cm H_2O pressure balloon is reserved for bladder neck placement.
- For revision surgeries where the entire device is not being replaced, hand-ties rather than quick-connectors should be used to secure the tubing.

Complications

- Bleeding
- Infection
- Urethral perforation
- Urinary retention
- Recurrent/persistent stress incontinence
- Urethral atrophy
- Urethral erosion
- Mechanical failure

Template Operative Dictation

Preoperative diagnosis: *Moderate/severe* stress urinary incontinence
Postoperative diagnosis: Same
Procedure: Placement of an artificial urinary sphincter
Indications: The patient is a _____-year-old male with *moderate/severe* stress urinary incontinence secondary to _____ presenting for placement of an artificial urinary sphincter.
Description of Procedure: The indications, alternatives, benefits, and risks were discussed with the patient and informed consent was obtained.

The patient was brought onto the operating room table, positioned supine, and secured with a safety strap. Pneumatic compression devices were placed on the lower extremities.

After the administration of intravenous antibiotics and *general endotracheal/regional* anesthesia, the patient was repositioned in dorsal lithotomy using well-padded *universal (Allen)/candy cane* stirrups. A gel bolster was placed under the buttocks to support and rotate the pelvis. The genitalia, perineum, and lower abdomen were prepped and draped in the standard sterile manner.

A time-out was completed, verifying the correct patient, surgical procedure, and positioning, prior to beginning the procedure.

The three components of the artificial urinary sphincter were appropriately prepared according to the manufacturer's specifications and soaked in sterile *normal saline/antibiotic solution*. Rubber-shod hemostats were used on the tubing to avoid inadvertent injury to the device.

A 14 Fr urethral catheter was inserted to drain the bladder. A vertical midline perineal skin incision was made, extending from the base of the scrotum to 3 cm above the anus. Colles' fascia and the subcutaneous tissues were incised with electrocautery, exposing

the bulbospongiosus muscle. The muscle was sharply divided in the midline and gently dissected off the underlying corpus spongiosum, taking care not to perforate its thin tunica albuginea. A self-retaining retractor (e.g. Lone Star, Bookwalter) was appropriately positioned to optimize exposure.

The proximal bulbar urethra was carefully dissected circumferentially, freeing it dorsally from the corporal bodies for a distance of 2 cm. A 0.25 in. Penrose drain was placed through this tunnel to facilitate the urethra's mobility, and the urethral catheter was removed. The cuff-sizer was positioned snugly around the urethra at this level and measured at _____cm. A *4.0/4.5* cm urethral cuff was chosen and passed behind the urethra with the mesh surface on the outside. Using the tab, the urethral cuff was secured ventrally, confirming a snug fit. Hemostasis was achieved with judicious electrocautery.

The urethral catheter was reinserted, the bladder was fully drained, and the catheter was connected to a drainage bag.

A 3 cm transverse *right/left* inguinal incision was made following Langer's lines and carried down through to the external oblique aponeurosis. This was incised sharply and the underlying internal oblique and transversis abdominis muscles were gently separated, entering the prevesical space where a small pocket was created. The 61–70 cm H_2O pressure-regulating balloon was positioned in this space and filled with 23 ml of sterile normal saline. The tubing was occluded with a rubber-shod hemostat and the overlying abdominal wall fascia was closed around the exiting tubing to avoid herniation, using a running 2-0 polyglactin (Vicryl) suture.

A hemostat clamp was placed through the inguinal incision and guided inferiorly to the *right/left* hemiscrotum. A dartos pouch was created and the scrotal pump placed within this, away from the testis, with its deactivation button facing the skin.

Using a curved Adson (Tonsil) clamp, the urethral cuff tubing was passed from the perineal to the inguinal incision, staying close to the pubic bone. The excess tubing was trimmed and the ends flushed with sterile normal saline. The urethral cuff and pressure-regulating balloon tubing were connected to the scrotal pump tubing using the quick-connectors, and the rubber-shod hemostats were removed. The device was cycled through the activation and deactivation phases, ensuring a secure watertight connection and proper function.

The urethral catheter was again removed and cystourethroscopy performed using a flexible cystoscope. The urethra was noted to coapt during cycling of the device and there was no evidence of a urethral injury. The urethral catheter was then reinserted into the bladder.

Having completed the artificial urinary sphincter placement, hemostasis was obtained and the self-retaining retractor was removed. The perineal wound was irrigated with warm sterile normal saline and closed using a running 3-0 Vicryl suture to approximate the bulbospongiosus muscle and a 3-0 chromic suture for Colles' fascia. Interrupted 3-0 chromic sutures were used on the skin.

The inguinal incision was closed using running 3-0 chromic and 4-0 poliglecaprone (Monocryl) sutures to approximate Scarpa's fascia and the subcuticular layer, respectively.

The perineal incision was covered with a sterile dressing and gauze fluffs, and an athletic supporter applied to help minimize swelling. Sterile adhesive strips and a gauze dressing were used to secure the inguinal incision.

The patient was repositioned supine and the urethral catheter was connected to a drainage bag and taped to the abdominal wall.

At the end of the procedure, all counts were correct.

The patient tolerated the procedure well and was taken to the recovery room in satisfactory condition.

Estimated blood loss: Approximately _____ml

58

Augmented Anastomotic Urethroplasty

Indications

- Bulbar urethral strictures ≤3 cm

Essential Steps

1) Make a vertical midline perineal incision and expose the bulbar urethra.
2) Identify the stricture and transect the urethra at that level.
3) Excise the entire scar and calibrate both urethral ends to 30 Fr.
4) Harvest an appropriate size oral mucosal graft.
5) Mobilize the urethra distally off the corporal bodies and proximally away from its posterior attachments. In sexually active patients, the distal limit of the dissection should be at the suspensory ligament to avoid penile shortening and chordee.
6) Spatulate the urethral ends according to the chosen graft placement.
7) Measure the urethral defect and tailor the graft accordingly.
8) Place the graft as an onlay, either dorsally or ventrally.
9) Complete the repair over a urethral catheter.
10) Close the incision in several layers.

Note These Variations

- Longer strictures involving the most proximal bulbar segment may be reconstructed with an augmented anastomotic repair.
- Mid and distal bulbar strictures can be accessed by retracting the bulbospongiosus muscle inferiorly, rather than incising it.
- If there is a question as to whether the urethra is amenable to an augmented anastomotic repair, it should be incised vertically and the stricture length assessed prior to transecting the urethra.
- A hemostatic sealant (e.g. fibrin glue) can be used in conjunction with the anastomotic sutures to reinforce the repair.

Operative Dictations in Urologic Surgery, First Edition. Noel A. Armenakas, John A. Fracchia, and Ron Golan.
© 2019 John Wiley & Sons Ltd. Published 2019 by John Wiley & Sons Ltd.

Complications

- Bleeding
- Infection
- Urine leak
- Post-void dribbling
- Graft sacculation
- Penile shortening and chordee
- Decreased penile sensitivity
- Erectile/ejaculatory dysfunction
- Neuropraxia
- Urethrocutaneous fistula
- Oral (harvest-site) complications
- Recurrent stricture

Template Operative Dictation

Preoperative diagnosis: Bulbar urethral stricture
Postoperative diagnosis: Same
Procedure: Augmented anastomotic urethroplasty
Indications: The patient is a ____-year-old male with a ____cm *proximal/mid/distal* bulbar urethral stricture presenting for an augmented anastomotic urethroplasty.
Description of Procedure: The indications, alternatives, benefits, and risks were discussed with the patient and informed consent was obtained.

The patient was brought onto the operating room table, positioned supine, and secured with a safety strap. Pneumatic compression devices were placed on the lower extremities.

After the administration of intravenous antibiotics and general endotracheal anesthesia, the patient was repositioned in high dorsal lithotomy using well-padded *universal (Allen)/ candy cane* stirrups. The genitalia, perineum, and lower abdomen were prepped and draped in the standard sterile manner.

The radiographic images were in the room.

A time-out was completed, verifying the correct patient, surgical procedure, and positioning, prior to beginning the procedure.

Using optical magnification with surgical loupes, a vertical midline perineal skin incision was made extending from the base of the scrotum to just above the anus. Colles' fascia and the subcutaneous tissues were incised with electrocautery, exposing the bulbospongiosus muscle. The muscle was sharply divided in the midline and carefully dissected off the underlying corpus spongiosum, taking care not to perforate its thin tunica albuginea. A self-retaining retractor (e.g. Lone Star, Bookwalter) was appropriately positioned to optimize exposure.

A 20 Fr red rubber catheter was advanced per the urethral meatus to the stricture. The urethra was dissected circumferentially distal to stricture, freeing it dorsally from the corporal bodies. The urethra was sharply transected at the level of the stricture, and the entire fibrotic scar excised. 4-0 chromic stay sutures were placed at the 3 o'clock and 9 o'clock positions of both severed healthy urethral ends for traction. Bougie-à-boule dilators were used to progressively calibrate the urethra to 30 Fr.

Cystourethroscopy was performed, using a *flexible/____Fr rigid* cystoscope, confirming the absence of any proximal urethral or bladder pathology.

Using a combination of sharp and blunt dissection, the distal bulbar urethra was mobilized to the suspensory ligament of the penis, releasing it from the tunica albuginea of the corpora cavernosa. The dissection was carried proximally, freeing the bulbar urethra from its posterior midline attachments. Care was taken to preserve the bulbar arteries. Meticulous hemostasis was achieved with electrocautery.

Dorsal onlay: After completing the urethral mobilization, the distal and proximal urethral ends were spatulated dorsally for 1cm. The urethral ends were brought together ventrally and the length of the defect was measured at ____cm.

Add graft harvest; see Chapter 60.

The harvested oral mucosal graft was tailored and placed dorsally where it was spread-fixed onto the corporal bodies with several 4-0 chromic quilting sutures. The proximal and distal apical edges of the graft were sutured to the corresponding spatulated dorsal wall of the corpus spongiosum using interrupted full-thickness 5-0 polydioxanone (PDS) sutures. Ventrally, the urethral ends were anastomosed in two layers using 5-0 PDS. The inner layer included only the urethral mucosa, whereas the outer layer incorporated the tunica albuginea of the corpus spongiosum, limiting injury to the spongiosal blood supply. The lateral edges of corpus spongiosum were then secured to the lateral aspect of the graft, incorporating the underlying tunica albuginea of the corpora, using a running 5-0 PDS suture on each side. Prior to completion, an *18/20* Fr urethral catheter was easily advanced into the bladder.

Ventral onlay: After completing the urethral mobilization, the distal and proximal urethral ends were spatulated ventrally for 1 cm. The urethral ends 1were brought together dorsally and the length of the defect was measured at ____cm.

Add graft harvest; see Chapter 60.

The urethral anastomosis was begun dorsally by placing several full-thickness interrupted 5-0 PDS sutures, incorporating the entire spongiosum and urethral mucosa. The harvested oral mucosal graft was tailored to fit the diamond-shaped ventral urethral defect and sutured to the urethral mucosal edges at the apices with 5-0 interrupted PDS. The lateral edges of graft were secured to the lateral aspect of the urethral mucosa using a running 5-0 PDS suture on each side. The corpus spongiosum was approximated over the graft using superficially placed sutures to limit injury to the spongiosal blood supply. Prior to completion, an *18/20* Fr urethral catheter was easily advanced into the bladder.

Having completed a tension-free urethral anastomosis and achieved adequate hemostasis, the self-retaining retractor was removed. The perineal wound was irrigated with sterile normal saline and the bulbospongiosus muscle closed with a running 3-0 polyglactin (Vicryl) suture. Two running 3-0 chromic sutures were used to approximate the subcutaneous tissue and Colles' fascia, separately, obliterating any dead space. The skin was closed with interrupted 3-0 chromic sutures.

The incision was covered with a sterile dressing and gauze fluffs, and an athletic supporter was applied to help minimize swelling.

The patient was repositioned supine, and the urethral catheter was connected to a drainage bag and taped to the abdominal wall.

At the end of the procedure, all counts were correct.

The patient tolerated the procedure well and was taken to the recovery room in satisfactory condition.

Estimated blood loss: Approximately _____ml

59

Augmented Urethroplasty Using a Buccal Mucosal Graft

Indications

- Penile and long bulbar urethral strictures

Essential Steps

1) Expose the urethra through the appropriate incision.
2) Identify the stricture and incise the urethra longitudinally along the entire length of the stricture.
3) Calibrate the urethra to 26 or 28 Fr.
4) Harvest an appropriate size oral mucosal graft.
5) Measure the urethral defect and tailor the graft accordingly.
6) Place the graft as an onlay, either dorsally or ventrally.
7) Complete the repair over a urethral catheter.

Note These Variations

- Exposure of penile urethral strictures can be accomplished through a longitudinal ventral penile incision over the median raphe, rather than a degloving incision.
- In patients who lack suitable buccal mucosa, lingual, penile, or posterior auricular skin grafts can be used for urethral augmentation.
- When placing the graft ventrally in the penile urethra, the overlying spongiosum cannot be adequately closed. In those instances, a "pseudospongioplasty" should be performed using the dartos and superficial Buck's fascias to cover and immobilize the graft.
- An additional option for graft placement is a dorsal inlay (Asopa). The urethra is incised ventrally and dorsally for exposure and placement, respectively.
- A hemostatic sealant (e.g. fibrin glue) can be used in conjunction with the anastomotic sutures to reinforce the repair.

Operative Dictations in Urologic Surgery, First Edition. Noel A. Armenakas, John A. Fracchia, and Ron Golan.
© 2019 John Wiley & Sons Ltd. Published 2019 by John Wiley & Sons Ltd.

Complications

- Bleeding
- Infection
- Urine leak
- Post-void dribbling
- Graft sacculation
- Erectile/ejaculatory dysfunction
- Neuropraxia
- Urethrocutaneous fistula
- Oral (harvest-site) complications
- Recurrent stricture

Template Operative Dictation

Preoperative diagnosis: *Penile/bulbar* urethral stricture
Postoperative diagnosis: Same
Procedure: Buccal graft urethroplasty
Indications: The patient is a ____-year-old male presenting with a ____cm *penile/bulbar* urethral stricture presenting for an augmentation urethroplasty using buccal mucosa.
Description of Procedure: The indications, alternatives, benefits, and risks were discussed with the patient and informed consent was obtained.

The patient was brought onto the operating room table, positioned supine, and secured with a safety strap. Pneumatic compression devices were placed on the lower extremities.

After the administration of intravenous antibiotics and general endotracheal anesthesia, the patient was repositioned in dorsal lithotomy using well-padded *universal (Allen)/candy cane* stirrups. *(Alternatively: If the stricture is limited to the penile urethra, the patient may be left supine.)* The genitalia, perineum, and lower abdomen were prepped and draped in the standard sterile manner.

The radiographic images were in the room.

A time-out was completed, verifying the correct patient, surgical procedure, and positioning, prior to beginning the procedure.

> ***For penile urethral exposure***: A 2-0 polypropylene (Prolene) stay suture was placed through the anterior mid glans for traction. Using optical magnification with surgical loupes, a circumferential penile skin incision was made 1 cm below the coronal sulcus and carried down through the dartos fascia. The penis was carefully degloved, using sharp and blunt dissection, exposing the penile urethra. A self-retaining retractor (e.g. Lone Star) was appropriately positioned to optimize exposure. Meticulous hemostasis was achieved with electrocautery.

> ***For bulbar urethral exposure***: Using optical magnification with surgical loupes, a vertical midline perineal skin incision was made extending from the base of the scrotum to just above the anus. Colles' fascia and the subcutaneous tissues were incised with electrocautery, exposing the bulbospongiosus muscle. The muscle

was sharply divided in the midline and carefully dissected off the underlying corpus spongiosum, taking care not to perforate its thin tunica albuginea. A self-retaining retractor (e.g. Lone Star, Bookwalter) was appropriately positioned to optimize exposure. Meticulous hemostasis was achieved with electrocautery.

Dorsal onlay: An 18 Fr red rubber catheter was advanced per the urethral meatus to the stricture. The lateral urethra was dissected from the corpora cavernosa and rotated 120°, remaining partially attached on its contralateral border to limit its vascular disruption. The urethra was incised over the distal tip of the catheter on its dorsal surface. The midline incision was extended proximally into healthy tissue, exposing the entire area of stricture. 4-0 chromic stay sutures were placed on the lateral edge of the incised urethra for traction. Bougie-à-boule dilators were used to progressively calibrate the urethra to 26/28 Fr.

Cystourethroscopy was performed using a *flexible/___ Fr rigid* cystoscope, confirming the absence of any proximal urethral or bladder pathology.

The urethral defect was measured at _____ cm. The harvested buccal mucosal graft was tailored and placed dorsally, where it was spread-fixed to the corporal bodies with several 4-0 chromic quilting sutures. The proximal and distal apical edges of the graft were sutured to the corresponding dorsal wall of the corpus spongiosum using interrupted full-thickness 5-0 polydioxanone (PDS) sutures. The lateral edges of corpus spongiosum were then secured to the lateral aspect of the graft and the underlying tunica albuginea of the corpora, using a running 5-0 PDS suture on each side allowing the urethra to rotate to its original position. Prior to completion, a *16/18* Fr urethral catheter was advanced easily into the bladder.

Having completed a tension free repair and achieved adequate hemostasis, the wound was irrigated with sterile normal saline and the self-retaining retractor was removed.

Ventral onlay: An 18 Fr red rubber catheter was advanced per the urethral meatus to the stricture. The urethra was incised over the distal tip of the catheter on its ventral surface. The midline incision was extended proximally into healthy tissue, exposing the entire area of stricture. 4-0 chromic stay sutures were placed on the lateral edges of the incised urethra for traction. Bougie-à-boule dilators were used to progressively calibrate the urethra to 26/28 Fr.

Cystourethroscopy was performed using a *flexible/___ Fr rigid* cystoscope, confirming the absence of any proximal urethral or bladder pathology.

The urethral defect was measured at _____ cm. The harvested buccal mucosal graft was tailored to fit the ventral urethral defect and sutured to the urethral mucosal edges at the apices with 5-0 interrupted polydioxanone (PDS). The lateral edges of graft were secured to the lateral aspect of the urethral mucosa using a running 5-0 PDS suture on each side. The corpus spongiosum was approximated over the graft using superficially placed sutures to limit injury to the spongiosal blood supply.

(Alternatively, for penile urethral reconstruction where spongiosal tissue is usually inadequate for graft coverage: A flap comprised of dartos and Buck's fascias was carefully mobilized and advanced over the graft, where it was secured with several interrupted 4-0 chromic sutures.)

Prior to completion, a *16/18* Fr urethral catheter was advanced easily into the bladder. Having completed a tension-free repair and achieved adequate hemostasis, the wound was irrigated with sterile normal saline and the self-retaining retractor was removed.

Penile skin closure: The penile skin was advanced distally and sutured to the subcoronal border with four-quadrant 3-0 chromic sutures. Similar interrupted sutures were placed between these in a circumferential manner, approximating the remainder of the incision. The mid-glans traction suture was removed.

The incision was covered with a sterile dressing and the penis wrapped loosely with a self-adherent (Coban) dressing.

Perineal skin closure: The bulbospongiosus muscle was closed with a running 3-0 polyglactin (Vicryl) suture. Two running 3-0 chromic sutures were used to approximate the subcutaneous tissue and Colles' fascia, separately, obliterating any dead space. The skin was closed with interrupted 3-0 chromic sutures.

The incision was covered with a sterile dressing and gauze fluffs, and an athletic supporter was applied to help minimize swelling.

The patient was repositioned supine, and the urethral catheter was connected to a drainage bag and taped to the abdominal wall.

At the end of the procedure, all counts were correct.

The patient tolerated the procedure well and was taken to the recovery room in satisfactory condition.

Estimated blood loss: Approximately _____ml

60

Buccal Mucosal Graft Harvest

Indications

- Urethral reconstruction necessitating tissue transfer

Essential Steps

1) Place an oral retractor and stay sutures for exposure.
2) Identify the parotid (Stensen's) duct at the level of the second upper molar.
3) Hydrodissect the buccal mucosa using injectable 1% lidocaine containing 1:100000 epinephrine.
4) Incise a 2 cm wide segment of buccal mucosa with the appropriate length, depending on the extent of the urethral defect.
5) Elevate the mucosa by dissecting it from the buccinator muscle, avoiding Stensen's duct.
6) Temporarily pack the donor site and allow the oral defect to heal by secondary intention.
7) Defat the graft and place it in sterile normal saline.

Note These Variations

- The donor site may be closed primarily with absorbable sutures.
- For long donor site defects, additional buccal grafts can be harvested from the contralateral cheek and inner lip.

Complications

- Bleeding
- Injury to Stensen's duct
- Oral pain and numbness
- Mouth tightness due to oral adhesions/fibrosis
- Infection
- Cheek granuloma

Operative Dictations in Urologic Surgery, First Edition. Noel A. Armenakas, John A. Fracchia, and Ron Golan.
© 2019 John Wiley & Sons Ltd. Published 2019 by John Wiley & Sons Ltd.

Template Operative Dictation

Preoperative diagnosis: Urethral stricture
Postoperative diagnosis: Same
Procedure: Buccal mucosal graft harvest
Indications: The patient is a __-year-old male with a _____cm *bulbar/penile/glanular* urethral stricture presenting for a buccal mucosal graft harvest.
Description of Procedure: The indications, alternatives, benefits, and risks were discussed with the patient and informed consent was obtained.

The patient was brought onto the operating room table, positioned supine, and secured with a safety strap. All pressure points were carefully padded and pneumatic compression devices were placed on the lower extremities.

After the administration of intravenous antibiotics and general endotracheal anesthesia, the endotracheal tube was taped to the patient's *right/left* side and the mouth was gently prepped using chlorohexidine wash.

A time-out was completed, verifying the correct patient, surgical procedure, and positioning, prior to beginning the procedure.

The mouth was opened using an oral retractor (e.g. Kilner-Doughty, McIvor mouth gag), taking care not to damage any teeth. A tongue depressor was used to retract the tongue. Three 2-0 silk sutures were placed at the *right/left* oral commissure for traction.

Using a ruler and marking pen, an area of buccal mucosa 2 cm wide by ___cm long was outlined on the inner *right/left* cheek, 1 cm proximal to the vermilion border. Stensen's duct was identified at the level of the second superior molar, away from the harvest site.

The delineated mucosa was hydrodissected with injectable 1% lidocaine containing 1:100 000 epinephrine to aid in hemostasis. A #15 blade was used to incise the oral mucosa along the markings. Two 4-0 polyglactin (Vicryl) stay sutures were placed at the distal graft edge for traction.

The buccal graft was dissected carefully off the underlying buccinator muscle, using fine scissors. The dissection proceeded proximally to the previously marked area. Once again, care was taken not to injure Stensen's duct. The proximal graft attachments were cut completely, freeing the graft, which was placed in sterile normal saline.

Meticulous hemostasis was achieved with electrocautery and the harvest site was compressed with a lidocaine and epinephrine-soaked gauze.

The entire mouth was inspected, confirming that the teeth, tongue, and Stensen's duct were intact, prior to removing the oral retractor, tongue depressor, and silk traction sutures.

Attention was then directed to the graft, which was measured at 2 cm by ____ cm. The inner surface of the graft was defatted using fine scissors, and was tagged with a 5-0 polydioxanone (PDS) suture before placing it back in sterile normal saline.

The oral gauze was removed and the donor site was inspected, confirming the absence of any bleeding.

At the end of the procedure, all counts were correct.

The patient tolerated the procedure well and was taken to the recovery room in satisfactory condition.

Estimated blood loss: Approximately _____ml

61

Excision and Primary Anastomotic Urethroplasty

Indications

- Bulbar urethral strictures ≤2 cm

Essential Steps

1) Make a vertical midline perineal incision and expose the bulbar urethra.
2) Identify the stricture and transect the urethra at that level.
3) Excise the entire scar and calibrate both urethral ends to 30 Fr.
4) Mobilize the urethra distally off the corporal bodies and proximally from its posterior attachments. In sexually active patients, the distal limit of the dissection should be at the suspensory ligament to avoid penile shortening and chordee.
5) Spatulate the urethra on opposite ends.
6) Create a tension-free urethral anastomosis using a one-layer closure dorsally and a two-layer closure ventrally.
7) Place a urethral catheter to stent the repair.
8) Close the incision in several layers.

Note These Variations

- Longer strictures involving the most proximal bulbar segment may be reconstructed with an excision and primary anastomotic repair.
- Mid- and distal bulbar strictures can be accessed by retracting the bulbospongiosus muscle inferiorly, rather than incising it.
- If there is a question as to whether the urethra is amenable to an excision and primary anastomotic repair, it should be incised vertically and the stricture length assessed prior to transecting the urethra. In a situation where the urethra has been transected and only the dorsal or ventral urethral wall can be anastomosed without tension, an augmented anastomotic urethroplasty should be performed.

Operative Dictations in Urologic Surgery, First Edition. Noel A. Armenakas, John A. Fracchia, and Ron Golan.
© 2019 John Wiley & Sons Ltd. Published 2019 by John Wiley & Sons Ltd.

Complications

- Bleeding
- Infection
- Urine leak
- Penile shortening and chordee
- Decreased penile sensitivity
- Erectile/ejaculatory dysfunction
- Neuropraxia
- Recurrent stricture

Template Operative Dictation

Preoperative diagnosis: Bulbar urethral stricture
Postoperative diagnosis: Same
Procedure: Excision and primary anastomotic urethroplasty
Indications: The patient is a _____-year-old male with a _____cm *proximal/mid/distal* bulbar urethral stricture presenting for an excision and primary anastomotic urethroplasty.
Description of Procedure: The indications, alternatives, benefits, and risks were discussed with the patient and informed consent was obtained.

The patient was brought onto the operating room table, positioned supine, and secured with a safety strap. Pneumatic compression devices were placed on the lower extremities.

After the administration of intravenous antibiotics and *general endotracheal/regional* anesthesia, the patient was repositioned in high dorsal lithotomy using well-padded *universal (Allen)/candy cane* stirrups. A gel bolster was placed under the buttocks to support and rotate the pelvis. The genitalia, perineum, and lower abdomen were prepped and draped in the standard sterile manner.

The radiographic images were in the room.

A time-out was completed, verifying the correct patient, surgical procedure, and positioning, prior to beginning the procedure.

Using optical magnification with surgical loupes, a vertical midline perineal skin incision was made extending from the base of the scrotum to just above the anus. Colles' fascia and the subcutaneous tissues were incised with electrocautery, exposing the bulbospongiosus muscle. The muscle was sharply divided in the midline and carefully dissected off the underlying corpus spongiosum, taking care not to perforate its thin tunica albuginea. A self-retaining retractor (e.g. Lone Star, Bookwalter) was appropriately positioned to optimize exposure.

A 20 Fr red rubber catheter was advanced per the urethral meatus to the stricture. The urethra was dissected circumferentially distal to the stricture, freeing it dorsally from the corporal bodies. The urethra was then sharply transected at the level of the stricture, and the entire fibrotic scar excised. 4-0 chromic stay sutures were placed at the 3 o'clock and 9 o'clock positions of both severed healthy urethral ends for traction. Bougie-à-boule dilators were used to progressively calibrate the urethra to 30 Fr.

Cystourethroscopy was performed, using a *flexible/___Fr rigid* cystoscope, confirming the absence of any proximal urethral or bladder pathology.

Using a combination of sharp and blunt dissection, the distal bulbar urethra was mobilized to the suspensory ligament of the penis, releasing it from the tunica albuginea of the corpora cavernosa. The dissection was carried proximally, freeing the bulbar urethra from its posterior midline attachments. Care was taken to preserve the bulbar arteries. Hemostasis was achieved with judicious electrocautery.

After completing the urethral mobilization, the distal and proximal urethral ends were spatulated for 1 cm ventrally and dorsally, respectively. The urethral anastomosis was begun dorsally by placing several full-thickness interrupted 5-0 polydioxanone (PDS) sutures, incorporating the entire spongiosum and urethral mucosa. Ventrally, a two-layer closure was performed with identical interrupted sutures. The inner layer approximated the urethral mucosa, whereas the outer layer incorporated only the tunica albuginea of the corpus spongiosum, limiting injury to the spongiosal blood supply. Prior to completion of the ventral anastomosis, an *18/20* Fr urethral catheter was easily advanced into the bladder.

Having completed a tension-free urethral anastomosis and achieved adequate hemostasis, the self-retaining retractor was removed. The perineal wound was irrigated with sterile normal saline and the bulbospongiosus muscle was closed with a running 3-0 polyglactin (Vicryl) suture. Two running 3-0 chromic sutures were used to approximate the subcutaneous tissue and Colles' fascia, separately, obliterating any dead space. The skin was closed with interrupted 3-0 chromic sutures.

The incision was covered with a sterile dressing and gauze fluffs, and an athletic supporter applied to help minimize swelling.

The patient was repositioned supine, and the urethral catheter was connected to a drainage bag and taped to the abdominal wall.

At the end of the procedure, all counts were correct.

The patient tolerated the procedure well and was taken to the recovery room in satisfactory condition.

Estimated blood loss: Approximately _____ml

62

Male Urethral Sling

Indications

- Mild to moderate stress urinary incontinence

Essential Steps

1) Make a vertical midline perineal incision to expose the bulbar urethra.
2) Incise the central tendon to allow for proximal urethral mobility.
3) Make a stab incision in each groin crease 2 cm below the adductor longus tendon, and use a spinal needle to identify the obturator foramen.
4) Insert the helical needle passer through the groin incision following the spinal needle's trajectory. Perforate the endopelvic fascia and guide the needle passer into the perineal incision, medial to the corpus cavernosum.
5) Position the urethral sling in the midline and pull the ends through the ipsilateral obturator foramen and out each groin incision.
6) Fix the sling to the ventral bulbar urethra, proximally.
7) Perform flexible cystoscopy to confirm integrity of the bladder and urethra, ureteral efflux, and adequate urethral mobility without obstruction.
8) Individually close each incision.

Note These Variations

- After positioning the sling, the distal ends can be tunneled back into the perineal incision and sutured together.
- Additional types of slings include bone anchor and quadratic fixation devices.

Complications

- Bleeding
- Urinary retention
- Infection

Operative Dictations in Urologic Surgery, First Edition. Noel A. Armenakas, John A. Fracchia, and Ron Golan.
© 2019 John Wiley & Sons Ltd. Published 2019 by John Wiley & Sons Ltd.

- Perineal pain
- Neuropraxia
- Persistent or worsening urinary incontinence
- Erosion

Template Operative Dictation

Preoperative diagnosis: Stress urinary incontinence
Postoperative diagnosis: Same
Procedure: Insertion of a male urethral sling
Indications: The patient is a _____-year-old male with _____(*post-prostatectomy*)____ stress urinary incontinence presenting for insertion of a male urethral sling.
Description of Procedure: The indications, alternatives, benefits, and risks were discussed with the patient and informed consent was obtained.

The patient was brought onto the operating room table, positioned supine, and secured with a safety strap. Pneumatic compression devices were placed on the lower extremities.

After the administration of intravenous antibiotics and *general endotracheal/regional* anesthesia, the patient was repositioned in high dorsal lithotomy using well-padded *universal (Allen)/candy cane* stirrups. The genitalia, perineum, anteromedial thighs, and lower abdomen were prepped and draped in the standard sterile manner.

A time-out was completed, verifying the correct patient, surgical procedure, and positioning, prior to beginning the procedure.

An 14 Fr urethral catheter was advanced into the bladder.

A 5 cm vertical midline perineal skin incision was made below the scrotum and taken down through Colles' fascia and the subcutaneous tissues to the bulbospongiosus muscle, using electrocautery. The muscle was sharply divided in the midline and carefully dissected off the underlying corpus spongiosum. A self-retaining retractor (e.g. Lone Star, Bookwalter) was appropriately positioned to optimize exposure.

The central tendon was identified at the midline and sharply incised mobilizing the proximal bulbar urethra. A sterile marking pen was used to highlight this level for subsequent sling placement.

Attention was then directed to the *right/left* groin crease where a small stab incision was made with a #15 blade, 2 cm below the adductor longus tendon.

The helical needle passer was inserted outside-in through the stab incision, and guided lateral to the ipsilateral ischiopubic ramus into the obturator foramen. With the bulbar urethra retracted medially, the endopelvic fascia was perforated and the needle passer guided between the lateral edge of the corpus spongiosum and the medial border of the corpus cavernosum.

The polypropylene urethral sling, which had been previously bathed in *betadine/ antibiotic solution*, was brought into the perineal field and connected to the tip of the needle passer. Using reverse rotation, the sling was pulled through the obturator foramen and brought out loosely through the groin incision. The connector and distal sling were cut above the skin level and the end of the sling grasped with a hemostat.

The identical procedure was repeated on the patient's contralateral side, making sure that the center of the mesh was positioned at the urethral midline.

The sling was laid flat on the ventral bulbar urethral surface with its proximal edge at the previously marked site. Its four corners were fixed to the superficial corpus spongiosum, using 4-0 polyglactin (Vicryl) sutures. Both arms of the sling were pulled tight, evenly displacing the urethra proximally.

The urethral catheter was removed and a flexible cystoscope was advanced to the bulbomembranous junction. Both arms of the sling were elevated under direct cystoscopic vision, confirming adequate proximal bulbar mobility without urethral obstruction. On cystoscopy the bladder was noted to be intact with clear ureteral efflux bilaterally. The cystoscope was removed and replaced with the urethral catheter.

The wound was irrigated with sterile *antibiotic solution/normal saline.*

The self-retaining retractor was removed and the perineum inspected, confirming correct sling placement without injury to the corpus spongiosum. The perineal incision was closed using a running 3-0 Vicryl suture to approximate the bulbospongiosus muscle. Two running 3-0 chromic sutures were used on the subcutaneous tissues and Colles' fascia, separately, obliterating any dead space. The perineal incision was closed with interrupted 3-0 chromic sutures and the groin incisions were approximated with a 4-0 subcuticular poliglecaprone (Monocryl) suture. Sterile adhesive strips were used to reinforce the groin incisions.

The perineal incision was covered with a sterile dressing and gauze fluffs, and an athletic supporter was applied to help minimize swelling. Sterile adhesive strips and a small gauze dressing were placed on each groin incision.

The patient was repositioned supine, and the urethral catheter was connected to a drainage bag.

At the end of the procedure, all counts were correct.

The patient tolerated the procedure well and was taken to the recovery room in satisfactory condition.

Estimated blood loss: Approximately _____ml

63

Perineal Urethrostomy

Indications

- Refractory or extensive urethral strictures
- Temporary access to the bladder and prostate (rarely used)

Essential Steps

1) Create a full-thickness infrascrotal inverted-U skin flap, ensuring a viable blood supply.
2) Make a 4 cm ventral urethrotomy in the proximal bulb.
3) Suture the perineal skin to the urethral mucosa and tunica albuginea of the corpus spongiosum, preserving the spongiosal tissue.
4) Close the lateral edges of the perineal skin flap in two layers.
5) Place a urethral catheter through the urethrostomy to drain the bladder.

Note These Variations

- There are several additional techniques for the creation of a perineal urethrostomy with comparable results (e.g. "7-flap" and inverted Y-flap).
- In obese patients, additional exposure can be obtained by extending the inverted-U incision cephalad at the midline.
- In cases where the dorsal urethral wall is extensively scarred, it can be replaced with a buccal graft placed as an onlay.

Complications

- Bleeding
- Infection
- Stomal stenosis
- Obstructive uropathy

Operative Dictations in Urologic Surgery, First Edition. Noel A. Armenakas, John A. Fracchia, and Ron Golan.
© 2019 John Wiley & Sons Ltd. Published 2019 by John Wiley & Sons Ltd.

Template Operative Dictation

Preoperative diagnosis: Refractory urethral stricture
Postoperative diagnosis: Same
Procedure: Perineal urethrostomy
Indications: The patient is a ____-year-old male with a refractory ____cm *bulbar/penile/ glanular* urethral stricture presenting for a perineal urethrostomy.
Description of Procedure: The indications, alternatives, benefits, and risks were discussed with the patient and informed consent was obtained.

The patient was brought onto the operating room table, positioned supine, and secured with a safety strap. Pneumatic compression devices were placed on the lower extremities.

After the administration of intravenous antibiotics and *general endotracheal/regional* anesthesia, the patient was repositioned in exaggerated dorsal lithotomy using well-padded *universal (Allen)/candy cane* stirrups. A gel bolster was placed under the buttocks to support and rotate the pelvis. The genitalia, perineum, and lower abdomen were prepped and draped in the standard sterile manner.

A time-out was completed, verifying the correct patient, surgical procedure, site, and positioning, prior to beginning the procedure.

The right and left ischial tuberosities were palpated, and an infrascrotal inverted-U incision was made between these and taken down to the bulbospongiosus muscle using electrocautery. The bulbospongiosus muscle was sharply divided in the midline and carefully dissected off the underlying corpus spongiosum, taking care not to perforate the tunica albuginea. A self-retaining retractor (e.g. Lone Star, Bookwalter) was appropriately positioned to optimize exposure.

The bulbar urethra was grasped with two pairs of DeBakey forceps and a 4 cm longitudinal incision was made ventrally between these. Several 4-0 chromic stay sutures were placed on the lateral edges of the incised urethra for traction. Bougie-à-boule dilators were used to calibrate the urethra to 30 Fr.

Cystourethroscopy was performed, using a *flexible/___Fr rigid* cystoscope, confirming the absence of any proximal urethral or bladder pathology.

Interrupted 2-0 polyglactin (Vicryl) sutures were used to approximate the perineal skin to the incised ventral urethral edges bilaterally. Spongiosal preservation was achieved by incorporating only the urethral mucosa and tunica albuginea of the corpus spongiosum within the urethral sutures. The apex of the perineal skin flap was sutured to the proximal urethral apex in a similar fashion. The lateral edges of the flap were closed in two layers using interrupted 2-0 Vicryl sutures. Meticulous hemostasis was achieved with electrocautery and the viability of the flap confirmed. A 20 Fr urethral catheter was easily advanced into the bladder through the urethrostomy.

The wound was covered with a sterile dressing and gauze fluffs, and an athletic supporter was applied to help minimize swelling.

The patient was repositioned supine and the urethral catheter was connected to a drainage bag.

At the end of the procedure, all counts were correct.

The patient tolerated the procedure well and was taken to the recovery room in satisfactory condition.

Estimated blood loss: Approximately _____ml

64

Posterior Urethral Reconstruction

Indications

- Posterior urethral disruption

Essential Steps

1) Make a vertical midline perineal incision and expose the bulbar urethra.
2) Identify the stricture distally and transect the urethra at that level.
3) Mobilize the urethra distally off the corporal bodies and proximally away from its posterior attachments. In sexually active patients, the distal limit of the dissection should be at the suspensory ligament to avoid penile shortening and chordee.
4) Consider additional maneuvers when needed to achieve a tension-free anastomosis.
5) Identify the proximal scar using a curved metal sound placed through the suprapubic cystostomy.
6) Excise the entire scar and calibrate both urethral ends to 28 or 30 Fr.
7) Spatulate the urethra on opposite ends.
8) Create a tension-free urethral anastomosis using 8–12 sutures.
9) Place a urethral catheter prior to tying all the anastomotic sutures.
10) Close the incision in several layers.

Note These Variations

- An inverted-Y incision (also referred to as a "lambda" incision) can be used to expose the urethra.
- If the proximal urethra is not palpable using a sound placed through the suprapubic cystostomy tract, an abdominoperineal approach may be required.
- The anastomotic distance can be further shortened by rerouting the anterior urethra around the left corporal body.

Operative Dictations in Urologic Surgery, First Edition. Noel A. Armenakas, John A. Fracchia, and Ron Golan.
© 2019 John Wiley & Sons Ltd. Published 2019 by John Wiley & Sons Ltd.

Complications

- Bleeding
- Infection
- Urine leak
- Penile shortening and chordee
- Urinary incontinence
- Erectile/ejaculatory dysfunction
- Neuropraxia
- Stricture formation

Template Operative Dictation

Preoperative diagnosis: Posterior urethral disruption
Postoperative diagnosis: Same
Procedure: Posterior urethral reconstruction
Indications: The patient is a ____-year-old male with an approximate ____cm pelvic fracture urethral disruption presenting for posterior urethral reconstruction.
Description of Procedure: The indications, alternatives, benefits, and risks were discussed with the patient and informed consent was obtained.

The patient was brought onto the operating room table, positioned supine, and secured with a safety strap. Pneumatic compression devices were placed on the lower extremities.

After the administration of intravenous antibiotics and *general endotracheal/regional* anesthesia, the patient was repositioned in high dorsal lithotomy using well-padded *universal (Allen)/candy cane* stirrups. A gel bolster was placed under the buttocks to support and rotate the pelvis. The genitalia, perineum, and lower abdomen were prepped and draped in the standard sterile manner.

The radiographic images were in the room.

A time-out was completed, verifying the correct patient, surgical procedure, and positioning, prior to beginning the procedure.

Using optical magnification with surgical loupes, a vertical midline perineal skin incision was made extending from the base of the scrotum to just above the anus. Colles' fascia and the subcutaneous tissues were incised with electrocautery, exposing the bulbospongiosus muscle. The muscle was sharply divided in the midline and carefully dissected off the underlying corpus spongiosum, taking care not to perforate its thin tunica albuginea. A self-retaining retractor (e.g. Lone Star, Bookwalter) was appropriately positioned to optimize exposure.

An 18 Fr red rubber catheter was advanced per the urethral meatus to the distal scar. The mid-bulbar urethra was dissected circumferentially, freeing it dorsally from the corporal bodies. The urethra was transected at the level of the scar tissue and mobilized distally to the penoscrotal junction, releasing it from the tunica albuginea of the corpora cavernosa. The dissection was carried proximally, freeing the proximal bulbar urethra from its posterior midline attachments. Care was taken to preserve the bulbar arteries. Meticulous hemostasis was achieved with electrocautery.

An 18 Fr curved-metal urethral sound (Van Buren) was placed into the cystostomy and gently manipulated into the bladder neck and advanced to the area of proximal obstruction. The bulbomembranous scar was sufficiently excised, allowing palpation of the metal sound. The obliterated proximal urethra was incised over the sound and the remaining fibrosis entirely excised down to healthy tissue.

The sound was withdrawn and cystourethroscopy performed using a *flexible/___ Fr rigid* cystoscope, confirming the absence of a false passage or any bladder pathology.

Both healthy severed urethral ends were tagged with 4-0 chromic sutures and progressively calibrated to *28/30* Fr with bougie-à-boule dilators.

> ***For longer defects***: The intracrural space was developed, down to the inferior surface of the pubis, by sharply separating the crura for a distance of 5 cm. Care was taken not to enter the tunica albuginea of the corpus cavernosa. A small self-retaining retractor (e.g. Gelpi, Weitlaner) was used to optimize exposure. The dorsal penile vein was identified at this level, ligated with 3-0 Vicryl and divided.
>
> Next, an inferior pubectomy was performed by removing a 2 cm wedge of bone, using an osteotome and bone rongeur. Bone wax was placed on the raw surface to limit bleeding.

The anterior urethra was brought to the proximal urethral stump, confirming a tension-free approximation. The distal and proximal urethral ends were spatulated for 1 cm dorsally and ventrally, respectively.

The urethral anastomosis was begun proximally by placing full-thickness interrupted 5-0 polydioxanone (PDS) sutures, outside-in, in a clockwise fashion, starting at the 12 o'clock position. The sutures were then passed inside-out through the distal urethral lumen incorporating the spongiosum and urethral mucosa. Each suture was secured with a rubber-shod mosquito clamp that was appropriately numbered to maintain orientation. After placing half of the distal sutures, an *18/20* Fr urethral catheter was easily advanced into the bladder. Once all the sutures were in place, they were individually tied, in a clockwise fashion, starting at 12 o'clock.

Having completed a tension-free urethral anastomosis and achieved adequate hemostasis, the self-retaining retractor was removed. The perineal wound was irrigated with sterile normal saline and the bulbospongiosus muscle closed with a running 3-0 polyglactin (Vicryl) suture. Two running 3-0 chromic sutures were used to approximate the subcutaneous tissue and Colles' fascia, separately, obliterating any dead space. The skin was closed with interrupted 3-0 chromic sutures. The cystostomy site was left to close by secondary intent and covered with a sterile dressing.

The perineal incision was covered with a sterile dressing and gauze fluffs, and an athletic supporter was applied to help minimize swelling.

The patient was repositioned supine and the urethral catheter was connected to a drainage bag and taped to the abdominal wall.

At the end of the procedure, all counts were correct.

The patient tolerated the procedure well and was taken to the recovery room in satisfactory condition.

Estimated blood loss: Approximately _____ ml

65

Transsphincteric Rectourethral Fistula Repair (York-Mason Procedure)

Indications

- Small, post-surgical rectourethral fistulas

Essential Steps

1) Perform a cystoscopy and pass a small catheter across the fistula.
2) Reposition the patient in prone jackknife.
3) Make an incision from the tip of the coccyx to the anal verge.
4) Divide the anal sphincter muscles at the midline, placing paired sutures at each level to facilitate realignment.
5) Incise the posterior rectal wall longitudinally and identify the fistula anteriorly.
6) Excise the entire fistulous tract and separate the urethra from the rectal wall.
7) Close the urethra in one and the anterior rectal wall in two perpendicular layers.
8) Reapproximate the posterior rectal wall in two layers.
9) Place a drain and maintain a urethral catheter.

Note These Variations

- A colonoscopy can be performed, in addition to the cystoscopy, at the onset of the procedure.
- Fecal (bowel) diversion may be performed at the time of the repair.
- The incision can be extended superiorly to the left of the coccyx for improved visualization.
- With a concomitant urethral stricture, the fistula can be addressed through an anterior transsphincteric approach, with the patient in dorsal lithotomy position.

Complications

- Infection
- Fecal/urinary incontinence
- Recurrent/persistent fistula

Operative Dictations in Urologic Surgery, First Edition. Noel A. Armenakas, John A. Fracchia, and Ron Golan.
© 2019 John Wiley & Sons Ltd. Published 2019 by John Wiley & Sons Ltd.

- Increased flatulence
- Anal stenosis
- Urethral stricture

Template Operative Dictation

Preoperative diagnosis: Rectourethral fistula
Postoperative diagnosis: Same
Procedure: Transsphincteric posterior rectourethral fistula repair
Indication: The patient is a _____-year-old male with a post-prostatectomy rectourethral fistula presenting for reconstruction.
Description of Procedure: The indications, alternatives, benefits, and risks were discussed with the patient and informed consent was obtained.

The patient was brought into the operating room positioned supine on the stretcher, and secured with a safety strap. Pneumatic compression devices were placed on the lower extremities.

Intravenous antibiotics and general endotracheal anesthesia were administered and a time-out was completed, verifying the correct patient, surgical procedure, and positioning, prior to beginning the procedure.

A *flexible/22 Fr rigid* cystoscope was advanced into the bladder and the fistula identified at the bladder neck. A 5 Fr open-ended catheter was used to intubate the fistula. The cystoscope was removed and replaced with an 18 Fr urethral catheter, which was connected to a drainage bag.

The patient was transferred from the stretcher onto the operating table and carefully positioned prone with two chest rolls. The arms were brought overhead with the elbows flexed at 90°. The table was maximally flexed, raising the hips and lowering the head and body in a jackknife position. All extremities were carefully padded, and the patient was well secured to the table with 3 in. tape and safety straps. The lower back, buttocks and upper thighs were prepped and draped in the standard sterile manner.

The radiographic images were in the room.

A vertical incision was made from the coccyx to the anal verge and taken down through the subcutaneous tissue using electrocautery. A self-retaining retractor (e.g. Lone Star, Parks) was appropriately positioned to optimize exposure.

The posterior anal sphincter was identified and the muscular layers individually divided at the midline, layer-by-layer. Paired 3-0 polyglactin (Vicryl) sutures were placed systematically at each level to facilitate subsequent realignment. The posterior rectal wall was exposed, incised longitudinally in the midline and retracted laterally. The open-ended catheter was identified exiting the fistula from the anterior rectal wall. The fistula was dissected circumferentially and mobilized proximally. The entire fistulous tract and surrounding inflammatory tissue were excised and the open-ended catheter removed. The urethra was further separated from the rectal wall using sharp dissection and closed with a running 4-0 poliglecaprone (Monocryl) suture over the previously placed urethral catheter. The anterior rectal wall was closed in two perpendicular layers, using interrupted 2-0 Vicryl sutures. The deep layer incorporated the rectal muscularis and submucosa, whereas the superficial layer imbricated the anterior rectal mucosa over the first layer in a "vest-over-pants" configuration.

The posterior rectal wall was closed in two layers using running 2-0 Vicryl sutures. The previously placed anal sphincter sutures were individually tied, anatomically restoring the muscle components. A surgical drain (e.g. Jackson-Pratt, 0.25 in. Penrose) was positioned under the presacral fascia, brought out through a separate stab incision and secured at the skin with a 2-0 silk suture.

The incision was closed using a running 3-0 chromic suture on Colles' fascia and interrupted 2-0 chromic sutures on the skin. A sterile dressing was applied and the patient was repositioned supine on the stretcher.

At the end of the procedure, all counts were correct.

The patient tolerated the procedure without difficulty and was taken to the recovery room in satisfactory condition.

Estimated blood loss: Approximately _____ml

66

Transverse Circular Penile Fasciocutaneous Flap Urethroplasty (McAninch Procedure)

Indications

- Long penile urethral strictures

Essential Steps

1) Mark a 2 cm wide area of penile skin circumferentially, 5 mm proximal to the corona.
2) Using the markings, create a thick, well-vascularized fasciocutaneous flap by degloving the penis above the dartos muscle proximally and below the superficial Buck's fascia distally. Maintain the subdermal plexus with the penile skin to avoid necrosis.
3) Divide the penile skin island and its pedicle, either ventrally or dorsally, preserving the healthier blood supply.
4) Rotate the skin island 90° and position it ventrally, parallel to the urethra, without tension.
5) Incise the entire length of the urethral stricture ventrally and calibrate the urethra to 26 or 28 Fr.
6) Invert the skin island over the incised urethra, tailor it appropriately, and suture it to the corpus spongiosum.
7) Complete the penile skin closure.

Note These Variations

- For shorter strictures or strictures limited to the glanular urethra, a rectangular ventrally based penile fasciocutaneous flap can be created, limiting circumferential penile dissection.
- Another option is to create a longitudinal penile flap (Orandi, Turner-Warwick); however, this should not be extended proximally into hair-bearing penile skin.
- For longer defects, the transverse circular fasciocutaneous flap can be modified as a Q-flap incorporating an additional mid-ventral longitudinal extension (Quartey procedure).
- In an uncircumcised patient, the inner prepuce, rather than penile skin, should be used for the flap.
- A hemostaic sealant (e.g. fibrin glue) can be used in conjunction with the anastomotic sutures to reinforce the repair.

Operative Dictations in Urologic Surgery, First Edition. Noel A. Armenakas, John A. Fracchia, and Ron Golan.
© 2019 John Wiley & Sons Ltd. Published 2019 by John Wiley & Sons Ltd.

Complications

- Bleeding
- Infection
- Urine leak
- Penile torsion
- Postvoid dribbling
- Flap sacculation
- Decreased penile sensitivity
- Erectile/ejaculatory dysfunction
- Neuropraxia
- Urethrocutaneous fistula
- Penile skin necrosis
- Recurrent stricture

Template Operative Dictation

Preoperative diagnosis: Penile urethral stricture
Postoperative diagnosis: Same
Procedure: Penile circular fasciocutaneous flap urethroplasty
Indications: The patient is a ____-year-old male with a ____cm penile urethral stricture presenting for a penile circular fasciocutaneous flap for urethral reconstruction.
Description of Procedure: The indications, alternatives, benefits, and risks were discussed with the patient and informed consent was obtained.

The patient was brought onto the operating room table, positioned supine, and secured with a safety strap. Pneumatic compression devices were placed on the lower extremities.

After the administration of intravenous antibiotics and *general endotracheal/regional* anesthesia, the genitalia, perineum, and lower abdomen were prepped and draped in the standard sterile manner.

The radiographic images were in the room.

A time-out was completed, verifying the correct patient, surgical procedure, and positioning, prior to beginning the procedure.

A 2-0 nylon (Ethilon) traction suture was placed through the anterior mid glans and the penis placed on stretch. Using optical magnification with surgical loupes, the penile skin was marked circumferentially 5 mm proximal to the corona. A second circumferential mark was made exactly 2 cm proximal to this, outlining the circular flap.

An incision was made over the distal skin marking and taken down through the dartos and superficial Buck's fascias. A second *superficial* circumferential skin incision was made over the proximal marking, staying above the dartos fascia. The dissection was continued proximally to the base of the penis, maintaining the subdermal plexus with the penile skin. The penis was degloved to the penoscrotal junction, creating a 2 cm circular ring of penile skin supported by a robust well-vascularized pedicle. Meticulous hemostasis was achieved using bipolar electrocautery.

The penile skin island and its pedicle were sharply divided *ventrally/dorsally*, rotated 90°, and transposed without tension adjacent to the urethra.

A self-retaining retractor (e.g. Lone Star) was appropriately positioned to optimize exposure and an 18 Fr red rubber catheter was advanced per the urethral meatus to the stricture. The urethra was incised over the distal tip of the catheter on its ventral surface. The midline urethrotomy was extended proximally into healthy tissue, exposing the entire area of stricture. Multiple 4-0 chromic stay sutures were placed on the lateral edges of the incised urethra for traction. Bougie-à-boule dilators were used to progressively calibrate the urethra to 26/28 Fr.

Cystourethroscopy was performed, using a *flexible/___Fr rigid* cystoscope, confirming the absence of any proximal urethral or bladder pathology.

The urethral defect was measured at _____cm and the skin island tailored accordingly to fit the defect. The skin island was inverted over the incised urethra and its pedicle edge secured to the corresponding lateral border of the corpus spongiosum using a running 5-0 polydioxanone (PDS) suture. The proximal and distal apical edges of the skin island were sutured to the corresponding ventral wall of the corpus spongiosum using interrupted full-thickness 5-0 PDS sutures. The remaining free edge of the skin island was then sutured to the contralateral border of the corpus spongiosum with a running 5-0 PDS suture. Prior to completing the anastomosis, a *16/18* Fr urethral catheter was easily advanced into the bladder.

Having completed a tension-free urethral repair, the penis was thoroughly inspected and hemostasis obtained. The wound was irrigated with sterile normal saline and the self-retaining retractor was removed.

The penile skin was advanced distally and sutured to the subcoronal border with four-quadrant 3-0 chromic sutures. Similar interrupted sutures were placed between these in a circumferential manner, approximating the remainder of the incision.

The subcoronal incision was covered with a sterile dressing and the penis wrapped loosely with a self-adherent (Coban) dressing, prior to removing the glans suture.

The urethral catheter was connected to a drainage bag and taped to the abdominal wall to limit postoperative swelling.

At the end of the procedure, all counts were correct.

The patient tolerated the procedure well and was taken to the recovery room in satisfactory condition.

Estimated blood loss: Approximately _____ml

67

Urethrectomy (Male)

Indications

- Primary urethral carcinoma
- Urothelial carcinoma involving the prostatic urethra
- Urethral recurrence after radical cystectomy

Essential Steps

1) Make a vertical midline perineal incision to expose the bulbar urethra.
2) Dissect the urethra circumferentially and mobilize it distally to the base of the glans penis.
3) Circumscribe the urethral meatus and dissect it down through the entire glanular portion to liberate the urethra distally.
4) Continue the dissection proximally, freeing the proximal bulbar and membranous urethral segments. In patients who have had a cystectomy, this dissection should be performed very carefully with limited electrocoagulation to avoid injury to potentially adherent bowel.
5) Remove the entire urethra *en bloc*.
6) Complete a multilayer closure.

Note these Variations

- Often, a urethrectomy is performed *en bloc* with a cystectomy.
- In females, a total urethrectomy is performed almost exclusively in conjunction with an anterior exenteration through a periurethral circumscribing or horseshoe incision.
- An inverted-U or -Y incision (also referred to as a "lambda" incision) can be used to expose the bulbar urethra.
- Placement of a tourniquet at the base of the penis may limit bleeding during the glanular urethral dissection.
- The use of a drain is optional.

Operative Dictations in Urologic Surgery, First Edition. Noel A. Armenakas, John A. Fracchia, and Ron Golan.
© 2019 John Wiley & Sons Ltd. Published 2019 by John Wiley & Sons Ltd.

Complications

- Bleeding
- Infection
- Abscess
- Bowel injury
- Erectile dysfunction

Template Operative Dictation

Preoperative diagnosis: Urethral carcinoma
Postoperative diagnosis: Same
Procedure: Total urethrectomy
Indications: The patient is a ____-year-old male with *a ____cm urethral carcinoma/a urothelial carcinoma involving the prostate/positive urethral washings* presenting for a total urethrectomy.
Description of Procedure: The indications, alternatives, benefits, and risks were discussed with the patient and informed consent was obtained.

The patient was brought onto the operating room table, positioned supine, and secured with a safety strap. Pneumatic compression devices were placed on the lower extremities.

After the administration of intravenous antibiotics and *general endotracheal/regional* anesthesia, the patient was repositioned in high dorsal lithotomy using well-padded universal (Allen) stirrups. A gel bolster was placed under the buttocks to support and rotate the pelvis. The genitalia, perineum, and lower abdomen were prepped and draped in the standard sterile manner.

A time-out was completed, verifying the correct patient, surgical procedure, and positioning, prior to beginning the procedure.

A vertical midline perineal skin incision was made, extending from the base of the scrotum to just above the anus. Colles' fascia and the subcutaneous tissues were incised with electrocautery, exposing the bulbospongiosus muscle. The muscle was sharply divided in the midline and carefully dissected off the underlying corpus spongiosum. A self-retaining retractor (e.g. Lone Star, Bookwalter) was appropriately positioned to optimize exposure.

An 18 Fr urethral catheter was advanced into the bladder and clamped. The mid-bulbar urethra was dissected circumferentially, freeing it dorsally from the corporal bodies. A 0.25 in. Penrose drain was placed around the urethra at this level for traction.

Using a combination of sharp and blunt dissection, the bulbar urethra was mobilized distally to the suspensory ligament of the penis, releasing it from the tunica albuginea of the corpora cavernosa.

The penis was invaginated providing exposure of the penile urethra, which was similarly dissected off the cavernosal tunica albuginea to the base of the glans penis. Care was taken to not perforate the tunica albuginea of the corpus cavernosa.

The penis was returned to its normal position and attention directed to the urethral meatus. A perimeatal circumscribing incision was made, including a cuff of glanular skin. This was taken down through the entire glans, completely freeing the terminal

anterior urethra, which was tunneled inferiorly through the perineal incision. The defect in the glans was closed in two layers using interrupted 2-0 polyglactin (Vicryl) sutures.

Having freed the urethra distally, attention was directed proximally. The proximal bulbar urethra was freed from its posterior midline and central tendon attachments dorsally and ventrally, respectively. The paired bulbar arteries were encountered at this level, ligated with 3-0 silk ties, and divided. The dissection was continued proximally through the deep perineal space and the membranous urethra circumferentially freed from the pelvic floor using sharp and blunt dissection. Electrocautery was used very judiciously at this level to avoid thermal injury to the underlying rectum.

The urethra was removed *en bloc* and the wound was copiously irrigated with warm sterile water. Meticulous hemostasis was achieved throughout the entire procedure using electrocautery.

The self-retaining retractor was removed and the perineal wound was closed using a running 3-0 Vicryl suture to approximate the bulbospongiosus muscle. Two running 3-0 chromic sutures were used to approximate the subcutaneous tissues and Colles' fascia, separately, obliterating any dead space. The skin was closed with interrupted 3-0 chromic sutures.

The penis was wrapped with a self-adherent (Coban) dressing. The perineal incision was covered with a sterile dressing and gauze fluffs, and an athletic supporter applied to help minimize swelling. The patient was repositioned supine.

At the end of the procedure, all counts were correct.

The patient tolerated the procedure well and was taken to the recovery room in satisfactory condition.

Estimated blood loss: Approximately _____ml

Urinary Diversion

68

Appendicovesicostomy (Mitrofanoff Procedure)

Indications

- Nonurethral catheterizable continent urinary diversion in patients with a neuropathic bladder, prune belly syndrome, posterior urethral valves, etc.

Essential Steps

1) Mark out the abdominal wall skin catheterizable stoma site in advance of the procedure.
2) Identify the appendix on the posteromedial cecal wall.
3) Separate the appendix from the cecum, preserving the appendiceal arterial mesentery.
4) Mobilize the appendix with a cuff of cecum on a wide pedicle.
5) Mobilize the bladder, open it anteriorly, and create a submucosal tunnel to implant the distal end of the appendix and its mesentery.
6) Maneuver the proximal (cecal) end of the appendix to the umbilicus as a catheterizable stoma.
7) Prior to closure, irrigate the appendicovesicostomy to ensure a watertight repair; similarly ensure that the cystotomy is watertight.
8) Place a drain.

Note These Variations

- A preoperative bowel prep is optional.
- A suprapubic longitudinal skin incision (modified Pfannenstiel) may be used for the procedure.
- If preferred, the appendiceal stoma can be brought out of the abdominal wall through the right lower quadrant instead of the umbilicus.
- If the appendix is too short, a tubularized cuff of cecum can be used to increase its length. Alternatively, a psoas hitch can be performed to shorten the distance.

Operative Dictations in Urologic Surgery, First Edition. Noel A. Armenakas, John A. Fracchia, and Ron Golan.
© 2019 John Wiley & Sons Ltd. Published 2019 by John Wiley & Sons Ltd.

- In cases where the appendix is not available the Yang-Monti technique can be applied to construct a catheterizable tube, incorporating a 2 cm segment of ileum opened horizontally and tubularized longitudinally,

Complications

- Bleeding
- Infection
- Ileus/bowel obstruction
- Urinary extravasation (appendicovesical anastomosis)
- Bowel injury/leak
- Stomal stenosis/stricture
- Angulation/kinking of the catheterizable channel
- Incontinence
- Parastomal hernia
- Stone formation

Template Operative Dictation

Preoperative diagnosis: *Neuropathic bladder/Prune belly syndrome/Posterior urethral valves,* etc.
Postoperative diagnosis: Same
Procedure: Appendicovesicostomy
Indications: The patient is a _____-year-old *male/female* with *a neuropathic bladder/ prune belly syndrome/posterior urethral valves,* etc. presenting for a non-urethral catheterizable continent urinary diversion.
Description of Procedure: The indications, alternatives, benefits, and risks were discussed with the *patient/patient's family* and informed consent was obtained.

The patient was brought onto the operating room table, positioned supine (*If a child: frog leg*) and secured with a safety strap. All pressure points were carefully padded.

After the administration of intravenous antibiotics and general endotracheal anesthesia, the abdomen was prepped and draped in the standard sterile manner.

A time-out was completed, verifying the correct patient, surgical procedure, and positioning, prior to beginning the procedure.

A ___Fr urethral catheter was inserted into the bladder and connected to a drainage bag. The previously marked site for the placement of the stoma was identified.

A midline abdominal incision was made from just below the umbilicus to the pubic symphysis. The subcutaneous tissue was incised with electrocautery, exposing the underlying rectus abdominis aponeurosis. This was incised at the linea alba and the rectus abdominis muscles were separated at the midline and retracted laterally, taking care not to injure the underlying inferior epigastric vessels.

The peritoneal cavity was entered sharply, avoiding injury to the bowel. A self-retaining retractor (e.g. Bookwalter, Omni-Tract, Balfour) was appropriately positioned to optimize exposure, using padding on each retractor blade.

The cecum was identified in the right lower quadrant and carefully dissected, exposing the appendix posteromedially. The appendix was grasped with a Babcock clamp and dissected to its base. Its length was felt to be adequate for the Mitrofanoff procedure. The parietal peritoneum was incised on the white line of Toldt, and the cecum and entire ascending colon were mobilized and reflected medially to allow the cecum and appendix to reach the bladder without tension.

The appendiceal artery was identified and its mesentery preserved. The appendix, with a small cuff of adjacent cecum, was sharply separated from the cecum. The cecal opening was closed in two layers, using running and interrupted 3-0 polyglactin (Vicryl) sutures for the mucosal and seromuscular layers, respectively.

The distal end of the appendix was sharply opened, irrigated with sterile normal saline and intubated with a 12 Fr red rubber catheter, ensuring an adequate luminal size.

Attention was turned to the bladder, which was mobilized to reach the previously marked stomal site at the umbilicus without tension. The anterior aspect of the bladder was opened and a 3 cm submucosal tunnel was created using sharp dissection. The distal end of the appendix was passed through the bladder hiatus into the submucosal tunnel and spatulated. The appendix was anchored to the detrusor wall with four full-thickness interrupted 4-0 Vicryl sutures. The appendicovesical anastomosis was completed using 4-0 chromic sutures, securing the appendix to the bladder mucosa. The bladder was anchored to the posterior abdominal wall to ensure that the appendix remains properly positioned, avoiding angulation. A 12 Fr red rubber catheter was used to catheterize the channel, confirming its proper unobstructed orientation.

A U-shaped skin incision was made at the umbilicus for stomal placement and dissected inferiorly to the underlying rectus fascia. The fascia was opened using a cruciate incision, permitting the passage of an index finger without difficulty. The appendix was gently grasped with a Babcock clamp and brought through the fascial and umbilical skin openings. The appendix was sutured to the posterior fascial wall with 3-0 Vicryl sutures, taking care not to compromise its mesentery.

The cecal end of the appendix was spatulated on its antimesenteric border and sutured to the skin and subcuticular edges of the stoma with interrupted 4-0 Vicryl sutures. The appendicovesicostomy was again intubated with the 12 Fr red rubber catheter, which was secured to the skin with a 2-0 silk suture.

The bladder was closed in two layers using 3-0 and 2-0 Vicryl sutures on the mucosal and muscularis and adventitial layers, respectively. The patency of the repair was confirmed by irrigating the urethral catheter with sterile normal saline.

The abdomen and pelvis were irrigated with warm sterile saline and inspected for any bleeding. Meticulous hemostasis was achieved with electrocautery. A surgical drain (e.g. Jackson-Pratt, 0.25 in. Penrose) was placed posterior to the bladder repair and brought out through a right lower quadrant stab wound where it was secured at the skin with a 3-0 silk suture. Prior to closure, the bowel, mesentery, ureters, bladder, appendiceal stoma, and abdominal wall were inspected and found to be intact.

The self-retaining retractor was removed and the abdominal incision was closed using a running 2-0 chromic to approximate the rectus muscles and 1-0 polydioxanone (PDS) for the rectus aponeurosis. 3-0 chromic sutures were used on Scarpa's fascia and the skin approximated with a subcuticular 4-0 poliglecaprone (Monocryl)

suture. The incision was reinforced with sterile adhesive strips and a sterile dressing was applied.

A stomal appliance was placed over the appendiceal stoma and the 12 Fr red rubber catheter.

At the end of the procedure, all counts were correct.

The patient tolerated the procedure well and was taken to the recovery room in satisfactory condition.

Estimated blood loss: Approximately _____ ml

69

Ileal Conduit

Indications

- Urinary diversion following extirpative pelvic surgery
- End-stage neurogenic bladder
- Total urinary incontinence
- Obstructive uropathy (e.g. secondary to radiation therapy for a pelvic malignancy, etc.)

Essential Steps

1) Mark out the abdominal skin stoma site in advance of the procedure.
2) Isolate and divide a 20–25 cm segment of distal ileum approximately 15–20 cm from the ileocecal valve. Use transillumination to identify the vascular arcades.
3) Perform a functional end-to-end ileoileal anastomosis, restoring bowel continuity.
4) Mobilize the ureters with their adventitia so the ureteral anastomoses rest without tension on the ileal loop.
5) Spatulate the distal ureters to create individual wide end-to-side ureteroileal anastomoses (Bricker).
6) Create a urinary stoma ideally suitable for the patient's body habitus.
7) Ensure that all suture lines are watertight.
8) Place a drain.

Note These Variations

- A preoperative bowel prep is optional.
- The ileoileal anastomosis and "butt" end of the loop may be hand sewn, using a two-layer technique.
- A conjoined end-to-end (Wallace) ureteroileal anastomosis can be performed.
- In obese patients with a short mesentery, an end-loop stoma can be created, positioning the defunctionalized short-limb cephalad.

Operative Dictations in Urologic Surgery, First Edition. Noel A. Armenakas, John A. Fracchia, and Ron Golan.
© 2019 John Wiley & Sons Ltd. Published 2019 by John Wiley & Sons Ltd.

Complications

- Bleeding
- Infection
- Ileus/bowel obstruction
- Urinary leak (conduit, ureteroileal anastomoses)
- Bowel injury/leak
- Ureteral obstruction/stricture
- Parastomal hernia
- Stomal stenosis
- Pyelonephritis
- Stone formation
- Metabolic abnormalities (hypokalemic, hyperchloremic metabolic acidosis)
- Vitamin B_{12} deficiency and bile salt malabsorption
- Renal failure

Template Operative Dictation

Preoperative diagnosis: Need for urinary diversion *(e.g. following extirpative pelvic surgery, neuropathic bladder, total urinary incontinence, obstructive uropathy)*
Postoperative diagnosis: Same
Procedure: Ileal conduit
Indications: The patient is a _____-year-old *male/female* with *a neuropathic bladder/ total urinary incontinence/obstructive uropathy/* _____ presenting for an ileal conduit.
Description of Procedure: The indications, alternatives, benefits, and risks were discussed with the patient and informed consent was obtained.

The patient was brought onto the operating room table, positioned supine, and secured with a safety strap. All pressure points were carefully padded and pneumatic compression devices were placed on the lower extremities.

After the administration of intravenous antibiotics and general endotracheal anesthesia, the entire abdomen was prepped and draped in the standard sterile manner.

A time-out was completed, verifying the correct patient, surgical procedure, and positioning, prior to beginning the procedure. *(A 16 Fr urethral catheter was inserted into the bladder and connected to a drainage bag.)* The preoperatively marked stomal site was identified on the *right/left* lower abdominal quadrant.

A midline abdominal incision was made starting just above the umbilicus and carried down to the pubic symphysis. The subcutaneous tissue was incised with electrocautery, exposing the underlying rectus abdominis aponeurosis. This was incised at the linea alba and the rectus abdominis muscles separated at the midline and retracted laterally, taking care not to injure the underlying inferior epigastric vessels.

The peritoneal cavity was entered sharply, avoiding any injury to the bowel. A self-retaining retractor (e.g. Bookwalter, Omni-Tract, Balfour) was appropriately positioned to optimize exposure, using padding on each retractor blade. The peritoneal contents were examined. There was no evidence of any inflammatory ileal or metastatic disease. The ileal mesentery appeared to be of sufficient length to reach the stomal site without tension.

The bowel contents were packed superiorly and the posterior peritoneum was incised at the level of the pelvic inlet over the iliac vessels, exposing both ureters. The ureters were carefully mobilized, preserving their blood supply, and transected close to the bladder between large hemoclips.

> ***In patients with a history of irradiation or urothelial cancer:*** A small segment of each distal ureter was sent to pathology for frozen section evaluation.

A 3-0 chromic tag suture was placed on the end of each severed ureter to aid in manipulation of the ureter to the subsequently created ileal conduit.

The bowel packing was removed, and attention was focused on isolating an appropriate ileal segment. The distal ileum was inspected and a 25 cm segment of ileum was chosen, 15–20 cm from the ileocecal valve and marked with a silk suture. With the aid of transillumination, the ileocolic and right colic arteries were identified. An avascular mesenteric window was opened on each side of the desired ileal segment using an electrothermal bipolar tissue sealing device (LigaSure) to incise and ligate the mesentery on both sides, avoiding injury to the main intestinal vasculature. *(Alternatively, the mesentery can be incised and its blood vessels individually clamped, divided and doubly ligated with chromic or silk ties.)* Additional hemostasis was achieved using 3-0 *chromic/silk* ties. Sufficient mesenteric length was obtained to allow the distal end of the ileal conduit to reach the stomal site without tension.

The isolated ileal segment was transected at its proximal and distal antimesenteric borders, using a GIA60 stapler. The "butt" end of the ileal conduit was marked and the conduit placed caudal to the defect in the small intestine.

The continuity of the ileum was restored using a stapled technique as follows: The antimesenteric corners of the proximal and distal ileal segments were identified, and a small segment of tissue was resected off each end of the stapled suture lines. One limb of the GIA60 stapler was inserted into the proximal and the other into the distal ileal segment with care taken not to injure the bowel mesentery. The ileal segments were rotated ensuring that the antimesenteric bowel walls faced each other prior to firing the stapler. Four small clamps were then placed on the ends of the transected bowel. The two clamps on the lines of the original bowel transection were held together, while the others were spread apart, creating a wide opening. A TA55 stapler was used to complete the functional end-to-end ileoileal anastomosis. The staple line was checked confirming its integrity, and was additionally reinforced with interrupted 3-0 silk sutures. The mesenteric window was closed with a running 4-0 chromic to avoid internal herniation.

The left ureter was identified with its tagged suture and mobilized cephalad taking care not to injure the ureteral vessels. The sigmoid mesentery was elevated superiorly and the posterior peritoneum was identified. An avascular space anterior to the great vessels was identified and created. The left ureteral tag suture was grasped with a right-angle clamp and brought to the right lower quadrant adjacent to the ileal conduit, without tension, through an opening created in the sigmoid mesocolon. Similarly, the right ureter was identified, carefully mobilized cephalad and placed adjacent to the ileal conduit. Both ureters were spatulated on the medial surface for a distance of 5–6 mm.

The conduit was irrigated with sterile normal saline until the returns were clear. A 1 cm seromuscular incision was made in the wall of the ileal conduit and the underlying

mucosa excised with a Potts scissors. A tonsil clamp was passed through the distal end of the ileal conduit and the ipsilateral ureteral tag suture individually grasped positioning the ureter at the ileal opening. Each ureteroileal anastomosis was completed using full-thickness 4-0 interrupted chromic sutures. Several additional sutures were placed in the ureteral adventitia and ileal muscular layer to reinforce the anastomosis.

Note: If desired, the ureteroileal anastomosis can be completed over single-J stents or infant feeding tubes, which exit through the stoma. These can be guided through the conduit using either a Kelly clamp or a suction tip catheter.

The stoma was created by making a 2.5 cm opening in the skin *(with the aid of an outline from the plunger of a 20 cc luer lock syringe)* at the previously determined stomal site. The underlying fascia was identified and opened using a cruciate incision. Two fingers were inserted through the fascia and the distal end of the conduit was brought through the skin, for a distance of 4–5 cm, with the aid of a Babcock clamp. 3-0 polyglactin (Vicryl) sutures were placed into each quadrant of the fascia and into the seromuscular ileum to anchor the conduit to the underlying fascia. Interrupted 3-0 chromic sutures were placed through the distal conduit's seromuscular bowel layer and the subcutaneous tissue, everting the stoma.

A 16 Fr multieyed catheter was advanced into the lumen of the conduit and its proximal end positioned near the "butt" end. Gentle irrigation confirmed the absence of any leaks. The catheter was secured to the abdominal wall, adjacent to the stoma, with a 3-0 silk suture.

> ***For stented anastomoses:*** The ureteral stents were affixed to the stomal mucosa using 3-0 *chromic/plain gut* sutures.

Having completed the ileal conduit, the abdomen was irrigated with warm sterile normal saline and examined for any bleeding. Meticulous hemostasis was obtained with electrocautery. A surgical drain (e.g. Jackson-Pratt) was placed in the retroperitoneum and brought out at the skin through a separate stab incision, where it was secured with a 2-0 silk suture. Prior to closure, the ureters, bowel, mesentery, conduit, stoma, and abdominal wall were inspected and found to be intact without any evidence of bleeding or injury.

The self-retaining retractor was removed and the abdominal incision was closed using a running 2-0 chromic to approximate the rectus muscles and 1-0 polydioxanone (PDS) for the rectus aponeurosis. The subcutaneous tissue was approximated with 3-0 chromic sutures and the skin was closed with staples.

The incision was covered with a sterile dressing and a stomal appliance fitted in a watertight fashion.

At the end of the procedure, all counts were correct.

The patient tolerated the procedure without difficulty and was taken to the recovery room in satisfactory condition.

Estimated blood loss: Approximately _____ml

70

Ileocecal Reservoir (Indiana Pouch)

Indications

- Urinary diversion following extirpative pelvic surgery or in patients with intractable urinary incontinence or fistula, without renal or hepatic dysfunction.

Essential Steps

1) Carefully select patients (i.e. motivated and diligent to perform timely catheterizations and irrigations as well as adhere to initially frequent postoperative visits). The serum creatinine should be below 2.0 ng/ml with a creatinine clearance >60 cc/min.
2) Mark out the abdominal skin catheterizable stoma site in advance of the procedure. During the procedure, confirm that the ileal efferent limb reaches in a straight, tension-free, easily catheterizable position.
3) Isolate and divide an ileocolonic segment, incorporating 25–30 cm of right colon and 7–10 cm of terminal ileum. Use transillumination to identify the vascular arcades.
4) Perform a functional end-to-end ileocolonic anastomosis, restoring bowel continuity.
5) Taper the terminal ileum and imbricate the ileocecal valve to assist with continence.
6) Close the reservoir by folding the anterior colonic wall.
7) Perform antirefluxing ureterocolonic anastomoses by tunneling each ureter in a tenial groove.
8) Position the efferent limb through the selected abdominal site and complete the stoma.
9) Ensure that all suture lines are watertight.
10) Place a drain.

Note These Variations

- A preoperative bowel prep is optional.
- The ileocolonic anastomosis can be hand-sewn using a two-layer technique.

Operative Dictations in Urologic Surgery, First Edition. Noel A. Armenakas, John A. Fracchia, and Ron Golan.
© 2019 John Wiley & Sons Ltd. Published 2019 by John Wiley & Sons Ltd.

- If the reservoir is too short or narrow, consider augmenting the cecum with an ileal patch.
- The umbilicus may be used as the stomal site in select patients.

Complications

- Bleeding
- Infection
- Ileus/bowel obstruction
- Urinary leak (reservoir, ureterocolonic anastomosis)
- Bowel injury/leak
- Difficulty catheterizing with/without mucus plugs
- Incontinence
- Ureteral obstruction/stricture
- Stomal stenosis
- Parastomal hernia
- Pyelonephritis
- Stone formation
- Metabolic abnormalities (hypokalemic, hyperchloremic metabolic acidosis)
- Vitamin B_{12} deficiency and bile salt malabsorption
- Chronic diarrhea
- Renal failure

Template Operative Dictation

Preoperative diagnosis: Need for urinary diversion due to _____.
Postoperative diagnosis: Same
Procedure: Ileocecal reservoir
Indications: The patient is a ____-year-old *male/female* with _____ presenting for an ileocecal reservoir.
Description of Procedure: The indications, alternatives, benefits, and risks were discussed with the patient and informed consent was obtained.

The patient was brought onto the operating room table, positioned supine, and secured with a safety strap. All pressure points were carefully padded and pneumatic compression devices were placed on the lower extremities.

After the administration of intravenous antibiotics and general endotracheal anesthesia, the entire abdomen was prepped and draped in the standard sterile manner.

A time-out was completed, verifying the correct patient, surgical procedure, and positioning, prior to beginning the procedure. The previously identified stomal site was marked on the *right/left* lower abdominal quadrant.

A midline abdominal incision was made, starting 4 cm above the umbilicus and carried down to the pubic symphysis. The subcutaneous tissue was incised with electrocautery, exposing the underlying rectus abdominis aponeurosis. This was incised at the linea alba and the rectus abdominis muscles were separated at the midline and retracted laterally, taking care not to injure the underlying inferior epigastric vessels.

The peritoneal cavity was entered sharply, avoiding injury to the bowel. A self-retaining retractor (e.g. Bookwalter, Omni-Tract, Balfour) was appropriately positioned to optimize exposure, using padding on each retractor blade. The peritoneal contents were examined. There was no evidence of any inflammatory bowel or metastatic disease.

The bowel contents were packed superiorly and the posterior peritoneum was incised at the level of the pelvic inlet over the iliac vessels, exposing both ureters. The ureters were carefully mobilized maintaining their blood supply, and transected close to the bladder between large hemoclips.

> ***In patients with a history of irradiation or urothelial cancer:*** A small segment of each distal ureter was sent to pathology for frozen-section evaluation.

A 3-0 chromic tag suture was placed on the end of each severed ureter to aid in manipulation of the ureters to the subsequently created ileal neobladder.

The bowel packing was removed, and attention was focused on isolating an appropriate bowel segment. The terminal ileum and right colon were inspected and an ileocolonic segment incorporating approximately 10 cm of terminal ileum and 25 cm of right colon was chosen from proximal to the ileocecal valve to the hepatic flexure. With the aid of transillumination, the vascular arcades were identified. An avascular mesenteric window was opened on each side of the desired ileocolonic segment using an electrothermal bipolar tissue sealing device (LigaSure) to incise and ligate the mesentery on both sides, avoiding injury to the main intestinal vasculature. *(Alternatively, the mesentery can be incised and its traversing blood vessels individually clamped, divided and doubly ligated with chromic or silk ties.)* Additional meticulous hemostasis was achieved using 3-0 *chromic/silk* ties. The isolated ileocolonic segment was transected at is proximal and distal antimesenteric border, using a GIA60 stapler.

The continuity of the bowel was restored using a stapled anastomosis as follows: The antimesenteric corners of the ileum and right colon were identified and a small segment of tissue was resected off each end of the stapled suture lines. One limb of the GIA60 stapler was inserted into the incised right colon and the other into the distal ileal segment, taking care not to injure the bowel mesentery. The bowel segments were rotated, ensuring that the antimesenteric bowel walls faced each other prior to firing the stapler. Four small clamps were then placed on the ends of the transected bowel. The two clamps on the lines of the original bowel transection were held together, while the others were spread apart, creating a wide opening. A TA55 stapler was used to complete the functional end-to-end ileocolonic anastomosis. The staple line was checked, confirming its integrity, and additionally reinforced with interrupted 3-0 silk sutures. The mesenteric window was closed with a running 4-0 chromic to avoid internal herniation. The ileocolonic anastomosis was returned to its natural position in the abdomen with the isolated bowel segment placed caudal to it.

The appendix was removed by dividing the appendiceal artery between 3-0 polyglactin (Vicryl) ties. A purse-string 2-0 Vicryl suture was placed around the base of the appendix at the cecum and the appendix sharply resected and sent for pathologic evaluation. The stump of the appendix was inverted into the cecum using a similar suture.

The isolated ileocolonic segment was irrigated clear with sterile normal saline and the right colon was incised on its antimesenteric border between the tinea proceeding toward to the cecum, sparing the cecal cap.

With the right colon open, attention was turned to tapering the ileum and plicating the ileocecal valve. The catheterizable efferent limb was tapered by placing a 12 Fr red rubber catheter through the ileum into the reservoir. Babcock clamps were used to create a snug fit around the catheter. A GIA75 stapler was placed adjacent to the Babcock clamps and fired, removing the redundant ileum up to its entrance into the cecum. Imbricating Lembert 2-0 silk sutures were placed to plicate the ileocecal valve. Upon completion of the efferent limb, the 12 Fr catheter was replaced with a 14 Fr red rubber catheter, ensuring that there was no obstruction. Continence was confirmed by distending the reservoir with sterile normal saline, without visible leakage through the efferent ileal limb.

The reservoir was closed utilizing the Heineke-Mikulicz technique by suturing the cephalad end of the detubularized right colon caudally to the apex of the antimesenteric incision, in one layer, using 3-0 Vicryl sutures. A 24-Fr Malecot catheter was placed in the cecal cap and anchored to the reservoir with a 2-0 chromic suture. The reservoir was irrigated and distended with sterile normal saline, confirming a watertight suture line.

Next, attention was focused on the ureteral anastomoses. Both ureters were identified and carefully mobilized. The left ureter and its investing tissue were passed underneath the mesentery and brought to the posterior aspect of the reservoir, taking care not to place the ureter under any tension. The right ureter was advanced directly to the posterior aspect of the reservoir. The reservoir was rotated cephalad and a small amount of adipose tissue on the posterior lateral aspect of the cecum was removed to facilitate the anastomoses. The ureters were spatulated and implanted into separate tenial tunnels. The sites of the neoureteral orifices were created by incising the colonic mucosa, and single-layer ureteromucosal anastomoses were completed using interrupted 4-0 chromic sutures. Additional serosal sutures were placed to reinforce the anastomoses. Each tenial tunnel was reapproximated, creating antirefluxing reimplantations. 7 Fr single-J ureteral stents were placed with their distal ends brought out through the reservoir wall. The stents were secured to the cecal wall with 4-0 chromic sutures to prevent dislocation.

The stoma was created at the preselected site in the *right/left* lower quadrant by making a 1.5 cm opening through the abdominal wall. A cruciate incision was made in the anterior rectus fascia and the efferent limb brought out through the abdominal defect. Four, 3-0 Vicryl sutures were placed to secure the efferent limb to the fascia. Additional similar sutures were used to approximate the efferent limb to the skin, creating a flush stoma.

The Malecot cecosotomy tube and the ureteral stents were brought out through a *right/left* lower abdominal stab incision caudal to the stoma. A surgical drain (e.g. Jackson-Pratt) was placed inferior to the reservoir and brought out through a separate incision in the contralateral lower quadrant. All tubes were secured at the abdominal skin with 2-0 silk sutures.

Having completed the reconstruction, the reservoir was again distended with sterile normal saline, ensuring the creation of a watertight reservoir without any clots. Prior to closure, the abdominal cavity was carefully inspected and irrigated with warm sterile water.

The ureters, bowel, mesentery, and abdominal wall were intact without any evidence of bleeding or injury.

The self-retaining retractor was removed and the abdominal incision was closed using a running 2-0 chromic to approximate the rectus muscles and 1-0 polydioxanone (PDS) for the rectus aponeurosis. The subcutaneous tissue was approximated with 3-0 chromic sutures and the skin was closed with staples. A sterile dressing was applied.

At the end of the procedure, all counts were correct.

The patient tolerated the procedure without difficulty and was taken to the recovery room in satisfactory condition.

Estimated blood loss: Approximately _____ml

The ureters, bowel, mesentery and abdominal wall were intact without any evidence of bleeding of injury.

The self-retaining retractor was removed and the abdominal incision was closed using a running 2-0 chromic to approximate the rectus muscles and 1-0 polydioxanone (PDS) for the rectus aponeurosis. The subcutaneous tissue was approximated with 3-0 chromic suture and the skin was closed with staples. A sterile dressing was applied.

At the end of the procedure, all counts were correct.

The patient tolerated the procedure without difficulty and was taken to the recovery room in stable condition.

71

Orthotopic Ileal Neobladder (Hautmann Pouch)

Indications

- Urinary diversion following extirpative pelvic surgery in motivated patients without renal or hepatic dysfunction.

Essential Steps

1) Carefully select patients (e.g. negative prostatic/bladder neck biopsies, absence of bladder CIS, adequate renal and hepatic function, no active inflammatory bowel disease or prior extensive bowel resection, proper motivation, compliance, and physical dexterity). The serum creatinine should be below 2.0 ng/ml with a creatinine clearance >60 cc/min.
2) Isolate and divide a 60 cm segment of distal ileum that will reach the urethral stump without tension. Use transillumination to identify the vascular arcades.
3) Perform a functional end-to-end ileoileal anastomosis, restoring bowel continuity.
4) Detubularize the ileum by incising it along its antimesenteric border, fashion it into a W-configuration, and suture the four limbs to one another, posteriorly.
5) Spatulate the ureters and anastomose them to the afferent limb of the neobladder.
6) Perform a mucosa-to-mucosa ileourethral anastomosis.
7) Fold the ileum, closing the anterior wall of the reservoir.
8) Ensure that all suture lines are watertight.
9) Place a drain.

Note These Variations

- A preoperative bowel prep is optional.
- There are many variations of ileal neobladders, including the Kock ileal reservoir (which incorporates an afferent intussuscepted nipple valve), the Studer ileal pouch (which uses a U-configuration with an isoperistaltic afferent limb), the Mainz ileocolonic reservoir (which additionally uses a 15 cm segment of cecum), and the T-pouch

Operative Dictations in Urologic Surgery, First Edition. Noel A. Armenakas, John A. Fracchia, and Ron Golan.
© 2019 John Wiley & Sons Ltd. Published 2019 by John Wiley & Sons Ltd.

(which incorporates a double folded U-configuration and a short ileal segment, which functions as a flap valve).
- The ileoileal anastomosis can be hand-sewn using a two-layer technique.

Complications

- Bleeding
- Infection
- Ileus/bowel obstruction
- Urine leak (reservoir, ureteroileal, and ileourethral anastomoses)
- Bowel injury/leak
- Ureteral obstruction/stricture
- Nocturnal enuresis/incontinence
- Pyelonephritis
- Stone formation
- Metabolic abnormalities (hypokalemic, hyperchloremic metabolic acidosis)
- Vitamin B12 deficiency and bile salt malabsorption
- Chronic diarrhea
- Renal failure
- Neobladder rupture (from mucous formation or prolonged infection)

Template Operative Dictation

Preoperative diagnosis: Need for urinary diversion following extirpative pelvic surgery
Postoperative diagnosis: Same
Procedure: Orthotopic ileal neobladder
Indications: The patient is a _____-year-old *male/female* following extirpative pelvic surgery for _____ presenting for an orthotopic ileal neobladder.
Description of Procedure: The indications, alternatives, benefits, and risks were discussed with the patient and informed consent was obtained.

The patient was brought onto the operating room table, positioned supine, and secured with a safety strap. All pressure points were carefully padded and pneumatic compression devices were placed on the lower extremities.

After the administration of intravenous antibiotics and general endotracheal anesthesia, the entire abdomen and genitalia were prepped and draped in the standard sterile manner.

A time-out was completed, verifying the correct patient, surgical procedure, and positioning, prior to beginning the procedure.

A midline abdominal incision was made starting just above the umbilicus and carried down to the pubic symphysis. The subcutaneous tissue was incised with electrocautery, exposing the underlying rectus abdominis aponeurosis. This was incised at the linea alba and the rectus abdominis muscles separated at the midline and retracted laterally, taking care not to injure the underlying inferior epigastric vessels.

The peritoneal cavity was entered sharply, avoiding any injury to the bowel. A self-retaining retractor (e.g. Bookwalter, Omni-Tract, Balfour) was appropriately positioned

to optimize exposure, using padding on each retractor blade. The peritoneal contents were examined. There was no evidence of any inflammatory bowel or metastatic disease.

The bowel contents were packed superiorly and the posterior peritoneum was incised at the level of the pelvic inlet over the iliac vessels, exposing both ureters. The ureters were carefully mobilized, maintaining their blood supply, and transected close to the bladder between large hemoclips.

> *In patients with a history of irradiation or urothelial cancer*: A small segment of each distal ureter was sent to pathology for frozen-section evaluation.

A 3-0 chromic tag suture was placed on the end of each severed ureter to aid in manipulation of the ureters to the subsequently created ileal neobladder.

The bowel packing was removed, and attention was focused on isolating an appropriate ileal segment. A 70 cm segment of ileum was isolated 10–15 cm from the ileocecal valve, with the aid of transillumination. An avascular mesenteric window was opened on each side of the desired ileal segment using an electrothermal bipolar tissue sealing device (LigaSure) to incise and ligate the mesentery on both sides, avoiding injury to the main intestinal vasculature. *(Alternatively, the mesentery can be incised and its traversing blood vessels individually clamped, divided, and doubly ligated with chromic or silk ties.)* Additional meticulous hemostasis was achieved using 3-0 *chromic/silk* ties. The proximal mesenteric incision was kept short to preserve the vasculature to the neobladder. The distal portion was long enough to allow the isolated segment to reach the urethra comfortably. The isolated ileal segment was transected at its proximal and distal antimesenteric borders using a GIA60 stapler.

The continuity of the ileum was restored using a stapled anastomosis as follows: The antimesenteric corners of the proximal and distal segments were identified, and a small segment of tissue was resected off each end of the stapled suture lines. One limb of the GIA60 stapler was inserted into the proximal and the other into the distal ileal segment, with care taken not to injure the bowel mesentery. The ileal segments were rotated, ensuring that the antimesenteric bowel walls faced each other, prior to firing the stapler. Four small clamps were then placed on the ends of the transected bowel. The two clamps on the lines of the original bowel transection were held together, while the others were spread apart, creating a wide opening. A TA55 stapler was used to complete the functional end-to-end ileoileal anastomosis. The staple line was checked confirming its integrity, and additionally reinforced with interrupted 3-0 silk sutures. The mesenteric window was closed with a running 4-0 chromic to avoid internal herniation. The ileoileal anastomosis was returned to its natural position in the abdomen with the isolated ileal segment placed caudal to it.

After irrigating the ileal segment clear with normal sterile saline, it was arranged in a W-configuration with four equidistant segments and incised at its antimesenteric border. A U-shaped inferior flap was fashioned by curving the incision at the inferior border of the afferent limb and a full-thickness segment of bowel excised, creating an appropriate opening for the ileourethral anastomosis. The four equal ileal limbs were sutured together posteriorly using running polyglactin (Vicryl) sutures.

The ileal neobladder was positioned in the pelvis and the ileourethral anastomosis performed using *2-0 Vicryl/poliglecaprone (Monocryl)* sutures placed full thickness between the circular opening in the neobladder and the urethral stump. The sutures

were placed over a temporary catheter through the edges of the intestinal and urethral mucosa to ensure complete approximation of the neobladder to the urethra. A 20 Fr urethral catheter was inserted through the urethra into the neobladder before tying the sutures. The anastomosis was completed without tension.

Attention was turned to the ureteroileal anastomoses. Each distal ureter was spatulated for approximately 1 cm and pulled through a small incision in the afferent ileal wall. The ileal mucosa was incised to create a 3 cm sulcus into which each ureter was placed and secured to the ileal wall with 4-0 chromic sutures. The neoureteral orifices were fashioned using interrupted 4-0 chromic sutures and the overlying ileal mucosa similarly loosely approximated, creating an antirefluxing reimplantation. 7 Fr single-J ureteral stents were placed with their distal ends exiting the afferent limb of the neobladder. The stents were secured to the ileal mucosa using 4-0 chromic sutures.

The anterior neoileal borders were approximated with running 2-0 Vicryl sutures. Prior to completing the closure, a 14 Fr cystotomy tube was placed into the neobladder through the avascular peritoneal fat of the ileal mesentery. The neobladder was flushed with sterile normal saline, ensuring the absence of any clots and the creation of a watertight closure.

Having completed the neobladder, the abdomen was irrigated with warm sterile normal saline and examined for any bleeding. Meticulous hemostasis was obtained with electrocautery. A surgical drain (e.g. Jackson-Pratt) was placed in the retroperitoneum and brought out at the skin through a separate stab incision, where it was secured with a 2-0 silk suture. Prior to closure, the ureters, bowel, mesentery, neobladder, and abdominal wall were inspected and found to be intact without any evidence of bleeding or injury.

The self-retaining retractor was removed and the abdominal incision was closed using a running 2-0 chromic to approximate the rectus muscles and 1-0 polydioxanone (PDS) for the rectus aponeurosis. The subcutaneous tissue was approximated with 3-0 chromic sutures and the skin was closed with staples. A sterile dressing was applied.

At the end of the procedure, all counts were correct.

The patient tolerated the procedure without difficulty and was taken to the recovery room in satisfactory condition.

Estimated blood loss: Approximately _____ ml

72

Transverse Colon Conduit

Indications

- Urinary diversion following extirpative pelvic surgery in patients with potential irradiation damage to the small bowel and distal ureters
- Urinary incontinence in patients with complex vesicovaginal, enterovesical, prostato-rectal, or rectovesicovaginal fistulae after irradiation

Essential Steps

1) Mark out the abdominal skin stoma site in advance of the procedure.
2) Isolate and divide a 15–20 cm segment of transverse colon by mobilizing the right and left flexures. Use transillumination to identify the vascular arcades.
3) Perform a stapled functional end-to-end bowel anastomosis.
4) Mobilize the ureters with their adventitia so their anastomoses rest without tension on the conduit.
5) Spatulate the distal ureters to create individual wide end-to-side ureterocolonic anastomoses.
6) Create a urinary stoma ideally suitable for the patient's body habitus.
7) Ensure that all suture lines are watertight.
8) Place a drain.

Note These Variations

- A preoperative bowel prep is optional.
- The colonic anastomosis and "butt" end of the conduit may be hand-sewn, using a two-layer technique.
- Alternatively, a conjoined end-to-end (Wallace) ureterocolonic anastomosis can be performed.
- In children, the ureters can be reimplanted in an antirefluxing manner.

Operative Dictations in Urologic Surgery, First Edition. Noel A. Armenakas, John A. Fracchia, and Ron Golan.
© 2019 John Wiley & Sons Ltd. Published 2019 by John Wiley & Sons Ltd.

Complications

- Bleeding
- Infection
- Ileus/bowel obstruction
- Bowel injury/leak
- Urinary leak (conduit, uretercolonic anastomosis)
- Ureteral obstruction/stricture
- Parastomal hernia
- Stomal stenosis
- Pyelonephritis
- Stone formation
- Metabolic abnormalities (hypokalemic, hyperchloremic metabolic acidosis)
- Renal failure

Template Operative Dictation

Preoperative diagnosis: *History of irradiated pelvic malignancy/Urinary incontinence/ Urinary obstruction/_____*

Postoperative diagnosis: Same

Procedure: Transverse colon conduit

Indications: The patient is a _____-year-old *male/female* with _____ presenting for creation of a transverse colon conduit.

Description of Procedure: The indications, alternatives, benefits, and risks were discussed with the patient and informed consent was obtained.

The patient was brought onto the operating room table, positioned supine, and secured with a safety strap. All pressure points were carefully padded and pneumatic compression devices were placed on the lower extremities.

After the administration of intravenous antibiotics and general endotracheal anesthesia, the entire abdomen was prepped and draped in the standard sterile manner.

A time-out was completed, verifying the correct patient, surgical procedure, and positioning, prior to beginning the procedure.

A 16 Fr urethral catheter was inserted into the bladder and connected to a drainage bag.

The previously marked stomal site was identified on the *right/left* upper abdominal quadrant.

A midline abdominal incision was made starting 5 cm above the umbilicus and carried down to the pubic symphysis. The subcutaneous tissue was incised with electrocautery, exposing the underlying rectus abdominis aponeurosis. This was incised at the linea alba and the rectus abdominis muscles were separated at the midline and retracted laterally, taking care not to injure the underlying inferior epigastric vessels.

The peritoneal cavity was entered sharply, avoiding any injury to the bowel. A self-retaining retractor (e.g. Bookwalter, Omni-Tract, Balfour) was appropriately positioned to optimize exposure, using padding on each retractor blade. The peritoneal contents were examined. There was no evidence of any inflammatory bowel or metastatic disease.

The bowel contents were packed superiorly and the posterior peritoneum was incised at the level of the pelvic inlet over the iliac vessels, exposing both ureters. The ureters were carefully mobilized, maintaining their blood supply, and transected close to the bladder between large hemoclips.

In patients with a history of irradiation or urothelial cancer: A small segment of each distal ureter was sent to pathology for frozen-section evaluation.

A 3-0 chromic tag suture was placed on the end of each severed ureter to aid in manipulation of the ureter to the subsequently created colon conduit.

The bowel packing was removed, and attention was directed on isolating an appropriate transverse colon segment. The transverse colon was identified and the gastrocolic ligament and greater omentum were dissected free from its superior surface. The splenic and hepatic flexures were gently mobilized, allowing a 15–20 cm segment of transverse colon to be isolated. Several 3-0 chromic tag sutures were placed in the seromuscular layer of the transverse colon to mark out the segment.

The vascular arcades were identified with transillumination. An avascular mesenteric window was opened on each side of the isolated colonic segment using an electrothermal bipolar tissue sealing device (LigaSure) to incise and ligate the mesentery on both sides, avoiding injury to the main intestinal vasculature. *(Alternatively, the mesentery can be incised and its traversing blood vessels individually clamped, divided, and doubly ligated with chromic or silk ties.)* Additional hemostasis was achieved using 3-0 *chromic/silk* ties. Sufficient mesenteric length was obtained to allow the distal end of the transverse colon conduit to reach the stomal site without tension.

The isolated transverse colon segment was divided with the GIA60 stapler. The "butt" end of the colon conduit was marked with a 3-0 silk suture and the conduit placed caudal to the bowel defect.

The continuity of the bowel was restored using a stapled anastomosis as follows: The antimesenteric corners of the proximal and distal transverse colon segments were identified and a small segment of tissue was resected off each end of the stapled suture lines. One limb of the GIA60 stapler was inserted into the proximal and the other into the distal colonic segment, with care taken not to injure the bowel mesentery. The transverse colon segments were rotated, ensuring that the antimesenteric bowel walls faced each other prior to firing the stapler. Four small clamps were then placed on the ends of the transected bowel. The two clamps on the lines of the original bowel transection were held together, while the others were spread apart, creating a wide opening. A TA55 stapler was used to complete the functional end-to-end bowel anastomosis. The staple line was checked, confirming its integrity, and additionally reinforced with interrupted 3-0 silk sutures. The mesenteric window was closed with a running 4-0 chromic to avoid internal herniation.

Each ureter was carefully mobilized cephalad and placed adjacent to the transverse colon conduit. Care was taken to preserve the adventitial ureteral blood supply. Both ureters were spatulated on their medial surface for a distance of 5–6 mm.

The transverse colon conduit was irrigated with sterile normal saline until the returns were clear. The sites for the ureterocolic anastomoses were selected in the posterior wall of the conduit. Two parallel 4 cm incisions were made into the tenia lifting the muscular layer off the mucosa. 3-0 chromic stay sutures were placed to hold

the seromuscular layers apart and the underlying colonic mucosa was incised for approximately 1 cm.

The left ureter was gently pulled through the bowel mesentery medial to the descending colon and reimplanted using interrupted 4-0 chromic sutures. The anastomosis was performed around a single-J ureteral stent, which was advanced to the renal pelvis and brought out through the stomal end of the conduit, where it was secured with a 3-0 chromic suture. The seromuscular layer was closed over the ureter with interrupted 4-0 chromic sutures avoiding any constriction.

The right ureter was reimplanted into the appropriate tenia in a similar fashion.

The creation of the conduit stoma was performed by excising a circular area of skin, 3 cm in diameter, at the previously determined stomal site. The underlying fascia was identified and opened using a cruciate incision. Two fingers were inserted through the fascia and the distal end of the conduit and both ureteral stents were brought through the skin, for a distance of 4–5 cm, with the aid of Babcock clamps. Four seromuscular 3-0 polyglactin (Vicryl) sutures were used to anchor the conduit to the abdominal fascia. Multiple 4-0 Vicryl sutures were circularly placed through the distal conduit's mucosa and the subcutaneous tissue to evert the stoma. A 20 Fr multi-eyed catheter was inserted into the conduit and gently irrigated, confirming the absence of any leaks. The catheter and ureteral stents were affixed to the abdominal wall, adjacent to the stoma, with a 3-0 silk suture.

Having completed the transverse colon conduit, the abdomen was irrigated with warm sterile normal saline and examined for any bleeding. Meticulous hemostasis was obtained. A surgical drain (e.g. Jackson–Pratt) was placed in the retroperitoneum and brought out at the skin through a separate stab incision, where it was secured with a 2-0 silk suture. Prior to closure, the ureters, bowel, mesentery, conduit, stoma and abdominal wall were inspected and found to be intact without any evidence of bleeding or injury.

The self-retaining retractor was removed and the abdominal incision was closed using a running 2-0 chromic to approximate the rectus muscles and 1-0 polydioxanone (PDS) for the rectus aponeurosis. The subcutaneous tissue was approximated with 3-0 chromic sutures and the skin was closed with staples.

The incision was covered with a sterile dressing and a stomal appliance fitted in a watertight fashion.

At the end of the procedure, all counts were correct.

The patient tolerated the procedure without difficulty and was taken to the recovery room in satisfactory condition.

Estimated blood loss: Approximately _____ml

73

Ureterosigmoidostomy

Indications

- Patients with competent anal sphincter function and normal upper tracts desiring a continent rectosigmoid urinary diversion.
- Etiologies include lower urinary tract cancer, bladder exstrophy/epispadias, and intractable urinary incontinence.

Essential Steps

1) Carefully select patients (e.g. competent anal sphincter confirmed preoperatively; no history of inflammatory/malignant rectosigmoid disease; sigmoid diverticulosis or pelvic radiation; serum creatinine <1.5 mg/dl with a creatinine clearance >60 cc/min).
2) Mobilize the ureters with their adventitia so their anastomoses to the sigmoid colon are without tension.
3) Open the anterior rectosigmoid colon to expose the posterior wall.
4) Create individual submucosal tunnels for ureteral reimplantation.
5) Spatulate the distal ureters to create individual wide end-to-side ureterosigmoid anastomoses.
6) Close the rectosigmoid in two layers.
7) Ensure that all suture lines are watertight.
8) Place a drain.

Note These Variations

- A preoperative bowel prep is optional.
- Alternatively, the ureteral anastomoses can be performed to the anterior wall of the rectosigmoid.
- A sigmoid-rectal pouch (Mainz II) can be created but requires more extensive dissection.

Operative Dictations in Urologic Surgery, First Edition. Noel A. Armenakas, John A. Fracchia, and Ron Golan.
© 2019 John Wiley & Sons Ltd. Published 2019 by John Wiley & Sons Ltd.

Complications

- Bleeding
- Infection
- Ileus/bowel obstruction
- Bowel injury/leak
- Urinary leak (ureterosigmoid anastomoses)
- Ureteral obstruction/stricture
- Ureteral reflux
- Pyelonephritis
- Metabolic abnormalities (hypokalemic, hyperchloremic metabolic acidosis)
- Renal failure
- Secondary development of rectosigmoid malignancy

Template Operative Dictation

Preoperative diagnosis: *Bladder cancer//Exstrophy/epispadias*
Postoperative diagnosis: Same
Procedure: Ureterosigmoidostomy
Indications: The patient is a _____ -year-old *male/female* with _____
presenting for a ureterosigmoidostomy.
Description of Procedure: The indications, alternatives, benefits, and risks were discussed with the *patient/patient's family* and informed consent was obtained.

The patient was brought onto the operating room table, positioned supine, and secured with a safety strap. All pressure points were carefully padded and pneumatic compression devices were placed on the lower extremities.

After the administration of intravenous antibiotics and general endotracheal anesthesia, the entire abdomen and rectum was prepped and draped in the standard sterile manner.

A time-out was completed, verifying the correct patient, surgical procedure, and positioning, prior to beginning the procedure.

A rectal tube was placed transanally at the start of the procedure.

A midline abdominal incision was made starting at the umbilicus and carried down to the pubic symphysis. The subcutaneous tissue was incised with electrocautery, exposing the underlying rectus abdominis aponeurosis. This was incised at the linea alba and the rectus abdominis muscles were separated at the midline and retracted laterally, taking care not to injure the underlying inferior epigastric vessels.

The peritoneal cavity was entered sharply, avoiding any injury to the bowel. A self-retaining retractor (e.g. Bookwalter, Omni-Tract, Balfour) was appropriately positioned to optimize exposure, using padding on each retractor blade. The peritoneal contents were examined. There was no evidence of any inflammatory bowel or metastatic disease.

The bowel contents were packed superiorly and the posterior peritoneum was incised at the level of the pelvic inlet over the iliac vessels, exposing both ureters. The ureters were carefully mobilized, maintaining their blood supply, and transected close to the

bladder between large hemoclips. *(In patients with urothelial cancer, consider sending a distal segment of each ureter for frozen section.)* A 3-0 chromic tag suture was placed on the end of each severed ureter to aid in manipulation of the ureters to the rectosigmoid.

The anterior tenia of the sigmoid colon, just proximal to the transition into the rectum, was incised between 3-0 chromic stay sutures over a length of approximately 5 cm. The anterior bowel wall was entered, exposing the posterior mucosal wall of the rectosigmoid. There, four 3-0 chromic stay sutures were placed over a length of about 4 cm, for preparation of the *right/left* submucosal tunnel. Then 1–2 cc of sterile normal saline were injected submucosally to facilitate separation of the mucosa from the muscularis. A 1 cm longitudinal mucosal incision was made between the proximal and distal stay sutures and a 3 cm submucosal tunnel was fashioned between these using caudal blunt dissection. Next, a full-thickness buttonhole was created by excising the posterior rectosigmoid wall at the proposed entrance of the *right/left* ureter. The ureter was gently pulled into the rectosigmoid and guided submucosally from the proximal to distal mucosal openings. The ureter was spatulated on its medial surface, for a distance of 8–10 mm, and anchored distally with two 5-0 polyglactin (Vicryl) sutures placed through the bowel muscularis and mucosa. The anastomosis of the spatulated ureter was completed with ureteral mucosal interrupted 4-0 chromic sutures. Additional seromuscular sutures were placed to reinforce the ureterosigmoid anastomosis. A 7-Fr single-J ureteral stent was inserted and secured to the intestinal mucosa with a 4-0 chromic suture.

A second submucosal tunnel was positioned lateral and offset, and the contralateral ureter was reimplanted using the same nonrefluxing technique and stented.

Both ureteral stents were advanced into the side holes of the rectal tube, which was pulled back to bring out the stents and then reinserted transanally. The rectal tube and ureteral stents were secured to the perianal skin with 2-0 silk sutures.

The anterior incision of the rectosigmoid was closed in two layers, using 4-0 running and 3-0 interrupted Vicryl sutures on the mucosal and seromuscular layers, respectively. The posterior peritoneum was approximated over both ureters using a running 3-0 chromic suture. The rectal tube was gently irrigated, confirming the absence of any leaks.

At the completion of the ureterosigmoidostomy, the bowel packing was removed and the pelvis was irrigated with warm sterile normal saline and examined for bleeding. Meticulous hemostasis was obtained with electrocautery. A surgical drain (e.g. Jackson-Pratt) was placed in the retroperitoneum and brought out at the skin through a separate stab incision, where it was secured with a 2-0 silk suture. Prior to closure, the ureters, bowel, mesentery, and abdominal wall were inspected and found to be intact without any evidence of bleeding or injury.

The self-retaining retractor was removed and the abdominal incision was closed using a running 2-0 chromic to approximate the rectus muscles and 1-0 polydioxanone (PDS) for the rectus aponeurosis. The subcutaneous tissue was approximated with 3-0 chromic sutures and the skin was closed with staples. A sterile dressing was applied.

At the end of the procedure, all counts were correct.

The patient tolerated the procedure without difficulty and was taken to the recovery room in satisfactory condition.

Estimated blood loss: Approximately _____ml

NOTES

NOTES

SECTION II   ENDOSCOPIC SURGERY

74

Endopyelotomy (Ureteroscopic Approach)

Indications

- Ureteropelvic junction obstruction

Essential Steps

1) Assess preoperatively for the presence of a crossing vessel.
2) Perform a retrograde pyelogram to delineate the ureteral and renal pelvis anatomy.
3) Pass a 0.035 in. (safety) guidewire into the renal pelvis.
4) Insert a second stiff (working) guidewire into the renal pelvis and advance a ureteral access sheath over this.
5) Advance a flexible ureteroscope through the access sheath to the proximal healthy portion of the renal pelvis.
6) Use a 200 μm laser fiber to incise the entire fibrotic segment *laterally*. Repetitive full-thickness longitudinal incisions should be made extending proximally and distally into healthy renal pelvis and ureter, respectively.
7) Pass a 4 cm, 15–24 Fr dilating balloon across the incised area. Inflate the balloon to a pressure of 3 atm to calibrate the ureteropelvic junction and separate the cut edges.
8) Deflate and remove the balloon and access sheath, and insert a large diameter double-J stent.
9) Drain the bladder.

Note These Variations

- The use of a ureteral access sheath is optional.
- On occasion, ureteral dilation may be required at the ureterovesical junction or more proximally to allow passage of the ureteroscope. This is best accomplished using a 12 Fr radially expanding balloon dilator passed over a guidewire and inflated up to 14 atm for 3–5 minutes. Alternatively, a tapered (6–12 Fr × 70 cm) hydrogel coated ureteral dilator can be used. If the ureter remains tight, it may be preferable to leave an indwelling double-J stent and return at a later date.

Operative Dictations in Urologic Surgery, First Edition. Noel A. Armenakas, John A. Fracchia, and Ron Golan.
© 2019 John Wiley & Sons Ltd. Published 2019 by John Wiley & Sons Ltd.

- A semi-rigid ureteroscope can sometimes be utilized in patients of short stature.
- Alternatively, electrocautery or a cold-knife can be used to incise the ureteropelvic junction.

Complications

- Bleeding
- Infection
- Ureteral perforation/avulsion/intussusception
- Ureteropelvic junction obstruction/stricture

Template Operative Dictation

Preoperative diagnosis: *Right/left* ureteropelvic junction obstruction
Postoperative diagnosis: Same
Procedure: *Right/left* ureteroscopic endopyelotomy
Indications: The patient is a ____-year-old *male/female* who presents with a *congenital/acquired right/left* ureteropelvic junction obstruction presenting for ureteroscopic endopyelotomy.
Description of Procedure: The indications, alternatives, benefits, and risks were discussed with the patient and informed consent was obtained.

The patient was brought onto the operating room table, positioned supine, and secured with a safety strap. Pneumatic compression devices were placed on the lower extremities.

After the administration of intravenous antibiotics and general anesthesia, the patient was repositioned in the dorsal lithotomy using (Allen) universal stirrups and all pressure points were carefully padded. The genitalia were prepped and draped in the standard sterile manner.

The fluoroscopy unit was brought into the field, draped, and positioned appropriately. The radiographic images were in the room.

A time-out was completed, verifying the correct patient, surgical procedure, site, and positioning, prior to beginning the procedure.

Isotonic sodium chloride was used for irrigation.

A 22 Fr cystoscope with a 30° lens was inserted per meatus and advanced, under direct vision, into the urinary bladder. Urethroscopy revealed a normal urethra. *(In a male patient, comment on the prostate size, lobes, and degree of obstruction.)* On cystoscopy, with both the 30° and 70° lenses, the media was clear, the bladder capacity was normal, and the bladder wall noted to expand symmetrically in all dimensions. There were no tumors, stones, foreign bodies, or diverticula present. The bladder wall was *minimally/ moderately/significantly/not* trabeculated with a normal appearing mucosa. Both ureteral orifices were in the normal anatomic position with clear urinary efflux bilaterally.

A *right/left* retrograde pyelogram was performed using dilute contrast to delineate the anatomy of the upper collecting system. A ____ cm area of narrowing was identified at the ureteropelvic junction with associated pelvicaliectasis.

A 5 Fr open-ended catheter was placed through the cystoscopic working port and advanced to the *right/left* ureteral orifice. A 0.035 in. (Sensor) safety guidewire was passed through the catheter and advanced to the kidney, under fluoroscopic guidance. The open-ended catheter and cystoscope were removed and a 10 Fr ureteral dual lumen catheter was advanced over the guidewire under fluoroscopic guidance. A second stiff (Amplatz Super Stiff) working guidewire was advanced through this to the renal pelvis, and its position was confirmed cystoscopically. The dual lumen catheter was withdrawn, leaving both guidewires in place. A *11 Fr/13 Fr × 36 cm//12 Fr/14 Fr × 36 cm* ureteral access sheath and obturator were inserted over the working guidewire and positioned in the proximal ureter. The obturator and working guidewire were removed and a flexible ureteroscope was inserted through the access sheath and advanced under direct vision to the stenotic segment. A *single action pump syringe/pressure irrigation bag* was used for irrigation, ensuring a clear visual field.

The stenotic ureteropelvic junction was visually inspected. There were no pulsations seen to suggest a crossing vessel. A 200 μm laser fiber was passed through the scope adapter (e.g. UroLok) and advanced past the ureteropelvic narrowing and oriented laterally. The holmium: YAG laser was readied and the entire stricture was carefully lased laterally in a longitudinal fashion, using an energy range of 0.8–1.2 J at a maximal rate of 15 pulses per second, until periureteral fat was visualized. The incision extended for a distance of ____ cm traversing the diseased segment from healthy urothelium proximally to healthy urothelium distally. Several small bleeding points were gently cauterized with the laser fiber, obtaining meticulous hemostasis.

The laser fiber was removed and the incised ureteropelvic junction thoroughly inspected. The ureteroscope was then removed under direct vision and a 4-cm, 15–24 Fr dilating balloon was passed over the safety guidewire traversing the incised area. The balloon was inflated to 3 atm with dilute contrast material for several minutes, and its position was confirmed fluoroscopically. The balloon was seen to fully inflate at this low pressure, confirming adequate patency of the repair.

The guidewire was backloaded into the cystoscope, using the 5 Fr open-ended catheter, and the cystoscope was advanced into the bladder. A ____ Fr _____ cm double-J stent was advanced over the guidewire and its proximal and distal ends positioned in the renal pelvis and bladder, respectively. Fluoroscopy was used to confirm its proper placement. The guidewire and cystoscope were then withdrawn.

A 16 Fr urethral catheter was inserted in the bladder and connected to a drainage bag. The patient was repositioned supine.

At the end of the procedure, all counts were correct.

The patient tolerated the procedure well and was taken to the recovery room in satisfactory condition.

Estimated blood loss: Approximately _____ml

75

Percutaneous Nephrolithotomy

Indications

- Large renal calculus(i)
- Staghorn calculus(i)
- Cystine calculus(i)
- Calculus(i) within a calyceal diverticulum
- Impacted ureteropelvic junction calculus(i)

Essential Steps

1) Ensure the appropriate percutaneous access.
2) Use fluoroscopic guidance throughout the procedure to confirm adequate positioning of the instruments.
3) Place two guidewires through the percutaneous catheter into the bladder.
4) Dilate the fascia to 30 Fr and advance the working sheath into the renal pelvis.
5) Remove the balloon dilator leaving it inflated so that it can be rapidly re-inserted to tamponade if significant bleeding occurs.
6) Fragment and extract all stones, and perform flexible nephroureteroscopy for confirmation.
7) Insert a council-tip catheter into the renal pelvis over the guidewire. If an open-ended catheter is also used, ensure that its proximal end is positioned outside the council-tip catheter so it does not inadvertently migrate distally into the bladder.

Note These Variations

- Percutaneous access may be obtained using sonographic guidance.
- If the working sheath's valve cannot accommodate both guidewires, a dual lumen catheter may be used to pass the second guidewire into the kidney.
- Amplatz dilators, rather than the (NephroMax) balloon dilator, can be used to sequentially dilate the nephrostomy tract to 30 Fr.
- A nitinol stone basket or grasper may be passed through the flexible cystoscope to remove any fragments.

Operative Dictations in Urologic Surgery, First Edition. Noel A. Armenakas, John A. Fracchia, and Ron Golan.
© 2019 John Wiley & Sons Ltd. Published 2019 by John Wiley & Sons Ltd.

- If there is a suspicion of a ureteral calculus, antegrade or retrograde ureteroscopy should be performed to fragment or remove any ureteral stones.
- The use of a nephrostomy tube and/or ureteral stent for postoperative drainage is at the discretion of the surgeon.

Complications

- Bleeding
- Infection
- Renal pelvis perforation
- Intraabdominal organ injury
- Pneumothorax
- Ileus
- Retained stone fragments

Template Operative Dictation

Preoperative diagnosis: Renal *calculus(i)/staghorn*
Postoperative diagnosis: Same
Procedure: *Right/Left* percutaneous nephrolithotomy
Indications: The patient is a ____-year-old *male/female* with a _____ cm *right/left// staghorn/renal calculus(i)* presenting for a percutaneous nephrolithotomy.
Description of Procedure: The indications, alternatives, benefits, and risks were discussed with the patient and informed consent was obtained.

The patient was brought into the operating room supine on the stretcher. Pneumatic compression devices were placed on the lower extremities.

After the administration of intravenous antibiotics and general endotracheal anesthesia, a 16 Fr urethral catheter was inserted into the bladder and connected to a drainage bag. The patient was transferred from the stretcher onto the operating table and carefully positioned prone with two chest rolls. The arms were brought overhead with the elbows flexed at 90°, all extremities carefully padded, and the patient secured to the table with 3 in. tape and a safety strap. The *right/left* flank and back were prepped and draped in the standard sterile manner, with special emphasis on the previously placed percutaneous sheath. The fluoroscopy unit was brought into the field, draped and positioned appropriately.

The radiographic images were in the room.

A time-out was completed, verifying the correct patient, surgical procedure, site, and positioning, prior to beginning the procedure.

[If percutaneous access is obtained intraoperatively, describe the technique here].

An antegrade nephrostogram was performed through the percutaneous sheath to delineate the collecting system and renal pelvis. Two guidewires with hydrophilic tips (Amplatz Super Stiff and PTFE-Nitinol, Sensor) were individually inserted through the sheath's valve and advanced into the bladder under fluoroscopic guidance. The percutaneous sheath was removed.

Using a #11 scalpel blade, a 1 cm skin incision was made at the level of the percutaneous catheter and taken down through the subcutaneous fat to the latissimus dorsi fascia. This was sharply incised and the muscle bluntly dissected with a clamp.

A 30 Fr Amplatz working sheath was backloaded over the (NephroMax) balloon dilator, which was passed over the Super Stiff guidewire and advanced into the renal pelvis. Its proper location was confirmed fluoroscopically using the radiopaque markers and the balloon was inflated with 50% nonionic contrast to 14 atm for 3–5 minutes using the inflator. This was again checked fluoroscopically ensuring correct balloon placement and inflation. The working sheath was gently advanced through the dilated nephrostomy tract into the renal pelvis and its proper placement confirmed with fluoroscopy. The balloon dilator was left inflated and carefully removed leaving both guidewires and the working sheath in place.

The *long/short* 24 Fr rigid nephroscope was inserted through the working sheath and advanced to the stone(s) in the *renal pelvis//lower/mid/upper calyx*. Under direct vision the stone(s) *was/were* fragmented using the *pneumatic lithoclast/ultrasonic lithotripter/holmium:YAG laser*. All fragments were removed with the rigid grasping forceps and sent for chemical analysis. Nephroureteroscopy was performed with a flexible cystoscope to ensure removal of all stone fragments from the kidney, ureteropelvic junction, and ureter.

An antegrade pyelogram was performed through the working sheath confirming prompt drainage down the ureter to the bladder, and the absence of any extravasation. The urine output was *light tea/pink* colored, suggesting the absence of any significant bleeding. The Super Stiff guidewire was removed, leaving the Sensor guidewire as a safety.

A 5 Fr open-ended catheter was back loaded through a 16 Fr council-tip catheter and both were advanced over the Sensor guidewire. The catheter's balloon was inflated with 2 ml 50% nonionic contrast and fluoroscopic images taken to ensure that the balloon and distal ureteral catheter were positioned in the renal pelvis and mid-ureter, respectively, before removing the Sensor guidewire. The working sheath was incised and removed from the patient.

The council-tip catheter was secured to the skin with a 2-0 silk suture and the nephrostomy incision closed with one interrupted 3-0 polyglactin (Vicryl) suture. The council-tip and open-ended catheters were connected to a drainage bag. A sterile dressing was applied and the patient repositioned supine on the stretcher.

At the end of the procedure, all counts were correct.

The patient tolerated the procedure well and was taken to the recovery room in satisfactory condition.

Estimated blood loss: Approximately _____ml

76

Ureteral Stent Exchange

Indications

- Ureteral obstruction

Essential Steps

1) Gently pass a cystoscope into the bladder under direct vision and completely inspect the lower urinary tract.
2) Advance an alligator grasping forceps through the working port and retrieve the distal end of the existing ureteral stent.
3) Withdraw the stent under direct vision until the distal end can be grasped at the urethral meatus.
4) Pass a guidewire through the ureteral stent and advance it to the collecting system using fluoroscopy. Remove the ureteral stent while maintaining the guidewire in place.
5) Back load the wire through the cystoscope and advance the ureteral stent over the guidewire, using direct vision, and fluoroscopic guidance.
6) Remove the guidewire and check for proper stent placement.

Note These Variations

- Cystoscopic stent exchange may be performed in the office or at the bedside with a rigid or flexible cystoscope using a topical anesthetic (jelly) or intravenous sedation.
- A ureteral stent may be placed over a guidewire under fluoroscopic guidance without backloading through the cystoscope. Its position should be confirmed radiographically.
- A guidewire may be passed alongside rather than through the ureteral stent under fluoroscopic guidance prior to removing the ureteral stent. This is helpful in cases of ureteral stent encrustation or difficult ureteral stent exchanges.

Operative Dictations in Urologic Surgery, First Edition. Noel A. Armenakas, John A. Fracchia, and Ron Golan.
© 2019 John Wiley & Sons Ltd. Published 2019 by John Wiley & Sons Ltd.

- Ureteral stent encrustation may require mechanical stone fragmentation, cystoscopy or ureteroscopy with laser lithotripsy, or percutaneous nephrolithotomy to remove the ureteral stent.
- In cases of a narrow meatus or fossa navicularis, gentle sequential dilation using curved metal sounds (Van Buren) should be performed initially to avoid traumatic endoscopic urethral insertion.

Complications

- Bleeding
- Infection
- Urethral injury
- Ureteral/renal perforation
- Fragmentation of encrusted ureteral stent
- Inability to advance the new ureteral stent into the renal pelvis
- Pain/lower urinary tract symptoms
- Persistent ureteral obstruction

Template Operative Dictation

Preoperative diagnosis: _____
Postoperative diagnosis: Same
Procedure: Cystoscopy with *right/left/bilateral* ureteral stent exchange
Indications: The patient is a ____-year-old *male/female* with a history of _____ presenting for cystoscopic *right/left/bilateral* ureteral stent exchange.
Description of Procedure: The indications, alternatives, benefits, and risks were discussed with the patient and informed consent was obtained.

The patient was brought onto the operating room table, positioned supine, and secured with a safety strap. Pneumatic compression devices were placed on the lower extremities.

After the administration of intravenous antibiotics and *intravenous sedation// general/regional* anesthesia, the patient was repositioned in dorsal lithotomy using (Allen) universal stirrups and all pressure points were carefully padded. A *rectal/ pelvic* examination was performed ____(describe)____. The genitalia were prepped and draped in the standard sterile manner.

The radiographic images were in the room.

A time-out was completed, verifying the correct patient, surgical procedure, site, and positioning, prior to beginning the procedure.

Isotonic sodium chloride was used for irrigation.

A 22 Fr rigid cystoscope with a 30° lens was inserted per meatus and advanced under direct vision into the urinary bladder. Urethroscopy revealed a normal urethra. *(In a male patient, comment on the prostate size, lobes, and degree of obstruction.)* The bladder was evaluated with both the 30° and 70° lenses. The media was clear, the bladder capacity was normal, and the bladder wall noted to expand symmetrically in all dimensions. There were no tumors, stones, foreign bodies, or diverticula present. The bladder

wall was *minimally/moderately/significantly/not* trabeculated with a normal appearing mucosa. Both ureteral orifices were in the normal anatomic position. The ureteral stent was seen emanating from the *left/right* ureteral orifice.

An alligator grasping forceps was passed through the cystoscopic working port and the distal end of the ureteral stent was retrieved. The cystoscope was withdrawn with the grasped stent, which was brought out to the urethral meatus. A 0.038 in. (Sensor) guidewire with a hydrophilic tip was passed through the ureteral stent and advanced into the collecting system under fluoroscopic guidance. The previous stent was removed over the guidewire.

> ***If a retrograde pyelogram is performed:*** A *5 Fr* open-ended catheter was inserted over the wire to the *distal ureter/mid ureter/proximal ureter//renal pelvis* under fluoroscopic guidance and the wire was removed. ____cc of diluted contrast medium (e.g. Omnipaque) was gently instilled, demonstrating ____*(describe)*____. The guidewire was then reinserted under fluoroscopic guidance and the open-ended catheter removed.

The guidewire was backloaded through the cystoscopic working port and the cystoscope was again inserted into the bladder. A ____Fr ____cm double-J stent was advanced over the wire and its proximal and distal ends positioned in the renal pelvis and bladder, respectively. This was confirmed under direct vision and radiographically. The guidewire was removed and the bladder emptied. Fluoroscopy was used to verify proper stent placement.

The cystoscope was removed under direct vision, confirming the absence of any lower urinary tract injuries, and the patient was repositioned supine.

At the end of the procedure, all counts were correct.

The patient tolerated the procedure well and was taken to the recovery room in satisfactory condition

Estimated blood loss: None

77

Ureteral Stent Insertion

Indications

- Ureteral obstruction
- Intraoperative ureteral identification

Essential Steps

1) Gently pass a cystoscope into the bladder under direct vision and completely inspect the lower urinary tract.
2) Advance a guidewire into the collecting system under fluoroscopic guidance.
3) Pass the appropriate-size stent over the guidewire, using direct visualization, and fluoroscopic guidance.
4) Remove the guidewire and check for proper stent placement.

Note These Variations

- Cystoscopic stent placement may be performed in the office/bedside with a rigid or flexible cystoscope, using a topical anesthetic.
- A 5 Fr open-ended catheter can be used to position the guidewire into the appropriate ureteral orifice.
- For ureteral J-ing, a soft angiographic catheter (e.g. Berenstein Soft-Vu) can be used to intubate the obscured orifice.
- A ureteral stent may be placed under fluoroscopic guidance alone, once the position of the guidewire has been confirmed.
- In cases of a narrow meatus or fossa navicularis, gentle sequential dilation using curved metal sounds (Van Buren) should be performed initially to avoid traumatic endoscopic urethral insertion.

Complications

- Bleeding
- Infection
- Urethral injury

Operative Dictations in Urologic Surgery, First Edition. Noel A. Armenakas, John A. Fracchia, and Ron Golan.
© 2019 John Wiley & Sons Ltd. Published 2019 by John Wiley & Sons Ltd.

- Ureteral/renal perforation
- Pain/lower urinary tract symptoms
- Inability to properly place the ureteral stent

Template Operative Dictation

Preoperative diagnosis: _____
Postoperative diagnosis: Same
Procedure: Cystoscopy with *right/left* ureteral stent placement
Indications: The patient is a _____-year-old *male/female* with a history of _____ presenting for cystoscopic *right/left* ureteral stent placement.
Description of Procedure: The indications, alternatives, benefits, and risks were discussed with the patient and informed consent was obtained.

The patient was brought onto the operating room table, positioned supine, and secured with a safety strap. Pneumatic compression devices were placed on the lower extremities.

After the administration of intravenous antibiotics and *intravenous sedation// general/regional* anesthesia, the patient was repositioned in dorsal lithotomy using (Allen) universal stirrups and all pressure points were carefully padded. A *rectal/pelvic* examination was performed ___*(describe)*___. The genitalia were prepped and draped in the standard sterile manner.

The radiographic images were in the room.

A time-out was completed, verifying the correct patient, surgical procedure, and positioning, prior to beginning the procedure.

Isotonic sodium chloride was used for irrigation.

A 22 Fr rigid cystoscope with a 30° lens was inserted per meatus and advanced under direct vision into the urinary bladder. Urethroscopy revealed a normal urethra. *(In a male patient, comment on the prostate size, lobes, and degree of obstruction.)* The bladder was evaluated with both the 30° and 70° lenses. The media was clear, the bladder capacity was normal and the bladder wall noted to expand symmetrically in all dimensions. There were no tumors, stones, foreign bodies, or diverticula present. The bladder wall was *minimally/moderately/significantly/not* trabeculated with a normal-appearing mucosa. Both ureteral orifices were in the normal anatomic position.

A 0.038 in. (Sensor) guidewire with a hydrophilic tip was passed through the cystoscopic working port to the *right/left* ureteral orifice and advanced into the collecting system under fluoroscopic guidance.

> ***If a retrograde pyelogram is performed:*** A 5 Fr open-ended catheter was inserted over the guidewire to the *distal/mid/proximal ureter//renal pelvis* under fluoroscopic guidance and the guidewire was removed. ___cc of dilute contrast medium (e.g. Omnipaque) were gently instilled, demonstrating ___*(describe)*___. The guidewire was then reinserted under fluoroscopic guidance and the open-ended catheter removed.

A ___Fr ___cm double-J stent was advanced over the guidewire and its proximal and distal ends positioned in the renal pelvis and bladder, respectively. The guidewire

was removed and the bladder emptied. Fluoroscopy was used to verify proper stent placement.

The cystoscope was removed under direct vision confirming the absence of any lower urinary tract injuries, and the patient was repositioned supine.

At the end of the procedure, all counts were correct.

The patient tolerated the procedure well and was taken to the recovery room in satisfactory condition.

Estimated blood loss: None

78

Ureteral Stent Removal

Indications

- Resolved ureteral obstruction
- Postoperative ureteral stent removal following renal/ureteral/bladder surgery

Essential Steps

1) Gently pass a cystoscope into the bladder under direct vision and completely inspect the lower urinary tract.
2) Advance an alligator grasping forceps through the working port and retrieve the distal end of the stent.
3) Withdraw the stent under direct visualization.

Note These Variations

- Cystoscopic stent removal may be performed in the office or at the bedside with a rigid or flexible cystoscope, using a topical anesthetic (jelly).
- Stents with extraction strings allow removal without requiring cystoscopy.
- Ureteral stent encrustation may require mechanical stone fragmentation, cystoscopy or ureteroscopy with laser lithotripsy, or percutaneous nephrolithotomy to remove the ureteral stent.
- In cases of a narrow meatus or fossa navicularis, gentle sequential dilation using curved metal sounds (Van Buren) should be performed initially to avoid traumatic endoscopic urethral insertion.

Complications

- Bleeding
- Infection
- Urethral injury

Operative Dictations in Urologic Surgery, First Edition. Noel A. Armenakas, John A. Fracchia, and Ron Golan.
© 2019 John Wiley & Sons Ltd. Published 2019 by John Wiley & Sons Ltd.

- Ureteral perforation
- Inability to remove an encrusted stent in its entirety
- Pain/lower urinary tract symptoms

Template Operative Dictation

Preoperative diagnosis: _____
Postoperative diagnosis: Same
Procedure: Cystoscopy with *right/left* ureteral stent removal
Indications: The patient is a _____-year-old *male/female* with a history of _____ presenting for cystoscopic *right/left* ureteral stent removal.
Description of Procedure: The indications, alternatives, benefits, and risks were discussed with the patient and informed consent was obtained.

The patient was brought onto the operating room table, positioned supine, and secured with a safety strap. Pneumatic compression devices were placed on the lower extremities.

After the administration of intravenous antibiotics and *intravenous sedation//general/regional* anesthesia, the patient was repositioned in dorsal lithotomy using (Allen) universal stirrups and all pressure points were carefully padded. The genitalia were prepped and draped in the standard sterile manner.

The radiographic images were in the room.

A time-out was completed, verifying the correct patient, surgical procedure, site, and positioning, prior to beginning the procedure.

Isotonic sodium chloride was used for irrigation.

A *22 Fr rigid cystoscope with a 30° lens/flexible cystoscope* was inserted per meatus and advanced under direct vision into the urinary bladder. Urethroscopy revealed a normal urethra. *(In a male patient, comment on the prostate size, lobes, and degree of obstruction.)* The bladder was evaluated with *both the 30° and 70° lenses/flexible cystoscopy*. The media was clear, the bladder capacity was normal, and the bladder wall was noted to expand symmetrically in all dimensions. There were no tumors, stones, foreign bodies, or diverticula present. The bladder wall was *minimally/moderately/significantly/not* trabeculated with a normal appearing mucosa. Both ureteral orifices were in the normal anatomic position. The ureteral stent was seen emanating from the *right/left* ureteral orifice.

An alligator grasping forceps was passed through the cystoscopic working port and the distal end of the ureteral stent was retrieved. The cystoscope and stent were withdrawn under direct vision, confirming the absence of any lower urinary tract injury, and the patient was repositioned supine. The stent was examined and noted to be intact.

At the end of the procedure, all counts were correct.

The patient tolerated the procedure well and was taken to the recovery room in satisfactory condition.

Estimated blood loss: None

79

Ureteroscopy for Stones

Indications

- Upper urinary tract stone(s)

Essential Steps

1) Pass a guidewire cystoscopically and advance it into the renal pelvis.
2) Advance the ureteroscope to the stone under direct vision. With flexible ureteroscopy, the initial passage can be performed fluoroscopically.
3) Fragment or dust the stone(s) using the holmium:YAG laser with a 200 or 365 μm fiber. For the former procedure, retrieve the fragments using a nitinol stone retrieval basket.
4) Carefully inspect the ureter (as well as the renal pelvis and calyces during flexible ureteroscopy) for residual stones or trauma.

Note These Variations

- A retrograde pyelogram can be performed at the beginning and/or end of the procedure to delineate the ureteral and intrarenal anatomy.
- For narrow ureters, a smaller (0.035 in.) guidewire can be used.
- When there is difficulty advancing the ureteroscope due to ureteral narrowing or kinking, pass a second (working) guidewire, either through the scope adapter (e.g. UroLok) or a dual lumen catheter, and confirm its position within the kidney fluoroscopically. Carefully advance the ureteroscope over the working guidewire.
- On occasion, ureteral dilation may be required at the ureterovesical junction or more proximally to allow passage of the ureteroscope. This is best accomplished using a 12 Fr radially expanding balloon dilator passed over a guidewire and inflated up to 14 atm for 3–5 minutes. Alternatively, a tapered (6 Fr–12 Fr × 70 cm) hydrogel coated ureteral dilator can be used.
- For flexible ureteroscopy, instead of the two-wire technique, a ureteral access sheath (11 Fr/13 Fr × 36 cm, 12 Fr/14 Fr × 36 cm) can be used. This facilitates ureteroscopic re-entry and fragment retrieval and can decrease operative time. The sheath is passed

Operative Dictations in Urologic Surgery, First Edition. Noel A. Armenakas, John A. Fracchia, and Ron Golan.
© 2019 John Wiley & Sons Ltd. Published 2019 by John Wiley & Sons Ltd.

over a second (working) guidewire with the obturator in place. Once the sheath is positioned correctly in the mid to proximal ureter, the obturator and second guidewire are removed and the flexible ureteroscope advanced through the sheath.

- Stones can be dusted using low energy (0.2–0.5 J) and high frequency (15–60 Hz) or fragmented using high energy (0.6–2.0 J) and low frequency (10–15 Hz), depending on the stone location, upper urinary tract characteristics, and the surgeon's preference.
- The use of a ureteral stent is at the discretion of the surgeon.

Complications

- Bleeding
- Infection
- Inability to access or treat the stone(s)
- Pain/lower urinary tract symptoms
- Urethral/bladder/renal injury
- Ureteral perforation/avulsion/intussusception
- Basket breakage or entrapment

Template Operative Dictation

Preoperative diagnosis: *Right/left ureteral/renal pelvis/calyceal* stone
Postoperative diagnosis: Same
Procedure: *Right/left* ureteroscopy with laser lithotripsy, stone basketing, and double-J stent placement.
Indications: The patient is a _____-year-old *male/female* with a ____*mm/cm* stone(s) in the *right/left ureter/renal pelvis/calyx* presenting for *right/left* ureteroscopy and stone management.
Description of Procedure: The indications, alternatives, benefits, and risks were discussed with the patient and informed consent obtained.

The patient was brought onto the operating room table, positioned supine, and secured with a safety strap. Pneumatic compression devices were placed on the lower extremities.

After the administration of intravenous antibiotics and general anesthesia, the patient was repositioned in the dorsal lithotomy using (Allen) universal stirrups and all pressure points were carefully padded. The genitalia were prepped and draped in the standard sterile manner.

The fluoroscopy unit was brought into the field, draped, and positioned appropriately.

The radiographic images were in the room.

A time-out was completed, verifying the correct patient, surgical procedure, site, and positioning, prior to beginning the procedure.

Isotonic sodium chloride was used for irrigation.

A 22 Fr cystoscope with a 30° lens was inserted per meatus and advanced, under direct vision, into the urinary bladder. Urethroscopy revealed a normal urethra. *(In a male*

patient, comment on the prostate size, lobes, and degree of obstruction.) On cystoscopy, with both the 30° and 70° lenses, the media was clear, the bladder capacity was normal and the bladder wall noted to expand symmetrically in all dimensions. There were no tumors, stones, foreign bodies, or diverticula present. The bladder wall was *minimally/ moderately/significantly/not* trabeculated with a normal appearing mucosa. Both ureteral orifices were in the normal anatomic position.

For semirigid ureteroscopy: A 5 Fr open-ended catheter was placed through the cystoscopic working port and advanced to the *right/left* ureteral orifice. A 0.038 in. (Sensor) guidewire with a hydrophilic tip was passed through the catheter and advanced to the kidney, under fluoroscopic guidance. The open-ended catheter and cystoscope were withdrawn, leaving the guidewire in place.

A semirigid ureteroscope was passed per meatus and advanced following the guide wire into the bladder and up the ureter to the *proximal/mid/distal ureteral// renal pelvis* stone. Ureteral dilation and irrigation were accomplished using a *single action pump syringe/pressure irrigation bag,* ensuring a clear visual field.

For flexible ureteroscopy: A 5 Fr open-ended catheter was placed through the cystoscopic working port and advanced to the *right/left* ureteral orifice. A 0.038 in. (Sensor) guidewire was passed through the catheter and advanced to the kidney, under fluoroscopic guidance. The open-ended catheter and cystoscope were removed and a 10 Fr ureteral dual lumen catheter advanced over the guidewire under fluoroscopic guidance. A second (working) guidewire was advanced through the dual lumen catheter to the renal pelvis and its position confirmed fluoroscopically. The dual lumen catheter was withdrawn, leaving both guidewires in place.

A flexible ureteroscope was advanced over the working guidewire into the bladder and up the ureter. Once in the upper ureter, the working guidewire was removed and the ureteroscope advanced under direct vision. The stone was visualized in the *mid/proximal ureter//renal pelvis//upper/middle/lower calyx.* A *single-action pump syringe/pressure irrigation bag* was used for ureteral dilation and irrigation, ensuring a clear visual field.

A *200/365* µm laser fiber was passed through the scope adapter (e.g. UroLok) and advanced to the stone. The holmium:YAG laser was readied and the stone *fragmented/ dusted* using a maximal energy of ____Joules at a maximal rate of _____pulses/sec.

For stone fragmentation: Stone fragments were extracted with a nitinol *stone retrieval basket/extractor* and sent for chemical analysis.

Upon completion of the laser procedure, the *ureter/collecting system* was thoroughly inspected, confirming thorough treatment of all visible stone fragments. The ureteroscope was removed slowly under direct vision, confirming an intact mucosa and the absence of residual stones.

The guidewire was backloaded into the cystoscope, using the 5 Fr open-ended catheter, and the cystoscope was advanced into the bladder. A ___Fr ____cm double-J stent was advanced over the guidewire and its proximal and distal ends positioned in the renal pelvis and bladder, respectively. Fluoroscopy was used to confirm

its proper placement. The guidewire and cystoscope were then withdrawn under direct vision, confirming the absence of any lower urinary tract injury, and the patient was repositioned supine.

At the end of the procedure, all counts were correct.

The patient tolerated the procedure well and was taken to the recovery room in satisfactory condition.

Estimated blood loss: Approximately _____ml

80

Ureteroscopy for Tumors

Indications

- Upper urinary tract tumor(s)

Essential Steps

1) Pass a guidewire cystoscopically and advance it into the renal pelvis.
2) Pass a second (working) guidewire and position it, as above.
3) Advance the flexible ureteroscope over the working guidewire to the proximal ureter and remove the guidewire.
4) Perform a thorough ureteropyelocalycoscopy.
5) Biopsy and fulgurate the tumor(s).
6) Carefully inspect the ureter, renal pelvis, and calyces for bleeding or trauma.
7) Advance a double-J stent into the renal pelvis.

Note These Variations

- For narrow ureters, a small (0.035 in.) guidewire can be used.
- Lower ureteral tumors can be accessed using a rigid ureteroscope and a single guidewire.
- On occasion, ureteral dilation may be required at the ureterovesical junction or more proximally to allow passage of the ureteroscope. This is best accomplished using a 12 Fr radially expanding balloon dilator passed over a guidewire and inflated up to 14 atm for 3–5 minutes. Alternatively, a tapered (6 Fr–12 Fr × 70 cm) hydrogel coated ureteral dilator can be used.
- The second (working) guidewire can be passed cystoscopically alongside the first guidewire using a dual lumen catheter.
- For tumors being treated definitively with ureteroscopy, instead of the two-guidewire technique, a ureteral access sheath (11 Fr/13 Fr × 36 cm, 12 Fr/14 Fr × 36 cm) can be used. This facilitates ureteroscope re-entry and may decrease operative time. In order to avoid injury to the ureter, the smallest caliber access sheath should be used and passage should never be forced. The sheath is passed over a second (working)

Operative Dictations in Urologic Surgery, First Edition. Noel A. Armenakas, John A. Fracchia, and Ron Golan.
© 2019 John Wiley & Sons Ltd. Published 2019 by John Wiley & Sons Ltd.

guidewire with the obturator in place. Once the sheath is positioned correctly in the mid to proximal ureter, the obturator and second guidewire are removed and the flexible ureteroscope advanced through the sheath.

- The tumor can be biopsied using biopsy forceps, a nitinol stone extractor, or retrieval basket.
- A holmium:YAG laser can be used to ablate the tumor and to fulgurate bleeding.

Complications

- Bleeding
- Infection
- Inability to access, biopsy, or remove the tumor(s)
- Pain/lower urinary tract symptoms
- Urethral/bladder/renal injury
- Ureteral perforation/avulsion/intussusception
- Breakage of the fine working instruments

Template Operative Dictation

Preoperative diagnosis: *Right/Left ureteral/renal pelvis/calyceal* tumor(s)
Postoperative diagnosis: Same
Procedure: *Right/Left* ureteroscopy with tumor biopsy, fulguration, and placement of a double-J stent
Indications: The patient is a _____-year-old *male/female* with a *right/left ureter/renal pelvis/calyx* tumor presenting for a *right/left* ureteroscopy, biopsy, and fulguration.
Description of Procedure: The indications, alternatives, benefits, and risks were discussed with the patient and informed consent obtained.

The patient was brought onto the operating room table, positioned supine, and secured with a safety strap. Pneumatic compression devices were placed on the lower extremities.

After the administration of intravenous antibiotics and general anesthesia, the patient was repositioned in dorsal lithotomy using (Allen) universal stirrups and all pressure points were carefully padded. The genitalia were prepped and draped in the standard sterile manner.

The fluoroscopy unit was brought into the field, draped, and positioned appropriately. The radiographic images were in the room.

A time-out was completed, verifying the correct patient, surgical procedure, site, and positioning, prior to beginning the procedure. 1.5% glycine was used for irrigation.

A 22 Fr cystoscope with a 30° lens was inserted per meatus and advanced, under direct vision, into the urinary bladder. Urethroscopy revealed a normal urethra. *(In a male patient, comment on the prostate size, lobes, and degree of obstruction.)* On cystoscopy, with both the 30° and 70° lenses, the media was clear, the bladder capacity was normal and the bladder wall noted to expand symmetrically in all dimensions. There were no tumors, stones, foreign bodies, or diverticula present. The bladder wall was *minimally/*

moderately/significantly/not trabeculated with a normal appearing mucosa. Both ureteral orifices were in the normal anatomic position with clear urinary efflux bilaterally.

A 5 Fr open-ended catheter was placed through the cystoscopic working port and advanced up the *right/left distal/mid/proximal ureter//renal pelvis*. 10 cc of urine were collected and sent for cytology. A retrograde ureteropyelogram was performed by instilling ___ cc dilute contrast medium (e.g. Omnipaque), demonstrating ___*(describe)*___. A 0.038 in. (Sensor) guidewire was then passed through the catheter and advanced to the kidney, under fluoroscopic guidance. The open-ended catheter and cystoscope were removed and a 10 Fr ureteral dual lumen catheter advanced over the guidewire under fluoroscopic guidance. A second (working) guidewire was advanced through this to the renal pelvis and its position confirmed fluoroscopically. The dual lumen catheter was withdrawn, leaving both guidewires in place.

A flexible ureteroscope was advanced over the working guidewire into the bladder and up the ureter, using fluoroscopy. Once in the upper ureter, the working guidewire was removed and the ureteroscope was advanced under direct vision. A *papillary/sessile* tumor was visualized in the *proximal/mid/distal ureter//renal pelvis//upper/middle/ lower pole calyx*. A *single action pump syringe/pressure irrigation bag* was used for ureteral dilation and irrigation, ensuring a clear visual field.

A 3 Fr ureteroscopic biopsy forceps was passed through the scope adapter (e.g. UroLok) and advanced to the tumor. *A biopsy/multiple biopsies* of the tumor *was/were* taken under direct vision and sent to pathology for evaluation. Upon completion of the biopsy, hemostasis was achieved with a 2 Fr endoscopic monopolar electrode (Bugbee) at a coagulation power setting of 20 W. The ureteroscope was removed slowly, under direct vision, confirming an intact mucosa without evidence of undue bleeding.

The guidewire was back loaded into the cystoscope, using the 5 Fr open-ended catheter, and the cystoscope advanced into the bladder. A ___Fr ___cm double-J stent was advanced over the guidewire and its proximal and distal ends positioned in the renal pelvis and bladder, respectively. Fluoroscopy was used to confirm its proper placement. The guidewire and cystoscope were then withdrawn under direct vision, confirming the absence of any lower urinary tract injury, and the patient was repositioned supine.

At the end of the procedure, all counts were correct.

The patient tolerated the procedure well and was taken to the recovery room in satisfactory condition.

Estimated blood loss: Approximately _____ml

NOTES

SECTION III   TRANSURETHRAL SURGERY

81

Bladder Biopsy

Indications

- Bladder tumor
- Abnormal urine cytology and/or fluorescence in situ hybridization (FISH)
- Bladder wall abnormalities

Essential Steps

1) Gently pass a cystoscope into the bladder under direct vision.
2) Completely inspect the lower urinary tract with both the 30° and 70° lenses and identify any bladder wall abnormalities.
3) Biopsy the lesion(s) and fulgurate the site(s) carefully.
4) Inspect the bladder for adequacy of the biopsy and absence of bleeding or injury.

Note These Variations

- If available, "Blue Light" cystoscopy (with intravesical hexaminolevulinate hydrochloride) or "narrow-band imaging" technology can be used to increase the detection of nonmuscle invasive bladder tumors (especially carcinoma in situ) not visible with white light.
- In cases of a narrow meatus or fossa navicularis, gentle sequential dilation using curved metal sounds (Van Buren) should be performed initially to avoid traumatic endoscopic urethral insertion.
- The use of a urethral catheter following the procedure is optional.

Complications

- Bleeding
- Infection
- Bladder perforation
- Urethral/bowel injury
- Urethral stricture

Operative Dictations in Urologic Surgery, First Edition. Noel A. Armenakas, John A. Fracchia, and Ron Golan.
© 2019 John Wiley & Sons Ltd. Published 2019 by John Wiley & Sons Ltd.

Template Operative Dictation

Preoperative diagnosis: *Bladder tumor/abnormal cytology/FISH/bladder wall* abnormalities

Postoperative diagnosis: Same

Procedure: Cold-cup bladder biopsies and fulguration

Indications: The patient is a ____-year-old *male/female* with a *bladder tumor/abnormal cytology/bladder wall abnormality* presenting for bladder biopsy and fulguration.

Description of Procedure: The indications, alternatives, benefits, and risks were discussed with the patient and informed consent was obtained.

The patient was brought onto the operating room table, positioned supine, and secured with a safety strap. Pneumatic compression devices were placed on the lower extremities.

After the administration of intravenous antibiotics and *general/regional* anesthesia, the patient was repositioned in dorsal lithotomy using (Allen) universal stirrups and all pressure points were carefully padded. A *rectal/pelvic* examination was performed ____ *(describe)* ____. The genitalia were prepped and draped in the standard sterile manner.

A time-out was completed, verifying the correct patient, surgical procedure, and positioning, prior to beginning the procedure. 1.5% glycine was used for irrigation.

A 22 Fr rigid cystoscope with a 30° lens was inserted per meatus and advanced, under direct vision, into the urinary bladder. Urethroscopy revealed a normal urethra. *(In a male patient, comment on the prostate size, lobes, and degree of obstruction.)* The bladder was evaluated with both the 30° and 70° lenses. The media was clear, the bladder capacity was normal, and the bladder wall noted to expand symmetrically in all dimensions. The bladder wall was *minimally/moderately/significantly/not* trabeculated with a normal appearing mucosa. Both ureteral orifices were in the normal anatomic position with clear urinary efflux bilaterally. There were no stones, foreign bodies, or diverticula present. *(Describe the mucosal/bladder wall findings.)*

A *rigid/flexible* biopsy forceps was advanced through the cystoscope and positioned at the bladder mucosa overlying the lesion at ___ o'clock. A cold cup biopsy was taken under direct vision, and the specimen was sent to pathology for evaluation. *(Repeat procedure for additional biopsies.)* The biopsy forceps was removed and replaced with an endoscopic monopolar electrode (Bugbee). The biopsied area(s) *was/were* fulgurated ensuring meticulous hemostasis.

After completion of the procedure, the bladder was again inspected, verifying removal of the area(s) in question without bleeding or bladder injury.

The cystoscope was withdrawn under direct vision, and a ___Fr urethral catheter was inserted into the bladder and connected to a drainage bag. The irrigant was clear. The patient was repositioned supine.

At the end of the procedure, all counts were correct.

The patient tolerated the procedure well and was taken to the recovery room in satisfactory condition.

Estimated blood loss: Approximately _____ml

82

Cystolithotripsy

Indications

- Bladder calculus(i)

Essential Steps

1) Gently pass the cystoscope into the bladder under direct vision.
2) Completely inspect the lower urinary tract and identify the stone(s).
3) Change to a 26 or 28 Fr (continuous flow) resectoscope with a laser bridge and pass the appropriate size laser fiber (e.g. 1000 μm) through this.
4) Thoroughly fragment the stone(s) and remove the fragments with an Ellik evacuator.
5) Inspect the bladder for residual fragments and any inadvertent injury.
6) Place a urethral catheter.

Note These Variations

- In cases of a narrow meatus or fossa navicularis, gentle sequential dilation using curved metal sounds (Van Buren) should be performed initially to avoid traumatic endoscopic urethral insertion.
- Alternatively, a dual-action ultrasonic and mechanical energy system (ShockPulse Stone Eliminator) may be used to simultaneously fragment and suction stones.
- The procedure can be done in conjunction with a transurethral resection of the prostate.

Complications

- Bleeding
- Infection
- Bladder perforation
- Urethral/bowel injury

Operative Dictations in Urologic Surgery, First Edition. Noel A. Armenakas, John A. Fracchia, and Ron Golan.
© 2019 John Wiley & Sons Ltd. Published 2019 by John Wiley & Sons Ltd.

Template Operative Dictation

Preoperative diagnosis: Bladder calculus(i)
Postoperative diagnosis:
Procedure: Cystolithotripsy
Indications: The patient is a ____-year-old *male/female* a history of bladder stone(s) presenting for a cystolithotripsy.
Description of Procedure: The indications, alternatives, benefits, and risks were discussed with the patient and informed consent was obtained.

The patient was brought onto the operating room table, positioned supine, and secured with a safety strap. Pneumatic compression devices were placed on the lower extremities.

After the administration of intravenous antibiotics and *general/regional* anesthesia, the patient was repositioned in dorsal lithotomy using (Allen) universal stirrups and all pressure points were carefully padded. A *rectal/pelvic* examination was performed ____(describe)____. The genitalia were prepped and draped in the standard sterile manner.

A time-out was completed, verifying the correct patient, surgical procedure, and positioning, prior to beginning the procedure.

Isotonic sodium chloride was used for irrigation.

A *17/22* Fr rigid cystoscope with a 30° lens was inserted per meatus and advanced, under direct vision, into the urinary bladder. Urethroscopy revealed a normal urethra. *(In a male patient, comment on the prostate size, lobes, and degree of obstruction.)* The bladder was evaluated with both the 30° and 70° lenses. The media was clear, the bladder capacity was normal, and the bladder wall noted to expand symmetrically in all dimensions. There were no tumors, foreign bodies or diverticula present. The bladder wall was *minimally/moderately/significantly/not* trabeculated with a normal appearing mucosa. Both ureteral orifices were in the normal anatomic position with clear urinary efflux bilaterally. *(State the number and size of stones.)*

The cystoscope was removed, having left the bladder partially full, and a *26/28* Fr (continuous flow) resectoscope sheath with a *Timberlake/visual* obturator was advanced into the bladder. The obturator was removed and replaced by the laser bridge. A 1000 μm laser fiber was introduced through the working channel. The holmium:YAG laser was readied and the bladder stone(s) *was/were* again visualized. The stones(s) *was/were* thoroughly fragmented using a maximal energy of ____Joules at a maximal rate of ____pulses/sec. All stone fragments were removed using an Ellik evacuator and sent for chemical analysis.

After completion of the procedure, the bladder was inspected, confirming complete removal of all stone fragments and the absence of any significant mucosal trauma or bleeding.

The resectoscope was withdrawn under direct vision, and an 18 Fr urethral catheter was inserted into the bladder and connected to a drainage bag. The irrigant was *clear/ light pink-tinged.* The patient was repositioned supine.

At the end of the procedure, all counts were correct.

The patient tolerated the procedure well and was taken to the recovery room in satisfactory condition.

Estimated blood loss: None

83

Cystoscopy

Indications

- Evaluation of the lower urinary tract (e.g. hematuria, lower urinary tract symptoms, etc.)

Essential Steps

1) Gently pass the cystoscope into the bladder, under direct vision.
2) Completely inspect the lower urinary tract with both the 30° and 70° lenses.

Note These Variations

- Cystoscopy is often performed supine in the office or at the bedside with a flexible cystoscope using a topical anesthetic (jelly).
- In cases of a narrow meatus or fossa navicularis, gentle sequential dilation using curved metal sounds (Van Buren) should be performed initially to avoid traumatic endoscopic urethral insertion.

Complications

- Bleeding
- Infection
- Urethral injury

Template Operative Dictation

Preoperative diagnosis: _____
Postoperative diagnosis: _____

Operative Dictations in Urologic Surgery, First Edition. Noel A. Armenakas, John A. Fracchia, and Ron Golan.
© 2019 John Wiley & Sons Ltd. Published 2019 by John Wiley & Sons Ltd.

Procedure: Cystoscopy

Indications: The patient is a _____-year-old *male/female* a history of _____, presenting for cystoscopic evaluation.

Description of Procedure: The indications, alternatives, benefits, and risks were discussed with the patient and informed consent was obtained.

The patient was brought onto the operating room table, positioned supine, and secured with a safety strap. Pneumatic compression devices were placed on the lower extremities.

After the administration of intravenous antibiotics and *intravenous sedation//general/regional* anesthesia, the patient was repositioned in dorsal lithotomy using (Allen) universal stirrups and all pressure points were carefully padded. A *rectal/pelvic* examination was performed _____ *(describe)* _____. The genitalia were prepped and draped in the standard sterile manner.

A time-out was completed, verifying the correct patient, surgical procedure, and positioning, prior to beginning the procedure.

Isotonic sodium chloride was used for irrigation.

A *17/22* Fr rigid cystoscope with a 30° lens was inserted per meatus and advanced, under direct vision, into the urinary bladder. Urethroscopy revealed a normal urethra. *(In a male patient, comment on the prostate size, lobes, and degree of obstruction.)* The bladder was evaluated with both the 30° and 70° lenses. The media was clear, the bladder capacity was normal, and the bladder wall was noted to expand symmetrically in all dimensions. There were no tumors, stones, foreign bodies, or diverticula present. The bladder wall was *minimally/moderately/significantly/not* trabeculated with a normal appearing mucosa. Both ureteral orifices were in the normal anatomic position with clear urinary efflux bilaterally.

Having thoroughly evaluated the lower urinary tract, the bladder was emptied and the cystoscope removed under direct vision, confirming the absence of any lower urinary tract injuries. The patient was repositioned supine.

At the end of the procedure, all counts were correct.

The patient tolerated the procedure well and was taken to the recovery room in satisfactory condition.

Estimated blood loss: None

84

Direct Visual Internal Urethrotomy

Indications

- Short bulbar urethral stricture
- Anastomotic stricture post-urethral reconstruction

Essential Steps

1) A retrograde urethrogram should be performed prior to surgery to delineate and document the location and length of the stricture.
2) Place a guidewire or open-ended ureteral catheter into the bladder before initiating the urethrotomy.
3) Advance the urethrotome proximally to the stricture and make full-thickness incision(s) in the scar to adequately open the urethra.
4) Perform a complete cystourethroscopy.
5) Pass a council-tip or urethral catheter into the bladder.

Note These Variations

- In cases of a narrow meatus or fossa navicularis, gentle sequential dilation using curved metal sounds (Van Buren) should be performed initially to avoid traumatic endoscopic urethral insertion.
- A 24 Fr, 4 cm balloon dilation catheter (e.g. UroMax Ultra) may be used initially to dilate the stricture.
- Alternatively, the Direct Visual Internal Urethrotomy (DVIU) may be performed using a holmium:YAG laser, with a 200 µm fiber, through an adult or pediatric cystoscope or a semi-rigid ureteroscope.
- With dense urethral scarring, radial urethrotomies can be performed to open the stricture circumferentially. Avoid cutting at the 4 o'clock and 8 o'clock positions where the bulbar arteries usually course.
- At the completion of the procedure, 10 ml triamcinolone acetonide (Kenalog) (40 mg/ml) can be injected into the stricture using a 35 cm cystoscopic injection (Williams) needle.

Operative Dictations in Urologic Surgery, First Edition. Noel A. Armenakas, John A. Fracchia, and Ron Golan.
© 2019 John Wiley & Sons Ltd. Published 2019 by John Wiley & Sons Ltd.

- The size of the urethral catheter used postoperatively is dependent on the urethral lumen and the surgeon's preference. Larger catheters can be used to tamponade urethral bleeding, but may predispose to urethral stricture formation.
- The semilunar urethrotome sheath can be used to position a well-lubricated urethral catheter into the bladder.

Complications

- Bleeding
- Infection
- Rectal/cavernosal injury
- Incontinence
- Recurrent urethral stricture

Template Operative Dictation

Preoperative diagnosis: Urethral stricture
Postoperative diagnosis: Same
Procedure: Direct visual internal urethrotomy
Indications: The patient is a _____-year-old male with _____mm *proximal/mid/distal bulbar//penile* urethral stricture presenting for a direct visual internal urethrotomy.
Description of Procedure: The indications, alternatives, benefits, and risks were discussed with the patient and informed consent was obtained.

The patient was brought onto the operating room table, positioned supine, and secured with a safety strap. Pneumatic compression devices were placed on the lower extremities.

After the administration of intravenous antibiotics and *general/regional* anesthesia, the patient was repositioned in dorsal lithotomy using (Allen) universal stirrups and all pressure points were carefully padded. A rectal examination was performed _____*(describe)*_____.
The genitalia were prepped and draped in the standard sterile manner.

The radiographic images were in the room.

A time-out was completed, verifying the correct patient, surgical procedure, and positioning, prior to beginning the procedure.

Isotonic sodium chloride was used for irrigation.

A 17 Fr cystoscope with a 30° lens was advanced under direct vision to the *proximal/mid/distal bulbar//penile* urethral stricture. A 0.038 in. (Sensor) guidewire with a hydrophilic tip was passed through the working port and directed into the bladder.

The cystoscope was removed with the guidewire in place, and a 21 Fr Sachse urethrotome sheath and working element with a cold-knife and 0° lens were inserted per meatus and advanced under direct vision to the level of the stricture. The urethrotome knife was extended and an incision made at the 12 o'clock position. This was repeated at the _____ o'clock position(s) ensuring full-thickness opening of the fibrous urethral tissue.

Once the stricture was thoroughly incised, the urethrotome was easily advanced into the bladder and cystoscopy performed. The bladder capacity was normal and the bladder wall was noted to expand symmetrically in all dimensions. There were no tumors, stones,

foreign bodies, or diverticula present. The bladder wall was *minimally/moderately/significantly/not* trabeculated, with a normal appearing mucosa. Both ureteral orifices were in the normal anatomic position. Upon withdrawal of the instrument, the prostatic urethra was noted to be *unobstructing/obstructing with bilobar/trilobar hypertrophy*. The area of stricture was open with negligible bleeding.

The urethrotome was removed under direct vision, confirming the absence of any lower urinary tract injuries. A *16/18/20* Fr council-tip catheter was advanced over the guidewire into the bladder. The guidewire was removed and the catheter connected to a drainage bag. The irrigant was *clear/light pink-tinged*. The patient was repositioned supine.

At the end of the procedure, all counts were correct.

The patient tolerated the procedure well and was taken to the recovery room in satisfactory condition.

Estimated blood loss: Approximately _____ml

85

Intravesical Injection of Botulinum Toxin

Indications

- Overactive bladder refractory to medical therapy
- Urge urinary incontinence refractory to medical therapy
- Neurogenic detrusor overactivity

Essential Steps

1) Gently pass a cystoscope into the bladder under direct vision and completely inspect the lower urinary tract.
2) Prime the injection needle with the previously reconstituted botulinum toxin.
3) Inject the posterolateral bladder wall, sparing the trigone.
4) Drain the bladder and withdraw the needle under direct visualization.

Note These Variations

- This procedure may be performed in the office with a flexible cystoscope, using a topical anesthetic (jelly).
- The number of units injected, diluent volume, template utilized, number of injections, and depth of injection may vary by surgeon preference and patient disease characteristics.
- Methylene blue or indigo carmine may be added to the diluent to aid in the visualization of injection sites.

Complications

- Bleeding
- Infection
- Urethral injury
- Urinary retention
- Pain/lower urinary tract symptoms
- Generalized muscle weakness

Operative Dictations in Urologic Surgery, First Edition. Noel A. Armenakas, John A. Fracchia, and Ron Golan.
© 2019 John Wiley & Sons Ltd. Published 2019 by John Wiley & Sons Ltd.

Template Operative Dictation

Preoperative diagnosis: _____
Postoperative diagnosis: Same
Procedure: Cystoscopy with intravesical injection of botulinum toxin.
Indications: The patient is a ____-year-old *male/female* a history of _____,
presenting for cystoscopy with intravesical injection of botulinum toxin.
Description of Procedure: The indications, alternatives, benefits, and risks were discussed with the patient and informed consent was obtained.

The patient was brought onto the operating room table, positioned supine, and secured with a safety strap. Pneumatic compression devices were placed on the lower extremities.

After the administration of intravenous antibiotics and *intravenous sedation// general/regional* anesthesia, the patient was repositioned in dorsal lithotomy using (Allen) universal stirrups and all pressure points were carefully padded. The genitalia were prepped and draped in the standard sterile manner.

A time-out was completed verifying the correct patient, surgical procedure, and positioning, prior to beginning the procedure.

Isotonic sodium chloride was used for irrigation.

A *22 Fr* rigid cystoscope with a 30° lens was inserted per meatus and advanced under direct vision into the urinary bladder. Urethroscopy revealed a normal urethra. *(In a male patient, comment on the prostate size, lobes, and degree of obstruction.)* The bladder was evaluated with both the 30° and 70° lenses. The media was clear, the bladder capacity was normal, and the bladder wall noted to expand symmetrically in all dimensions. There were no tumors, stones, foreign bodies, or diverticula present. The bladder wall was *minimally/moderately/significantly/not* trabeculated with a normal appearing mucosa. Both ureteral orifices were in the normal anatomic position.

A cystoscopic injection needle (e.g. Williams) was inserted through the cystoscopic working channel. *100/200/300* units of botulinum toxin were reconstituted in *10/15/20/30 ml* of sterile injectable saline per the manufacturer's instructions prior to the start of the case. The injection needle was primed with the reconstituted solution. Starting on the *right/left/midline* above the interureteric ridge of the trigone, *10/20/30* injections were administered within the detrusor muscle 1 cm apart along the posterolateral bladder wall and sparing the trigone.

The bladder was emptied and the cystoscope was removed under direct vision, confirming the absence of any injuries. The patient was repositioned supine.

At the end of the procedure, all counts were correct.

The patient tolerated the procedure well and was taken to the recovery room in satisfactory condition.

Estimated blood loss: None

86

Laser Prostatectomy (Photoselective Vaporization)

Indications

- Symptomatic benign prostatic enlargement (usually up to 100 g)
- Silent urinary retention with adequate detrusor function, with/without azotemia

  Patients may be maintained on anticoagulation.

Essential Steps

1) Complete a thorough cystoscopy with both the 30° and 70° lenses.
2) Establish the anatomic landmarks prior to starting the resection (i.e. external sphincter, verumontanum, prostatic configuration, bladder neck, and ureteral orifices).
3) Vaporize the prostate in a circumferential pattern, preferably starting with two grooves at the median lobe at 5 o'clock and 7 o'clock. Excessive vaporization at the bladder neck may result in bladder undermining, perforation, and retrograde ejaculation. Limit direct tissue contact to avoid carbonization of the fiber tip.
4) Use a slow sweeping rotational motion of the fiber, starting at the bladder neck and advancing to the prostatic apex, optimizing tissue removal.
5) Obtain meticulous hemostasis.
6) Inspect the prostatic bed for bleeding and the ureteral orifices, bladder and external sphincter for injury, prior to completing the procedure.
7) Place a urethral catheter.

Note These Variations

- Besides the potassium titanyl phosphate (KTP:YAG) laser presented herein, the holmium:YAG and thulium:YAG lasers can be used to enucleate, vaporize, and resect prostatic tissue.
- In cases of a narrow meatus or fossa navicularis, gentle sequential dilation using curved metal sounds (Van Buren) should be performed initially to avoid traumatic endoscopic urethral insertion.
- Large glands may require more than one laser fiber to complete the vaporization.
- It is not always necessary to use continuous bladder irrigation postoperatively.

Operative Dictations in Urologic Surgery, First Edition. Noel A. Armenakas, John A. Fracchia, and Ron Golan.
© 2019 John Wiley & Sons Ltd. Published 2019 by John Wiley & Sons Ltd.

Complications

- Bleeding
- Infection
- Injury to the ureteral orifices
- Incontinence
- Persistent urinary tract symptoms/urinary retention
- Erectile dysfunction

Template Operative Dictation

Preoperative diagnosis: Benign prostatic enlargement
Postoperative diagnosis: Same
Procedure: Photoselective vaporization of the prostate (GreenLight laser)
Indications: The patient is a _____-year-old male with bladder outlet obstruction presenting for photoselective vaporization of the prostate.
Description of Procedure: The indications, alternatives, benefits, and risks were discussed with the patient and informed consent was obtained.

The patient was brought onto the operating room table, positioned supine, and secured with a safety strap. Pneumatic compression devices were placed on the lower extremities.

After the administration of intravenous antibiotics and *general/regional* anesthesia, the patient was repositioned in dorsal lithotomy using (Allen) universal stirrups and all pressure points were carefully padded. A rectal examination was performed ___*(describe)*___. The genitalia were prepped and draped in the standard sterile manner.

A time-out was completed, verifying the correct patient, surgical procedure, and positioning, prior to beginning the procedure.

Isotonic sodium chloride was used for irrigation. The GreenLight XPS laser system was used for the procedure.

A 22 Fr cystoscope with a 30° lens was advanced under direct vision into the bladder. The anterior urethra appeared normal in its entirety. The prostatic urethra was elongated with *bilobar/trilobar* hyperplasia. On cystoscopic evaluation, with both the 30° and 70° lenses, the media was clear. The bladder capacity was normal and the bladder wall noted to expand symmetrically in all dimensions. There were no tumors, stones, foreign bodies or diverticula present. The bladder wall was *minimally/moderately/significantly/not* trabeculated, with a normal appearing mucosa. Both ureteral orifices were in the normal anatomic position with clear urinary efflux noted bilaterally.

The cystoscope was withdrawn, having left the bladder partially full, and a 26 Fr continuous flow resectoscope sheath with a *Timberlake/visual* obturator was advanced into the bladder. The obturator was removed and replaced by the laser bridge and the side-firing laser fiber (GreenLight MoXy) introduced through the working channel. The location of the ureteral orifices and the configuration of the prostate were again assessed.

The GreenLight XPS laser was readied, set at a power of 80 W, and the laser beam checked prior to proceeding with the procedure. Prostatic vaporization was begun by establishing two grooves at the 5 o'clock and 7 o'clock positions, starting at the bladder neck proximally and carried distally to the verumontanum. The middle lobe was vaporized with special care taken at the bladder neck using a slow sagittal motion of the fiber

to avoid injury to the trigone and bladder wall. Attention was then turned to the *left/right* lateral lobe, which was vaporized using a slow sweeping rotational motion maintaining a fiber to tissue distance of approximately 1 mm. The power was increased progressively at 10–20 W intervals to *120/140/180* W. The limits of vaporization again were the bladder neck proximally and the verumontanum distally. The identical procedure was performed on the contralateral side. The adenoma was debulked to the level of the transverse capsular fibers, obtaining a large central prostatic defect. Lastly, the anterior prostatic tissue was vaporized from the 10 o'clock to 2 o'clock positions at lower power.

Meticulous hemostasis was achieved using a pulse coagulation setting of 30 W. The bladder was irrigated with an Ellik evacuator, ensuring removal of any free-floating ablated tissue.

The overall lasing time was _____minutes for a total of _____ Joules.

Upon completion of the procedure, the bladder and posterior urethra were reexamined confirming an open prostatic urethra and bladder neck with absence of bleeding or perforation, intact ureteral orifices and a patent external sphincter mechanism.

The resectoscope was withdrawn under direct, and a ____Fr urethral catheter with a 30 cc balloon inserted into the bladder. The balloon was inflated with ____ml sterile water and the catheter connected to a drainage bag. The catheter was irrigated, ensuring clear return of the fluid. The patient was repositioned supine.

At the end of the procedure, all counts were correct.

The patient tolerated the procedure well and was taken to the recovery room in satisfactory condition.

Estimated blood loss: Approximately _____ml

87

Prostate Cryotherapy

Indications

- Select patients with clinically localized prostate cancer

Essential Steps

1) Image the prostate using transrectal real-time sonography and place the cryo- and temperature probes appropriately.
2) Prior to initiating the freeze cycle, complete a thorough cystoscopy to rule out any probe intrusion into the bladder or urethra.
3) Activate the cryoprobes in the correct sequence and monitor the formation, extent, and thawing of the ice balls using real-time sonography.
4) Allow the urethral warmer to passively thaw for 20-plus minutes.
5) Repeat the freeze–thaw cycle.
6) Remove all probes and apply manual perineal pressure to the probe sites.

Note These Variations:

- Manual initiation of the freeze and thaw cycles can be performed.
- Localized lesions can be focally ablated using targeted magnetic resonance-sonographic fusion techniques.

Complications

- Bleeding
- Infection
- Urinary retention
- Urinary leakage
- Rectal pain

Operative Dictations in Urologic Surgery, First Edition. Noel A. Armenakas, John A. Fracchia, and Ron Golan.
© 2019 John Wiley & Sons Ltd. Published 2019 by John Wiley & Sons Ltd.

- Urethral injury
- Rectal injury
- Erectile dysfunction

Template Operative Dictation

Preoperative diagnosis: Prostate cancer
Postoperative diagnosis: Same
Procedure: Prostate cryotherapy
Indications: The patient is a _____-year-old male with a clinical stage T___, Gleason Score ____ prostate cancer presenting for prostate cryotherapy.
Description of Procedure: The indications, alternatives, benefits, and risks were discussed with the patient and informed consent was obtained.

The patient was brought onto the operating room table, positioned supine, and secured with a safety strap. Pneumatic compression devices were placed on the lower extremities.

After the administration of intravenous antibiotics and *general endotracheal/regional* anesthesia, the patient was repositioned in dorsal lithotomy using (Allen) universal stirrups and all pressure points were carefully padded. A digital rectal examination was performed, confirming the lack of fixation of the prostate.

The prostate brachytherapy cradle was used to support the biplanar transrectal ultrasound system and attached to the operating table.

The genitalia and perineum were prepped and draped in the standard sterile manner.

A time-out was completed, verifying the correct patient, surgical procedure, and positioning, prior to beginning the procedure.

A 20 Fr urethral catheter was inserted into the bladder and the bladder was distended with approximately 200 ml of normal sterile saline solution. The ultrasound probe was centered, assuring that the plane of the urethra and the plane of the transducer were parallel. The volume of the prostate was calculated as _____cc.

[*Note:* Prostate volume (cc) = Length × Width × Height × $\pi/6$]

Sonographic planning was accomplished by identifying and capturing the widest transverse image of the prostate. The perimeter of the prostate, urethra, and rectal wall were carefully outlined. Six cryoprobes were tested to assure their functionality prior to placement.

Placement of the cryoprobes and temperature probes was performed utilizing the perineal brachytherapy grid in the following sequence:

- Cryoprobe numbers 1 and 2 were placed in the anterior prostate.
- Temperature probe sensors were placed anteriorly, at the level of the external sphincter and in Denonvillier's fascia.
- Cryoprobe numbers 5 and 6 were placed posteromedially within the prostate.
- Cryoprobe numbers 3 and 4 were placed posterolaterally within the prostate.
- Temperature probe sensors were placed laterally, adjacent to the right and left neurovascular bundles.

The cryoprobes were carefully placed so that their distance from the prostatic capsule was ≤1 cm, and > 0.5 cm from both the rectal and urethral walls. The distance between each cryoprobe was ≤2 cm.

The urethral catheter was removed and flexible cystoscopy performed, confirming that none of the probes or sensors had penetrated the bladder or urethral walls. The cystoscope was removed and replaced with the urethral warming catheter.

The cryoprobes were activated in AutoFreeze mode proceeding in an anterior to posterior direction, starting with numbers 1 and 2, until the anterior temperature probe reached the target temperature of −40°C *and/or* the ice ball approximated probe numbers 3 and 4. This initial freeze took approximately 5 minutes. Cryoprobe numbers 3 and 4 were activated until the right and left neurovascular bundle sensors reached within 15°C of the targeted temperature (−40°C) and placed on thaw. Lastly, cryoprobe numbers 5 and 6 were activated until the Denonvillier's fascia probe reached the target temperature of −40°C, while carefully monitoring the ice ball to make sure that it did not extend to the rectal wall. The thaw cycle was initiated, and once the temperature probe sensors reached 0°C, the entire freezing and thawing cycle was repeated.

At the conclusion of the procedure, all probes were removed and manual pressure applied to the perineum to assist in hemostasis. A digital rectal exam confirmed the lack of ice within the rectum and a smooth anterior rectal wall. The urethral warmer was allowed to passively thaw for more than 20 minutes. The 20 Fr urethral catheter was reinserted into the bladder and connected to a drainage bag. The patient was repositioned supine.

At the end of the procedure, all counts were correct.

The patient tolerated the procedure well and was taken to the recovery room in satisfactory condition.

Estimated blood loss: Approximately _____ml

88

Transurethral Resection of Bladder Tumor

Indications

- New or recurrent bladder tumors

Essential Steps

1) Perform a bimanual evaluation.
2) Evaluate the bladder with a thorough cystoscopy using both the 30° and 70° lenses.
3) Resect all tumor(s), ensuring an adequately deep specimen that includes muscularis. Take extra care when resecting the lateral bladder walls to avoid an obturator reflex.
4) Achieve meticulous hemostasis.
5) Inspect the bladder for bleeding or injury.
6) Place a urethral catheter.

Note These Variations

- If available, "Blue Light" cystoscopy (with intravesical hexaminolevulinate hydrochloride) or "narrow-band imaging" technology can be used to increase the detection of nonmuscle invasive bladder tumors (especially carcinoma in situ) not visible with white light.
- The initial cystoscopy may be performed as a separate procedure using a 17–22 Fr cystoscope if a continuous flow resectoscope with a visual obturator is not available.
- In cases of a narrow meatus or fossa navicularis, gentle sequential dilation using curved metal sounds (Van Buren) should be performed initially to avoid traumatic endoscopic urethral insertion.
- A monopolar resectoscope may be used, with either 1.5% glycine or 3% sorbitol irrigation.
- For resection of lateral wall bladder tumors, a paralytic (anesthetic) agent may be administered to limit the obturator nerve reflex.
- In cases where the tumor is in close proximity or involving the ureteral orifice, methylene blue or indigo carmine may be administered intravenously. A ureteral stent may be necessary following the resection.

Operative Dictations in Urologic Surgery, First Edition. Noel A. Armenakas, John A. Fracchia, and Ron Golan.
© 2019 John Wiley & Sons Ltd. Published 2019 by John Wiley & Sons Ltd.

- The procedure can be partially or completely performed with a resection electrode button. Since it does not provide tissue for histologic diagnosis, it is best employed at the end of the resection for hemostasis.
- Small tumors may be managed with cold cup biopsies and fulguration, using the endoscopic monopolar electrode (Bugbee).
- A single intravesical instillation of Mitomycin C may be given immediately postoperatively to decrease the risk of bladder recurrence in patients with low grade urothelial tumors.

Complications

- Bleeding
- Infection
- Bladder perforation
- Resection/fulguration of the ureteral orifice
- Bowel injury
- Urinary retention

Template Operative Dictation

Preoperative diagnosis: *(Recurrent)* Bladder tumor
Postoperative diagnosis: Same
Procedure: Transurethral resection of bladder tumor(s)
Indications: The patient is a _____-year-old *male/female* with *a ____cm/multiple* bladder tumor(s) presenting for transurethral resection.
Description of Procedure: The indications, alternatives, benefits, and risks were discussed with the patient and informed consent was obtained.

The patient was brought onto the operating room table, positioned supine, and secured with a safety strap. Pneumatic compression devices were placed on the lower extremities.

After the administration of intravenous antibiotics and *general/regional* anesthesia, the patient was repositioned in dorsal lithotomy using (Allen) universal stirrups and all pressure points were carefully padded. A bimanual examination was performed, confirming the absence of a palpable mass or pelvic wall fixation. The genitalia were prepped and draped in the standard sterile manner.

A time-out was completed, verifying the correct patient, surgical procedure, and positioning, prior to beginning the procedure.

Isotonic sodium chloride was used for irrigation.

A *24/26* Fr (continuous flow) resectoscope sheath with a visual obturator and a 30° lens was advanced under direct vision into the bladder. The urethra appeared normal in its entirety. *(In a male patient, comment on the prostate size, lobes, and degree of obstruction.)*

On cystoscopic evaluation, with both the 30° and 70° lenses, the media was clear, the bladder capacity was normal, and the bladder wall was noted to expand symmetrically in all dimensions. There were no stones, foreign bodies, or diverticula present. The bladder wall was *minimally/moderately/significantly/not* trabeculated. Both ureteral orifices were in the normal anatomic position with clear urinary efflux noted bilaterally.

A ____cm bladder tumor was seen on the ___*(location)*___ wall. The remaining mucosa appeared normal.

The obturator was removed and replaced by the working element with a resection electrode loop. The location of the ureteral orifices was again confirmed.

The tumor(s) *was/were* visualized and thoroughly resected to the detrusor muscle incorporating muscularis propria, using a bipolar power setting of 200 and *(120–)*160 watts for cutting and coagulation, respectively. Meticulous hemostasis was achieved. The bladder was gently irrigated with an Ellik evacuator ensuring removal of all resected tissue, and the specimen(s) sent to pathology for evaluation. The bladder was again visualized, confirming complete tumor resection, absence of bleeding or perforation, and intact ureteral orifices.

The resectoscope was withdrawn under direct vision, and a ____Fr urethral catheter inserted into the bladder and connected to a drainage bag. The irrigant was *clear/light pink-tinged*. The patient was repositioned supine.

At the end of the procedure, all counts were correct.

The patient tolerated the procedure well and was taken to the recovery room in satisfactory condition.

Estimated blood loss: Approximately _____ml

89

Transurethral Resection of Ejaculatory Ducts

Indications

- Ejaculatory duct obstruction

Essential Steps

1) Perform transurethral sonography and inject 10 ml of diluted methylene blue or indigo carmine into the seminal vesicles.
2) Complete a thorough cystoscopy with both the 30° and 70° lenses.
3) Resect the entire verumontanum, preserving the bladder neck, prostate, and external sphincter.
4) Visualize milky fluid from the ducts to confirm an adequate resection.

Note These Variations

- The seminal vesicles can be aspirated and fluid examined using microscopy. Vasography may be considered if there is no sperm in the aspirate.
- In cases of a narrow meatus or fossa navicularis, gentle sequential dilation using curved metal sounds (Van Buren) should be performed initially to avoid traumatic endoscopic urethral insertion.
- A monopolar resectoscope may be used with either 1.5% glycine or 3% sorbitol irrigation.
- At the end of the procedure, vesiculography can be performed by placing a 5 Fr ureteral catheter through the opened ejaculatory ducts to confirm their patency.

Complications

- Hematuria
- Infection
- Urinary reflux

Operative Dictations in Urologic Surgery, First Edition. Noel A. Armenakas, John A. Fracchia, and Ron Golan.
© 2019 John Wiley & Sons Ltd. Published 2019 by John Wiley & Sons Ltd.

- Sphincteric injury
- Epididymitis
- Watery ejaculate
- Retrograde ejaculation
- Urethral stricture
- Infertility

Template Operative Dictation

Preoperative diagnosis: Ejaculatory duct obstruction
Postoperative diagnosis: Same
Procedure: Transurethral resection of the ejaculatory ducts
Indications: The patient is a ____-year-old male with imaging and semen analysis evidence of ejaculatory duct obstruction presenting for transurethral resection of the ejaculatory ducts.
Description of Procedure: The indications, alternatives, benefits, and risks were discussed with the patient and informed consent was obtained.

The patient was brought onto the operating room table, positioned supine, and secured with a safety strap. Pneumatic compression devices were placed on the lower extremities.

After the administration of intravenous antibiotics and *general endotracheal/regional* anesthesia, the patient was repositioned in dorsal lithotomy using (Allen) universal stirrups and all pressure points were carefully padded. A rectal examination was performed ____*(describe)*____. The genitalia were prepped and draped in the standard sterile manner.

A time-out was completed, verifying the correct patient, surgical procedure, and positioning prior to beginning the procedure.

Isotonic sodium chloride was used for irrigation.

Transrectal ultrasonography was performed and the seminal vesicles identified. A spinal needle was introduced into each seminal vesicle and 10 ml diluted *methylene blue/indigo carmine* were instilled under direct vision.

A rectal shield (O'Connor steri-drape) was placed, allowing placement of a finger in the rectum during the procedure to avoid a rectal injury.

A 24 Fr (continuous flow) resectoscope sheath with a visual obturator and a 30° oblique lens was advanced under direct vision into the bladder. The anterior urethra appeared normal in its entirety. The prostatic urethra was elongated with *bilobar/trilobar* hyperplasia. On cystoscopic evaluation with both the 30° and 70° lenses, the media was clear, the bladder capacity was normal, and the bladder wall noted to expand symmetrically in all dimensions. There were no tumors, stones, foreign bodies, or diverticula present. The bladder wall was *minimally/moderately/significantly/not* trabeculated, with a normal-appearing mucosa. Both ureteral orifices were in the normal anatomic position with clear urinary efflux noted bilaterally.

The obturator was removed and replaced by the working element with a 24 Fr resection electrode loop. The location of the ureteral orifices and the prostatic configuration was again confirmed.

The resectoscope was positioned just proximal to the verumontanum and transurethral resection of the verumontanum was started at the midline using a bipolar power setting of 200 W. The entire verumontanum was resected, confirming efflux of copious *methylene blue/indigo carmine*-tinted milky fluid. Meticulous hemostasis was achieved with judicious cautery at a power setting of 120 W.

Having completed the resection, the bladder, prostate, and urethra were visualized, confirming a patent bladder neck and intact external sphincter mechanism.

The resectoscope was withdrawn under direct vision, and a 16 Fr urethral catheter was placed into the bladder and connected to a drainage bag. The irrigant was *clear/light pink-tinged*. The patient was repositioned supine.

At the end of the procedure, all counts were correct.

The patient tolerated the procedure well and was taken to the recovery room in satisfactory condition.

Estimated blood loss: Approximately _____ml

90

Transurethral Resection of Prostate

Indications

- Symptomatic benign prostatic enlargement (usually up to 100 g)
- Silent urinary retention with adequate detrusor function, with/without azotemia

Essential Steps

1) Complete a thorough cystoscopy with both the 30° and 70° lenses.
2) Establish the anatomic landmarks prior to starting the resection (i.e. external sphincter, verumontanum, prostatic configuration, bladder neck, and ureteral orifices).
3) Systematically resect the prostate in a circumferential pattern. If the middle lobe is significantly enlarged, start the resection there to facilitate irrigation and the instrument's movement. Over-resection of the bladder neck may result in bladder undermining and perforation.
4) Fulgurate bleeding vessels and achieve meticulous hemostasis.
5) Remove all prostate chips using an Ellik evacuator.
6) Prior to completing the procedure, inspect the prostatic bed for bleeding and the ureteral orifices, bladder and external sphincter for injury.
7) Place a three-way urethral catheter and begin continuous bladder irrigation.

Note These Variations

- The initial cystoscopy may be performed as a separate procedure with a 17–22 Fr cystoscope if a continuous flow resectoscope with a visual obturator is not available.
- In cases of a narrow meatus or fossa navicularis, gentle sequential dilation using curved metal sounds (Van Buren) should be performed initially to avoid traumatic endoscopic urethral insertion.
- A monopolar resectoscope may be used, with either 1.5% glycine or 3% sorbitol irrigation.

Operative Dictations in Urologic Surgery, First Edition. Noel A. Armenakas, John A. Fracchia, and Ron Golan.
© 2019 John Wiley & Sons Ltd. Published 2019 by John Wiley & Sons Ltd.

- The procedure can be partially or completely performed with a resection electrode button. It does not provide tissue for histologic diagnosis; consequently, it may be best employed at the end of the resection to improve hemostasis.
- For small glands without bleeding, the use of traction may not be required.

Complications

- Bleeding
- Infection
- Dilutional hyponatremia
- Resection/fulguration of the ureteral orifices
- Incontinence
- Bladder or rectal perforation
- Persistent urinary tract symptoms/urinary retention
- Erectile dysfunction

Template Operative Dictation

Preoperative diagnosis: Benign prostatic enlargement
Postoperative diagnosis: Same
Procedure: Transurethral resection of prostate
Indications: The patient is a _____-year-old male with bladder outlet obstruction presenting for transurethral resection of the prostate.
Description of Procedure: The indications, alternatives, benefits, and risks were discussed with the patient and informed consent was obtained.

The patient was brought onto the operating room table, positioned supine, and secured with a safety strap. Pneumatic compression devices were placed on the lower extremities.

After the administration of intravenous antibiotics and *general/regional* anesthesia, the patient was repositioned in dorsal lithotomy using (Allen) universal stirrups and all pressure points were carefully padded. A rectal examination was performed, confirming a smooth, symmetrically enlarged gland. The genitalia were prepped and draped in the standard sterile manner.

A time-out was completed, verifying the correct patient, surgical procedure, and positioning prior to beginning the procedure.

Isotonic sodium chloride was used for irrigation.

A *24/26* Fr (continuous flow) resectoscope sheath with a visual obturator and a 30° lens was advanced under direct vision into the bladder. The anterior urethra appeared normal in its entirety. The prostatic urethra was elongated with *bilobar/trilobar* hyperplasia. On cystoscopic evaluation, with both the 30° and 70° lenses, the media was clear, the bladder capacity was normal, and the bladder wall noted to expand symmetrically in all dimensions. There were no tumors, stones, foreign bodies or diverticula present. The bladder wall was *minimally/moderately/significantly* trabeculated, with a normal appearing mucosa. Both orifices were in the normal anatomic position with clear urinary efflux noted bilaterally.

The obturator was removed and replaced by the working element with a resection electrode band. The location of the ureteral orifices and the prostatic configuration were again confirmed.

The resectoscope was positioned at the verumontanum and transurethral resection of the prostate performed using a bipolar power setting at 200 and 120 W for cutting and coagulation, respectively. The procedure began at the bladder neck at the 5 o'clock and 7 o'clock positions, and carried distally to the verumontanum, resecting the intervening prostatic adenoma. Using a rotational motion, the *left/right* lateral lobe was similarly resected to the level of the transverse capsular fibers. The identical procedure was performed on the contralateral lobe. Attention was then directed anteriorly and the resection completed from the 10 o'clock to 2 o'clock positions.

All bleeding vessels were fulgurated achieving meticulous hemostasis. The bladder was irrigated with an Ellik evacuator, ensuring removal of all prostatic chips, which were sent to pathology for evaluation.

Having completed the resection, the electrode band was exchanged for the electrode button. Irregular areas of residual prostatic adenoma were vaporized using a sweeping in-and-out motion to smooth out the prostate. Bleeding vessels were controlled using the coagulating current.

Upon completion of the entire procedure, the bladder and posterior urethra were re-examined, confirming an open prostatic urethra and bladder neck without evidence of bleeding or perforation. Both ureteral orifices and the external sphincter mechanism were intact.

The resectoscope was withdrawn under direct vision, and a ___Fr three-way urethral catheter with a 30 cc balloon was inserted into the bladder. The balloon was inflated with ____ml sterile water and the catheter was placed on gentle traction. After multiple manual irrigations ensuring light-pink return of the irrigant, the procedure was terminated. The catheter was attached to a drainage bag and continuous bladder irrigation was started with normal saline. The patient was repositioned supine.

At the end of the procedure, all counts were correct.

The patient tolerated the procedure well and was taken to the recovery room in satisfactory condition.

Estimated blood loss: Approximately _____ml

NOTES

SECTION IV TRANSVAGINAL SURGERY

91

Anterior Vaginal Prolapse Repair (Cystocele)

Indications

- Anterior vaginal prolapse with a central and lateral defect

Essential Steps

1) Place a urethral catheter and make sure the bladder is continually decompressed.
2) Through a midline longitudinal vaginal incision, create vaginal flaps and dissect these off of the pubocervical fascia. Extend the dissection laterally to the arcus tendineus fascia pelvis, bilaterally.
3) Reduce the bladder centrally and perform an anterior colporrhaphy.
4) Reduce the lateral defects by suturing the arcus tendineus fascia pelvis to the pubocervical fascia and inner vaginal flap.
5) Perform cystoscopy to confirm integrity of the bladder and urethra, ureteral efflux, and the absence of an intravesical suture.
6) Trim the excess vaginal mucosa and complete a midline vaginal closure.

Note These Variations

- The procedure alternatively can be performed through an inverted-U midline vaginal incision.
- Isolated central defects can be managed with an anterior colporraphy alone.
- A synthetic mesh can be placed over the midline plication to support the repair. There are many choices of mesh materials, including autologous or cadaveric fascias, xeno-grafts, and synthetics. Ultimately, the choice of mesh material is at the surgeon's discretion.
- In cases where there is associated stress urinary incontinence, a mid-urethral sling procedure can be performed concurrently.
- Prior to cystoscopy, indigo carmine or methylene blue can be injected intravenously to confirm ureteral patency.

Operative Dictations in Urologic Surgery, First Edition. Noel A. Armenakas, John A. Fracchia, and Ron Golan.
© 2019 John Wiley & Sons Ltd. Published 2019 by John Wiley & Sons Ltd.

- A suprapubic cystotomy catheter may be inserted, in addition to the urethral catheter, to assist in the subsequent voiding trial.
- Postoperatively the vagina may be packed with a sterile rolled gauze to aid in hemostasis.

Complications

- Bleeding
- Infection
- Bladder perforation
- Ureteral obstruction/laceration
- Urinary retention
- De-novo/worsening urge or stress urinary incontinence
- Dyspareunia/hispareunia
- Fistula
- Mesh erosion
- Recurrent prolapse

Template Operative Dictation

Preoperative diagnosis: Anterior vaginal prolapse
Postoperative diagnosis: Same
Procedure: Anterior vaginal prolapse repair
Indications: The patient is a _____-year-old female with an anterior vaginal prolapse presenting for surgical repair.
Description of Procedure: The indications, alternatives, benefits, and risks were discussed with the patient and informed consent was obtained.

The patient was brought onto the operating room table, positioned supine, and secured with a safety strap. Pneumatic compression devices were placed on the lower extremities.

After the administration of intravenous antibiotics and *general endotracheal/regional* anesthesia, the patient was repositioned in dorsal lithotomy using well-padded *universal (Allen)/candy cane* stirrups. The genitalia, perineum, and lower abdomen were prepped and draped in the standard sterile manner.

A time-out was completed, verifying the correct patient, surgical procedure, and positioning, prior to beginning the procedure.

A 16 Fr urethral catheter was inserted to drain the bladder. A weighted speculum was placed in the posterior vaginal wall and a self-retaining retractor (e.g. Lone Star, Bookwalter) was appropriately positioned to optimize exposure. The anterior vaginal mucosa was hydrodissected using injectable 1% lidocaine with 1:100000 epinephrine to facilitate the dissection and assist with hemostasis.

With the bladder decompressed, a midline incision was made in the anterior vaginal wall, 1 cm below the urethral meatus to the apex of the defect. Using a combination of sharp and blunt dissection, the lateral vaginal wall flaps were dissected off the periurethral and pubocervical fascias, exposing the central defect. The bladder was reduced into

the pelvis and an anterior colporraphy was performed by placing midline interrupted 2-0 polydioxanone (PDS) plication sutures approximating the vaginal muscularis and adventitia over the prolapsed bladder.

The bladder was retracted medially and the dissection continued laterally to the *right/left* arcus tendineus fascia pelvis, exposing the lateral bladder defect. Five 2-0 PDS sutures were placed through the arcus tendineus fascia pelvis and passed through the lateral edge of the pubocervical fascia and the inner vaginal flap. After placement, the sutures were individually tied, reducing the *right/left* lateral defect. During the entire dissection, care was taken to avoid entering the bladder and urethra. Hemostasis was achieved with electrocautery.

The identical procedure was performed at the level of the contralateral arcus tendineus fascia pelvis.

Having completed the prolapse repair, the urethral catheter was removed and cystourethroscopy was performed, using a *flexible cystoscope/___Fr rigid cystoscope with both the 30° and 70° lenses.* The proximal urethra and bladder were intact, and clear ureteral efflux was noted bilaterally. There were no intravesical sutures. The cystoscope was removed and replaced with the urethral catheter.

The wound was irrigated with sterile normal saline and hemostasis again confirmed. The edges of the vaginal epithelium were appropriately trimmed and the vaginal wall was closed with interrupted 2-0 polyglactin (Vicryl) sutures. The self-retaining retractor and weighted vaginal speculum were removed.

The urethral catheter was connected to a drainage bag and the patient was repositioned supine.

At the end of the procedure, all counts were correct.

The patient tolerated the procedure well and was taken to the recovery room in satisfactory condition.

Estimated blood loss: Approximately _____ml

92

Autologous Pubovaginal Sling

Indications

- Female stress urinary incontinence with internal sphincter deficiency
- Failed mid-urethral sling

Essential Steps

1) Harvest a 2 cm by 8 cm longitudinal segment of rectus fascia through a lower abdominal incision.
2) Place a urethral catheter and make sure the bladder is continually decompressed.
3) Incise the anterior vaginal wall and dissect the vaginal epithelium off the periurethral and endopelvic fascias, dorsally and laterally, respectively.
4) Sharply perforate the endopelvic fascia bilaterally.
5) Using blunt finger dissection, create a tunnel from the vagina to the posterior rectus abdominis fascia within the space of Retzius.
6) Perforate the rectus fascia just off midline above the pubis bilaterally, using a transvaginal needle. Guide the needle inferiorly, through each endopelvic incision, closely hugging the posterior aspect of the symphysis pubis.
7) Individually load the sling sutures onto the transvaginal needle and pull these through the rectus fascia.
8) Perform cystoscopy to confirm integrity of the bladder and urethra, ureteral efflux, and the absence of an intravesical suture.
9) Reapproximate the rectus fascia and loosely tie the sling sutures to each other.

Note These Variations

- There are many choices for sling materials, including autologous or cadaveric fascias, xenografts, and synthetics. Ultimately, the choice of sling material is at the surgeon's discretion.
- In cases where the rectus abdominis fascia is not adequate for sling harvest (such as in patients having had prior major abdominal surgery), the fascia lata is another autologous option and can be harvested from the lateral aspect of the thigh.

Operative Dictations in Urologic Surgery, First Edition. Noel A. Armenakas, John A. Fracchia, and Ron Golan.
© 2019 John Wiley & Sons Ltd. Published 2019 by John Wiley & Sons Ltd.

- The procedure alternatively can be performed through a midline vertical vaginal incision.
- Prior to cystoscopy, indigo carmine or methylene blue can be injected intravenously to confirm ureteral patency endoscopically.
- A cystotomy catheter may be placed in addition to the urethral catheter to assist in the subsequent voiding trial.
- Postoperatively the vagina may be packed with a sterile rolled gauze to aid in hemostasis.

Complications

- Bleeding
- Infection
- Bladder perforation
- Ureteral obstruction/laceration
- Urinary retention
- De-novo/worsening urge incontinence
- Recurrent/persistent stress incontinence
- Dyspareunia/hispareunia
- Fistula (vesicovaginal/urethrovaginal)
- Erosion

Template Operative Dictation

Preoperative diagnosis: Stress urinary incontinence with intrinsic sphincter deficiency
Postoperative diagnosis: Same
Procedure: Autologous pubovaginal sling
Indications: The patient is a ____-year-old female with stress urinary incontinence and intrinsic sphincter deficiency presenting for an autologous pubovaginal sling.
Description of Procedure: The indications, alternatives, benefits, and risks were discussed with the patient and informed consent was obtained.

The patient was brought onto the operating room table, positioned supine, and secured with a safety strap. Pneumatic compression devices were placed on the lower extremities.

After the administration of intravenous antibiotics and *general endotracheal/regional* anesthesia, the patient was repositioned in dorsal lithotomy using well-padded *universal (Allen)/candy cane* stirrups. The genitalia, perineum, and abdomen were prepped and draped in the standard sterile manner.

A time-out was completed, verifying the correct patient, surgical procedure, and positioning, prior to beginning the procedure.

A 10 cm suprapubic longitudinal incision was made 2 cm above the pubic symphysis (modified Pfannenstiel). A self-retaining retractor (e.g. Weitlaner, Denis-Browne) was appropriately positioned for exposure. The skin incision was carried down through the subcutaneous tissue to the underlying anterior rectus abdominis fascia, which was sharply incised longitudinally for a distance of 8 cm. A 2 cm × 8 cm sling was harvested

from the inferior fascial leaf by elevating the fascia off the underlying muscle. Hemostasis was achieved with electrocautery. A full-length 0 *polyglactin (Vicryl)/polypropylene (Prolene)* figure-of-eight suture was placed on each end of the harvested sling and individually clamped. The sling was stored in sterile normal saline.

The cut edges of the rectus abdominis fascia were mobilized and a tension free fascial closure completed using a running 1-0 polydioxanone (PDS) suture. The suprapubic incision was irrigated with sterile normal saline and the self-retaining retractor was removed.

Attention was then directed to the perineum. A 16 Fr urethral catheter was inserted to drain the bladder. A weighted speculum was placed in the posterior vaginal wall and a self-retaining retractor (e.g. Lone Star, Bookwalter) was appropriately positioned to optimize exposure. The anterior vaginal mucosa was hydrodissected using injectable 1% lidocaine with 1:100 000 epinephrine to facilitate the dissection and assist with hemostasis.

With the bladder decompressed, an inverted-U incision was made in the anterior vaginal wall 1 cm below the urethral meatus to the level of the bladder neck. Using a combination of sharp and blunt dissection, an anterior vaginal wall flap was dissected off the underlying periurethral and pubocervical fascias. The dissection was continued laterally to the ischiopubic rami, exposing the endopelvic fascia bilaterally. Metzenbaum scissors were used to perforate the endopelvic fascia at this level, entering the retropubic space below the inferior pubic margin. Blunt-finger dissection was utilized to further develop this plane, creating a tunnel from the vagina to the posterior rectus abdominis fascia through the space of Retzius. During the entire dissection, care was taken to hug the posterior aspect of the pubic symphysis to avoid injuring the bladder.

A transvaginal needle (e.g. Raz, Stamey) was used to perforate the rectus fascia just to the *right/left* of midline, above the pubis. Using a finger placed intravaginally into the space of Retzius, the needle was angled inferiorly and advanced through the ipsilateral endopelvic incision into the vagina, again closely hugging the posterior aspect of the pubic symphysis.

The sling was brought into the vaginal field and the *right/left* sling suture loaded on the transvaginal needle. The needle was pulled back into the suprapubic incision and the suture ends were clamped. Hemostasis was achieved with judicious electrocautery.

The identical procedure was performed on the contralateral side.

The urethral catheter was removed and cystourethroscopy was performed, using a *flexible cystoscope/___ Fr rigid cystoscope with both the 30° and 70° lenses*. The proximal urethra and bladder were intact, and clear ureteral efflux was noted bilaterally. There were no intravesical sutures. The cystoscope was removed and replaced with the urethral catheter.

Having confirmed proper suture placement, gentle traction was placed on both suture ends and the sling positioned at the level of the bladder neck and proximal urethra. The center of the sling was secured to the periurethral fascia using two 4-0 Vicryl sutures. The sutures at each end of the sling were loosely tied together above the rectus abdominis fascia.

Scarpa's fascia was approximated with 3-0 chromic sutures and the suprapubic incision was closed with a running subcuticular 4-0 poliglecaprone (Monocryl) suture. Sterile adhesive strips and a gauze dressing were applied.

The vaginal self-retaining retractor and weighted speculum were removed and the vaginal wall was approximated with interrupted 2-0 Vicryl sutures.

The urethral catheter was connected to a drainage bag and the patient was repositioned supine.

At the end of the procedure, all counts were correct.

The patient tolerated the procedure well and was taken to the recovery room in satisfactory condition.

Estimated blood loss: Approximately _____ml

93

Enterocele Repair with Uterosacral Ligament Fixation

Indications

- Enterocele and apical prolapse

Essential Steps

1) Place a urethral catheter and make sure the bladder is continually decompressed.
2) Grasp the prolapsed vaginal wall and bring it out through the vaginal introitus.
3) Incise the anterior vaginal wall along the length of the enterocele, and dissect it free from the underlying pubocervical fascia and enterocele sac.
4) Isolate the enterocele sac circumferentially, open it, and enter the peritoneal cavity.
5) Retract the intraabdominal contents and identify the uterosacral ligaments bilaterally.
6) Suspend the vaginal apex by placing two to three sutures through each uterosacral ligament and secure these to the ipsilateral pubocervical and rectovaginal fascias superiorly and inferiorly, respectively.
7) Perform cystoscopy to confirm integrity of the bladder and urethra, ureteral efflux and the absence of an intravesical suture.
8) Trim the excess vaginal mucosa and complete a midline vaginal closure.

Note These Variations

- Alternatively, the vaginal vault can be suspended to the sacrospinous ligament or iliococcygeus fascia.
- A synthetic mesh can be used to augment the repair.
- In cases where there is associated stress urinary incontinence or a rectocele, a mid-urethral sling or rectocele procedure can be performed concurrently.
- Prior to cystoscopy, indigo carmine or methylene blue can be injected intravenously to confirm ureteral patency.
- A percutaneous cystotomy may be inserted in addition to the urethral catheter, to assist in the subsequent voiding trial.
- Postoperatively, the vagina may be packed with a sterile rolled gauze to aid in hemostasis.

Operative Dictations in Urologic Surgery, First Edition. Noel A. Armenakas, John A. Fracchia, and Ron Golan.
© 2019 John Wiley & Sons Ltd. Published 2019 by John Wiley & Sons Ltd.

Complications

- Bleeding
- Infection
- Bladder/bowel/nerve/ureteral/vaginal injury
- Dyspareunia/hispareunia
- Erosion
- Fistula
- Recurrent prolapse

Template Operative Dictation

Preoperative diagnosis: Enterocele with apical prolapse
Postoperative diagnosis: Same
Procedure: Transvaginal enterocele repair with uterosacral ligament fixation
Indications: The patient is a _____-year-old female with an enterocele and apical prolapse presenting for a transvaginal enterocele repair with uterosacral ligament fixation.
Description of Procedure: The indications, alternatives, benefits, and risks were discussed with the patient and informed consent was obtained.

The patient was brought onto the operating room table, positioned supine, and secured with a safety strap. Pneumatic compression devices were placed on the lower extremities.

After the administration of intravenous antibiotics and *general endotracheal/regional* anesthesia, the patient was repositioned in dorsal lithotomy using well-padded *universal (Allen)/candy cane* stirrups. The genitalia, perineum, and lower abdomen were prepped and draped in the standard sterile manner.

A time-out was completed, verifying the correct patient, surgical procedure, and positioning, prior to beginning the procedure.

A 16 Fr urethral catheter was inserted to drain the bladder. A weighted speculum was placed in the posterior vaginal wall and a self-retaining retractor (e.g. Lone Star, Bookwalter) was appropriately positioned to optimize exposure. The anterior vaginal mucosa was hydrodissected using injectable 1% lidocaine with 1 : 100 000 epinephrine to facilitate the dissection and assist with hemostasis.

With the bladder completely decompressed, the prolapsed vaginal wall was grasped between two Allis clamps and brought out through the vaginal introitus. Using a #15 blade, a longitudinal midline incision was made in the anterior vaginal wall along the length of the enterocele. The vaginal wall was carefully dissected from the underlying pubocervical fascia and enterocele sac, staying superficially. Using sharp and blunt dissection, the enterocele sac was isolated circumferentially to its neck, opened distally, and the peritoneal cavity entered. A moist laparotomy pad and Deaver retractor were positioned anteriorly to reduce the intraabdominal contents.

The ischial spines were palpated bilaterally and the uterosacral ligaments identified posteromedially at the 4 o'clock and 8 o'clock positions along the pelvic sidewall. Three, double-armed interrupted 2-0 *polydioxanone (PDS)/polyester (Ethibond)* sutures were

passed from lateral-to-medial through each uterosacral ligament. One arm of each suture was placed in the pubocervical and the other in the rectovaginal fascia. The laparotomy pad and Deaver retractor were removed and each suture was individually tied, resuspending the vaginal apex. Care was taken to avoid injury to the bowel, ureters and bladder.

Having completed the repair, the urethral catheter was removed and cystourethroscopy performed, using a *flexible cystoscope/___Fr rigid cystoscope with both the 30° and 70° lenses.* The urethra and bladder were intact, and clear ureteral efflux noted bilaterally. There were no intravesical sutures. The cystoscope was removed and replaced with the urethral catheter.

The edges of the vaginal epithelium were appropriately trimmed and the vaginal wall approximated with a running 2-0 polyglactin (Vicryl) suture.

The self-retaining retractor and weighted vaginal speculum were removed.

The urethral catheter was connected to a drainage bag and the patient was repositioned supine.

At the end of the procedure, all counts were correct.

The patient tolerated the procedure well and was taken to the recovery room in satisfactory condition.

Estimated blood loss: Approximately _____ml

94

Midurethral Retropubic Sling

Indications

- Female stress urinary incontinence with urethral hypermobility and mild to moderate internal sphincter deficiency.

Essential Steps

1) Place a urethral catheter and make sure the bladder is continually decompressed.
2) Incise the anterior vaginal wall and dissect the vaginal epithelium off the periurethral and endopelvic fascias, dorsally and laterally, respectively.
3) Sharply perforate the endopelvic fascia bilaterally.
4) Using blunt finger dissection, create a tunnel from the vagina to the posterior rectus abdominis fascia within the space of Retzius.
5) Make two 1 cm skin incisions directly over the symphysis pubis, on each side of the midline. Place a transvaginal needle in each incision, perforate the rectus fascia, and guide the needle inferiorly through the endopelvic fascia, closely hugging the posterior aspect of the symphysis pubis.
6) Individually load the sling sutures onto the transvaginal needle and pull these through the rectus fascia into the suprapubic incisions.
7) Perform cystoscopy to confirm integrity of the bladder and urethra, ureteral efflux, and the absence of an intravesical suture.
8) Loosely tie the sling sutures individually and close each incision separately.

Note These Variations

- There are many choices for sling materials, including autologous or cadaveric fascias, xenografts, and synthetics. Ultimately, the choice of sling material is at the surgeon's discretion.
- Additional sling-anchoring options include prepubic and transobturator, and are accessible in a variety of commercially available kits.
- Alternatively, the procedure can be performed through an inverted-U vaginal incision.

Operative Dictations in Urologic Surgery, First Edition. Noel A. Armenakas, John A. Fracchia, and Ron Golan.
© 2019 John Wiley & Sons Ltd. Published 2019 by John Wiley & Sons Ltd.

- Prior to cystoscopy, indigo carmine or methylene blue can be injected intravenously to confirm ureteral patency endoscopically.
- A cystotomy catheter may be placed, in addition to the urethral catheter, to assist in the subsequent voiding trial.
- Postoperatively the vagina may be packed with a sterile rolled gauze to aid in hemostasis.

Complications

- Bleeding
- Infection
- Bladder perforation
- Ureteral obstruction/laceration
- Urinary retention
- De-novo/worsening urge incontinence
- Recurrent/persistent stress incontinence
- Dyspareunia/hispareunia
- Fistula (vesicovaginal/urethrovaginal)
- Erosion

Template Operative Dictation

Preoperative diagnosis: Stress urinary incontinence
Postoperative diagnosis: Same
Procedure: Midurethral retropubic sling
Indications: The patient is a _____-year-old female with stress urinary incontinence and *mild/moderate* intrinsic sphincter deficiency presenting for a midurethral retropubic sling.
Description of Procedure: The indications, alternatives, benefits, and risks were discussed with the patient and informed consent was obtained.

The patient was brought onto the operating room table, positioned supine, and secured with a safety strap. Pneumatic compression devices were placed on the lower extremities.

After the administration of intravenous antibiotics and *general endotracheal/regional* anesthesia, the patient was repositioned in dorsal lithotomy using well-padded *universal (Allen)/candy cane* stirrups. The genitalia, perineum and lower abdomen were prepped and draped in the standard sterile manner.

A time-out was completed verifying the correct patient, surgical procedure, and positioning, prior to beginning the procedure.

A 16 Fr urethral catheter was inserted to drain the bladder. A weighted speculum was placed in the posterior vaginal wall and a self-retaining retractor (e.g. Lone Star, Bookwalter) was appropriately positioned to optimize exposure. The anterior vaginal mucosa was hydrodissected using injectable 1% lidocaine with 1 : 100 000 epinephrine to facilitate the dissection and assist with hemostasis.

With the bladder completely empty, a midline incision was made in the anterior vaginal wall 1 cm below the urethral meatus to the level of the bladder neck. Using a

combination of sharp and blunt dissection, an anterior vaginal wall flap was dissected off the underlying periurethral and pubocervical fascias. The dissection was continued laterally to the ischiopubic rami, exposing the endopelvic fascia bilaterally. Metzenbaum scissors were used to perforate at this level, entering the retropubic space below the inferior pubic margin. Blunt finger dissection was utilized to further develop this plane, creating a tunnel from the vagina to the posterior rectus abdominis fascia through the space of Retzius. During the entire dissection, care was taken to hug the posterior aspect of the pubic symphysis to avoid injuring the bladder.

Paired 1 cm skin incisions were made directly over the symphysis pubis, on each side of the midline. A transvaginal needle (e.g. Raz, Stamey) was placed through the *right/left* skin incision and advanced hugging the posterior aspect of the pubic symphysis. Using a finger placed intravaginally into the space of Retzius, the needle was angled inferiorly and advanced through the ipsilateral endopelvic incision into the vagina.

[*Note:* If a commercially available sling is not available, a sling can be fashioned by cutting a 2 cm by 8 cm polypropylene mesh and placing a full-length figure-of-eight polyglactin (Vicryl)/polypropylene (Prolene) suture at each end].

The polypropylene mesh was brought into the vaginal field and the *right/left* sling suture was loaded on the transvaginal needle. The needle was pulled back into the suprapubic incision and the suture ends clamped. Hemostasis was achieved with judicious electrocautery.

The identical procedure was performed on the contralateral side, positioning the mesh as a hammock on the ventral urethral wall.

The urethral catheter was removed and cystourethroscopy performed, using a *flexible cystoscope/___Fr rigid cystoscope with both the 30° and 70° lenses.* The proximal urethra and bladder were intact, and clear ureteral efflux noted bilaterally. There were no intravesical sutures. The cystoscope was removed and replaced with the urethral catheter.

Having confirmed proper suture placement, gentle traction was placed on both suture ends and the sling was positioned at the level of the bladder neck and proximal urethra. The center of the sling was secured to the periurethral fascia using two 4-0 Vicryl sutures. The two sutures at the end of the sling were loosely tied individually, above the rectus abdominis fascia.

The incisions were irrigated with sterile normal saline. Hemostasis was again confirmed. The suprapubic incisions were closed using a 3-0 chromic suture on Scarpa's fascia and a 4-0 poliglecaprone (Monocryl) suture placed subcuticularly. Sterile adhesive strips and a gauze dressing were applied.

The vaginal wall was approximated with interrupted 2-0 Vicryl sutures and the self-retaining retractor and weighted vaginal speculum were removed.

The urethral catheter was connected to a drainage bag and the patient was repositioned supine.

At the end of the procedure, all counts were correct.

The patient tolerated the procedure well and was taken to the recovery room in satisfactory condition.

Estimated blood loss: Approximately _____ml

95

Rectocele Repair

Indications

- Symptomatic rectocele

Essential Steps

1) Place a urethral catheter and make sure the bladder is decompressed.
2) Excise a triangular segment of posterior vaginal epithelium and dissect this from the underlying perirectal fascia. Extend the dissection laterally to the rectovaginal fascia.
3) Plicate the rectovaginal fascia, starting at the apex and moving distally to the posterior fourchette.
4) If a perineorrhapy is indicated, excise an additional triangular piece of perineal and vaginal skin to create a diamond-shaped posterior vaginal defect. Plicate the bulbocavernosus and transverse perineal muscles at the midline.
5) Check the caliber of the vagina to avoid excessive narrowing. In a sexually active patient, it should accommodate at least two fingers.
6) Close the vaginal incision(s).

Note These Variations

- During dissection of the vaginal epithelium, a finger can be placed in the rectum to identify the proximity to the anterior rectal wall.
- With a high-grade prolapse, the levator musculature may be plicated in the midline; however, this may increase the likelihood of dyspareunia.
- A mesh can be used to reinforce the repair. Choices of mesh materials include autologous or cadaveric fascias, xenografts, and synthetic materials.
- In cases where there is associated stress urinary incontinence, a midurethral sling procedure can be performed concurrently.
- Postoperatively the vagina may be packed with a sterile rolled gauze to aid in hemostasis.

Operative Dictations in Urologic Surgery, First Edition. Noel A. Armenakas, John A. Fracchia, and Ron Golan.
© 2019 John Wiley & Sons Ltd. Published 2019 by John Wiley & Sons Ltd.

Complications

- Bleeding
- Infection
- Rectal injury
- Dyspareunia/hispareunia
- Constipation
- Defecatory pain
- Recurrent rectocele

Template Operative Dictation

Preoperative diagnosis: Rectocele
Postoperative diagnosis: Same
Procedure: Rectocele repair
Indications: The patient is a ____-year-old female with a rectocele presenting for rectocele repair.
Description of Procedure: The indications, alternatives, benefits, and risks were discussed with the patient and informed consent was obtained.

The patient was brought onto the operating room table, positioned supine, and secured with a safety strap. Pneumatic compression devices were placed on the lower extremities.

After the administration of intravenous antibiotics and *general endotracheal/regional* anesthesia, the patient was repositioned in dorsal lithotomy using well-padded *universal (Allen)/candy cane* stirrups. The genitalia, perineum, and lower abdomen were prepped and draped in the standard sterile manner.

A time-out was completed, verifying the correct patient, surgical procedure, and positioning, prior to beginning the procedure.

A 16 Fr urethral catheter was inserted to drain the bladder. A Deaver retractor was placed in the anterior vaginal wall and a self-retaining retractor (e.g. Lone Star, Bookwalter) was appropriately positioned to optimize exposure. The posterior vaginal mucosa was hydrodissected using injectable 1% lidocaine with 1:100 000 epinephrine to facilitate the dissection and assist with hemostasis.

Two Allis clamps were placed at the posterior vaginal fourchette along the lateral margins of the vaginal wall, and a third Allis clamp positioned at the proximal border of the rectocele at the midline. With the clamps as a guide, a triangular segment of vaginal wall epithelium was incised between these, with the base oriented distally. Using Metzenbaum scissors, the vaginal epithelium was carefully dissected off the underlying perirectal fascia away from the rectum. With downward traction on the rectum, the dissection was extended lateral to the rectocele, exposing the rectovaginal fascia. Interrupted 2-0 *polydioxanone (PDS)/polyglactin (Vicryl)* sutures were used to plicate the rectovaginal fascia, starting at the apex and moving distally to the posterior vaginal fourchette. Shallow bites were taken to avoid incorporating the rectum in the repair. Similarly, care was taken not to include the levator ani muscles. Once all the sutures were placed, they were individually tied in succession. The edges of the vaginal epithelium were appropriately trimmed and the midline incision approximated with a running 2-0 Vicryl suture.

If a perineorrhaphy is indicated: A triangular piece of vaginal epithelium was excised at the posterior commissure, exposing the attenuated perineal body. The bulbocavernosus and transverse perineal muscles ware approximated using vertical 2-0 *PDS/Vicryl* sutures. The overlying perineal skin was closed with a running 2-0 Vicryl suture.

Hemostasis was achieved throughout the procedure with judicious electrocautery. Adequate introital size was confirmed by placing three fingers intravaginally. At the end of the procedure, a finger was placed in the rectum, confirming an intact rectal wall and the absence of bleeding or palpable sutures.

The self-retaining and Deaver retractors were removed and the wound irrigated with sterile normal saline. Hemostasis was again confirmed.

The urethral catheter was connected to a drainage bag and the patient repositioned supine.

At the end of the procedure, all counts were correct.

The patient tolerated the procedure well and was taken to the recovery room in satisfactory condition.

Estimated blood loss: Approximately _____ml

96

Urethral Diverticulectomy

Indications

- Symptomatic urethral diverticulum

Essential Steps

1) Place a urethral catheter and make sure the bladder is decompressed.
2) Incise the anterior vaginal wall and dissect the vaginal epithelium off the periurethral fascia.
3) Make a transverse incision into the periurethral fascia and mobilize the fascia off the underlying urethral diverticulum.
4) Dissect the diverticulum circumferentially to its origin and excise it entirely.
5) Perform a ventral urethroplasty and close the periurethral fascia perpendicularly to limit suture overlap.
6) Close the vaginal wall as a third layer.

Note These Variations

- The procedure alternatively can be performed through a midline vertical or T- vaginal incision.
- Circumurethral diverticula require more extensive dissection and urethral reconstruction, possibly using an excision and anastomotic repair.
- A vascularized labial (Martius) flap can be used to reinforce the repair when the vaginal tissue is deficient or compromised.
- Select distal diverticula occasionally can be managed simply with marsupialization, creating a hypospadiac vaginal meatus.
- In cases where there is associated stress urinary incontinence, a midurethral sling can be performed concurrently.
- Postoperatively, the vagina may be packed with a sterile rolled gauze to aid in hemostasis.

Operative Dictations in Urologic Surgery, First Edition. Noel A. Armenakas, John A. Fracchia, and Ron Golan.
© 2019 John Wiley & Sons Ltd. Published 2019 by John Wiley & Sons Ltd.

Complications

- Bleeding
- Infection
- Urinary incontinence
- Urinary retention
- Urethral stricture
- Dyspareunia/hispareunia
- Recurrent diverticulum
- Pseudodiverticulum formation
- Fistula (urethrovaginal)

Template Operative Dictation

Preoperative diagnosis: Urethral diverticulum
Postoperative diagnosis: Same
Procedure: Urethral diverticulectomy
Indications: The patient is a _____-year-old female with a urethral diverticulum presenting for a diverticulectomy.
Description of Procedure: The indications, alternatives, benefits, and risks were discussed with the patient and informed consent was obtained.

The patient was brought onto the operating room table, positioned supine, and secured with a safety strap. Pneumatic compression devices were placed on the lower extremities.

After the administration of intravenous antibiotics and *general endotracheal/regional* anesthesia, the patient was repositioned in dorsal lithotomy using well-padded *universal (Allen)/candy cane* stirrups. The genitalia, perineum, and lower abdomen were prepped and draped in the standard sterile manner.

The radiographic images were in the room.

A time-out was completed, verifying the correct patient, surgical procedure, and positioning, prior to beginning the procedure.

A 14 Fr urethral catheter was inserted to drain the bladder. A weighted speculum was placed in the posterior vaginal wall and a self-retaining retractor (e.g. Lone Star, Bookwalter) was appropriately positioned to optimize exposure. The anterior vaginal mucosa was hydrodissected using injectable 1% lidocaine with 1 : 100 000 epinephrine to facilitate the dissection and assist with hemostasis.

With the bladder completely decompressed, an inverted-U incision was made in the anterior vaginal wall 1 cm below the urethral meatus to the level of the proximal urethra. Using a combination of sharp and blunt dissection, an anterior vaginal wall flap was dissected off the underlying periurethral fascia. The periurethral fascia was incised transversely and carefully dissected superiorly and inferiorly, avoiding entry into the urethral diverticulum. The urethral diverticulum was grasped with a Babcock clamp and dissected circumferentially to its urethral origin. The entire diverticulum was excised, exposing the urethral catheter on the ventral urethral wall. The urethra was reconstructed using vertically placed interrupted 5-0 polydioxanone (PDS) sutures to achieve a watertight, tension-free closure. The periurethral fascial flaps were closed

transversely with a running 4-0 polyglactin (Vicryl) suture, limiting interposing suture lines. Hemostasis was achieved with judicious electrocautery.

Upon completion of the repair, the urethral catheter was removed and cystourethroscopy performed, using a *flexible cystoscope/___Fr rigid cystoscope with both the 30° and 70° lenses.* The proximal urethra and bladder were intact, and clear ureteral efflux was noted bilaterally. The cystoscope was removed and replaced with the urethral catheter.

The edges of the vaginal epithelium were appropriately trimmed and the anterior vaginal wall was closed with interrupted 2-0 Vicryl sutures. The vaginal wound was irrigated with sterile normal saline, and the self-retaining retractor and weighted vaginal speculum were removed.

The urethral catheter was connected to a drainage bag and the patient repositioned supine.

At the end of the procedure, all counts were correct.

The patient tolerated the procedure well and was taken to the recovery room in satisfactory condition.

Estimated blood loss: Approximately _____ml

97

Vesicovaginal Fistula Repair

Indications

- Vesicovaginal fistula

Essential Steps

1) Perform cystoscopy to localize the fistula intravesically and identify its location in relation to the trigone and ureteral orifices.
2) Place a urethral catheter and make sure the bladder is decompressed.
3) Pass an 8 Fr urethral catheter across the fistula, transvaginally.
4) Circumscribe the fistula and create an inverted-U anterior vaginal wall flap, with its apex abutting the fistula.
5) Dissect and excise the fistulous tract posteriorly to the detrusor muscle, separating it from the vagina.
6) Close the fistula in two opposing layers to limit suture overlap.
7) Repeat the cystoscopy to confirm ureteral patency bilaterally, and check the repair by filling the bladder with dilute dye.
8) Advance the anterior vaginal wall flap to cover the repair as a third layer.

Note These Variations

- With a narrow introitus, vaginal exposure can be improved by making posterolateral episiotomies at the 5 o'clock and 7 o'clock positions.
- Visualization of the fistula can be enhanced with intravesical methylene blue or indigo carmine. If the fistula tract is narrow, it can be dilated carefully to accommodate an 8 Fr urethral catheter; alternatively, sutures can be placed on either side of the fistula for traction.
- If the fistula is near the ureteral orifice(s), the ureter(s) can be stented to reduce the incidence of inadvertent injury.
- In the event that the vaginal tissue is deficient or compromised (e.g. post-radiation therapy), the repair can be reinforced with a vascularized flap, using labial fat (Martius), peritoneum, or gracilis muscle.

Operative Dictations in Urologic Surgery, First Edition. Noel A. Armenakas, John A. Fracchia, and Ron Golan.

- A cystotomy catheter may be inserted in addition to the urethral catheter, to optimize drainage and assist in the subsequent voiding trial.
- Postoperatively, the vagina may be packed with a sterile rolled gauze to aid in hemostasis.

Complications

- Bleeding
- Infection
- Ureteral injury/obstruction
- Recurrent/persistent fistula
- Vaginal shortening
- Dyspareunia/hispareunia

Template Operative Dictation

Preoperative diagnosis: Vesicovaginal fistula
Postoperative diagnosis: Same
Procedure: Transvaginal vesicovaginal fistula repair
Indications: The patient is a ____-year-old female with a vesicovaginal fistula presenting for a transvaginal repair.
Description of Procedure: The indications, alternatives, benefits, and risks were discussed with the patient and informed consent was obtained.

The patient was brought onto the operating room table, positioned supine, and secured with a safety strap. Pneumatic compression devices were placed on the lower extremities.

After the administration of intravenous antibiotics and *general endotracheal/regional* anesthesia, the patient was repositioned in dorsal lithotomy using well-padded *universal (Allen)/candy cane* stirrups. The genitalia, perineum, and lower abdomen were prepped and draped in the standard sterile manner.

A time-out was completed, verifying the correct patient, surgical procedure, site, and positioning, prior to beginning the procedure.

A *17/22* Fr rigid cystoscope was inserted per meatus and advanced under direct vision into the urinary bladder. Cystoscopy was performed using the 30° and 70° lenses. The bladder was thoroughly inspected and both ureteral orifices visualized in the normal anatomic position with clear efflux noted bilaterally. The fistula was identified at the _____(location)_____. The cystoscope was removed under direct vision.

A 16 Fr urethral catheter was inserted to drain the bladder.

A weighted vaginal speculum was placed in the posterior vaginal wall and a self-retaining retractor (e.g. Lone Star, Bookwalter) was appropriately positioned to optimize exposure. The anterior vaginal mucosa was hydrodissected using injectable 1% lidocaine with 1:100 000 epinephrine to facilitate the dissection and assist with hemostasis.

Vaginally, the fistula was identified anteriorly at the *apex/vaginal cuff* and intubated with an 8 Fr Foley catheter. The balloon was inflated to 3 cc with sterile water. The vaginal mucosa around the fistula was circumferentially incised.

With the bladder completely decompressed, an inverted-U incision was made in the anterior vaginal epithelium, with the apex contiguous with the circumscribed fistula and the base extending to the bladder neck. Using a combination of sharp and blunt dissection, the vaginal mucosa was dissected from the underlying perivesical fascia, creating vaginal flaps anterior and posterior to the fistula.

With gentle traction on the catheter, the fistulous tract was dissected proximally to the level of the detrusor muscle. Having achieved adequate circumferential mobilization, the entire fistulous tract and surrounding inflammatory tissue were excised and the 8 Fr Foley catheter removed. The fistula was closed in two opposing layers using interrupted 3-0 polyglactin (Vicryl) sutures. The deep layer incorporated the edges of the fistula with the adjacent detrusor muscle, whereas the superficial layer imbricated the perivesical fascia over the first layer.

Upon completion of the repair, the urethral catheter was removed and thorough cystourethroscopy performed again. The proximal urethra and bladder were intact, and clear ureteral efflux noted bilaterally. The cystoscope was removed and replaced with the urethral catheter.

The bladder was filled with a dilute solution of *methylene blue/indigo carmine* in 300 ml sterile normal saline, confirming an intact watertight fistula closure.

The vaginal wall flap was advanced over the two-layer fistula repair and closed with a running interlocking 3-0 Vicryl suture. Hemostasis was achieved with judicious electrocautery throughout the procedure.

The wound was irrigated with sterile normal saline, and the self-retaining retractor and weighted vaginal speculum were removed.

The urethral catheter was connected to a drainage bag and the patient repositioned supine.

At the end of the procedure, all counts were correct.

The patient tolerated the procedure well and was taken to the recovery room in satisfactory condition.

Estimated blood loss: Approximately _____ml

NOTES

SECTION V LAPAROSCOPIC AND ROBOTIC SURGERY

- *Adrenal*
- *Bladder*
- *Kidney*
- *Lymphatics*
- *Prostate*

Adrenal

98

Laparoscopic Adrenalectomy

Indications

- Select adrenal tumors or metastases

Essential Steps

1) Perform the appropriate preoperative catecholamine blockade in patients with suspected pheochromocytoma.
2) Incise the white line of Toldt to reflect the colon medially.
3) Divide the surrounding renal attachments.
4) Identify and obtain early vascular control of the renal hilum and identify and divide the adrenal vein. With pheochromocytomas this should be done prior to any adrenal manipulation in order to limit hemodynamic instability from blood pressure changes caused by catecholamine release. The anesthesiologist should be informed prior to any adrenal manipulation in these instances.
5) Separate the adrenal gland and its surrounding fat from the superior pole of the kidney and ligate perforating vessels.

Note These Variations

- Access into the peritoneal cavity may be obtained with a Veress needle, the open Hasson technique, or with direct vision optical trocars.
- A retroperitoneal approach for the adrenalectomy may be undertaken. This is especially beneficial in patients with prior abdominal surgery or vascular/anatomic variations. The retroperitoneal space should be adequately developed prior to inserting instruments.
- This procedure may vary with regards to port placement and instruments. Hand-assistance may be utilized to improve tactile feedback for dissection, retraction, and hemostatic control. Robotic assistance may be utilized to improve visualization, dexterity, and surgical ergonomics.
- If there is any suspicion of lymphatic invasion, a regional lymphadenectomy can be performed from the level of the renal vessels to the diaphragmatic crus.

Operative Dictations in Urologic Surgery, First Edition. Noel A. Armenakas, John A. Fracchia, and Ron Golan.
© 2019 John Wiley & Sons Ltd. Published 2019 by John Wiley & Sons Ltd.

- The specimen may be retrieved through a periumbilical, Pfannenstiel, modified Gibson, or paramedian incision.
- The need for fascial closure of port sites depends on trocar size and design, patient characteristics, and surgeon preference. Fascial closures may be performed by a hand-sutured technique or with assistance of devices, under direct visualization, in order to minimize the risk of visceral injury.

Complications

- Bleeding
- Infection
- Hemodynamic instability
- Intraabdominal organ injury
- Pneumothorax
- Ileus
- Adrenal insufficiency

Template Operative Dictation

Preoperative diagnosis: Adrenal tumor
Postoperative diagnosis: Same
Procedure: Laparoscopic *right/left* adrenalectomy
Indications: The patient is a ___-year-old *male/female* with a *right/left* adrenal tumor presenting for a laparoscopic adrenalectomy.
Description of Procedure: The indications, alternatives, benefits, and risks were discussed with the patient and informed consent was obtained.

> *For pheochromocytoma*: The biochemical evaluation was consistent with a pheochromocytoma and the appropriate preoperative catecholamine blockade performed.

The patient was brought onto the operating room table, placed supine, and secured with a safety strap. Pneumatic compression devices were placed on the lower extremities.

After the administration of intravenous antibiotics and general endotracheal anesthesia, a 16 Fr urethral catheter was inserted to drain the bladder. The patient was repositioned in the *right/left* lateral decubitus position at a 45° angle with the lower leg flexed 90° and the upper leg extended. An axillary roll was positioned to protect the brachial plexus and a gel pad placed to support the back. Multiple pillows were used to pad beneath and between both the upper and lower extremities to ensure adequate cushioning. The patient was secured in place across the hips, chest, and legs with foam padding and cloth tape, and the table was flexed. The patient was prepped and draped in the standard sterile manner.

The radiographic images were in the room.

A time-out was completed, verifying the correct patient, surgical procedure, site, and positioning, prior to beginning the procedure.

Pneumoperitoneum was introduced by placing a Veress needle into the abdomen and insufflating with CO_2 to a pressure of 15 mmHg. The camera trocar was placed below the costal margin along the mid-clavicular line and the *0°/30°* lens was inserted under direct visualization. The abdominal cavity was examined for any sign of injury, adhesions, and identification of anatomic landmarks. The remainder of the trocars were placed, which included a *5/10* mm port cephalad to the camera trocar below the costal margin and a *5/10* mm port caudal to the camera trocar along the anterior axillary line. (*If retraction is required*: An additional assistant port was inserted to retract the *liver/ spleen.*)The parietal peritoneum was incised along the white line of Toldt and the colon reflected medially, exposing Gerota's fascia.

>   ***On the right*:** The hepatic flexure was mobilized by dividing the triangular and coronary ligaments, allowing for retraction of the liver. The duodenum was kocherized and the inferior vena cava was visualized. The retroperitoneal fascia overlying the renal vessels was carefully separated, exposing the underlying renal vein. The inferior vena cava was carefully dissected cephalad until the insertion of the adrenal vein was identified. The adrenal vein was dissected laterally and the adrenal gland was visualized. The adrenal vein was secured with polymer ligating clips (e.g. Hem-o-lok) and sharply divided.
>
>   ***On the left*:** The splenorenal and splenophrenic ligaments were incised to mobilize the spleen. The tail of the pancreas was mobilized medially. The gonadal vein was identified and the dissection carried cephalad toward the renal vein. The retroperitoneal fascia overlying the renal vein was carefully dissected, exposing the insertion of the adrenal vein. The adrenal vein was dissected laterally and the adrenal gland was visualized. The adrenal vein was secured with polymer ligating clips (e.g. Hem-o-lok) and sharply divided.

The adrenal gland was elevated and a circumferential dissection performed with a laparoscopic electrothermal bipolar tissue sealing device (LigaSure) to control and divide perforating vessels. The gland was maintained intact as it was circumferentially dissected off the superior pole of the kidney along with the suprarenal fat. The adrenal gland was placed into a specimen retrieval bag and set aside.

The operative field was inspected for bleeding or injury. The insufflation pressure was reduced, again confirming the absence of bleeding. The trocars were withdrawn under direct visualization. The camera trocar incision was extended and the specimen retrieval bag was removed. The specimen was sent to pathology for evaluation.

The anterior fascia at the specimen extraction site was carefully closed with a 1-0 polydioxanone (PDS) suture, and a total of __ ml of local anesthetic (*specify*) injected subcutaneously at the port sites. The skin incisions were closed with a 4-0 poliglecaprone (Monocryl) suture and reinforced with sterile adhesive strips. Sterile dressings were applied and the patient repositioned supine.

At the end of the procedure, all counts were correct.

The patient tolerated the procedure well and was taken to the recovery room in satisfactory condition.

Estimated blood loss: Approximately _____ml

Bladder

99

Robotic-Assisted Laparoscopic Abdominal Sacrocolpopexy

Indications

- Pelvic organ prolapse

Essential Steps

1) Retract the sigmoid and expose the anterior longitudinal ligament at or below the level of the sacral promontory. Avoid a more cranial dissection, which can injure the presacral vessels. Identify the course of the ureters prior to dissection.
2) Incise the peritoneum and dissect the rectum and bladder from the posterior and anterior vaginal wall, respectively.
3) Affix the lateral arms of the polypropylene Y-mesh to the anterior and posterior vaginal wall, avoiding the vaginal lumen.
4) Attach the tail of the mesh to the anterior longitudinal ligament, adjusting the tension appropriately using transvaginal retraction.
5) Retroperitonealize the mesh.

Note These Variations

- Access into the peritoneal cavity may be obtained with a Veress needle, the open Hasson technique or with direct vision optical trocars.
- A robotic-assisted laparoscopic hysterectomy with/without bilateral oophorectomy or salpingectomy may be performed, if indicated, prior to repair of the pelvic organ prolapse.
- A midurethral sling may be placed in patients with stress urinary incontinence. There are many choices of sling materials as well as a variety of available kits.
- Postoperatively, the vagina may be packed with a sterile rolled gauze to aid in hemostasis.
- The need for fascial closure of port sites depends on trocar size and design, patient characteristics, and surgeon preference. Fascial closures may be performed by a hand-sutured technique or with assistance of devices, under direct visualization in order to minimize the risk of visceral injury.

Operative Dictations in Urologic Surgery, First Edition. Noel A. Armenakas, John A. Fracchia, and Ron Golan.
© 2019 John Wiley & Sons Ltd. Published 2019 by John Wiley & Sons Ltd.

Complications

- Bleeding
- Infection
- Intraabdominal organ injury
- Ileus
- Dyspareunia/hispareunia
- Mesh erosion
- Recurrent prolapse
- Neuropraxia
- Fistula

Template Operative Dictation

Preoperative diagnosis: Pelvic organ prolapse
Postoperative diagnosis: Same
Procedure: Robotic-assisted laparoscopic sacrocolpopexy
Indications: The patient is a ___-year-old female with stage ___ pelvic organ prolapse presenting for robotic-assisted laparoscopic sacrocolpopexy.
Description of Procedure: The indications, alternatives, benefits, and risks were discussed with the patient and informed consent was obtained.

The patient was brought onto the operating room table, placed supine, and secured with a safety strap. All pressure points were carefully padded and pneumatic compression devices placed on the lower extremities.

After the administration of intravenous antibiotics and general endotracheal anesthesia, the patient was repositioned in dorsal lithotomy with well-padded universal (Allen) stirrups. The arms were tucked at the patient's side and secured with padding. The chest was secured in place with foam padding and cloth tape, and the table positioned in 30° Trendelenburg. The abdomen, genitalia, and upper thighs were prepped and draped in the standard sterile manner.

A time-out was completed, verifying the correct patient, surgical procedure, and positioning, prior to beginning the procedure.

A 16 Fr urethral catheter was inserted to drain the bladder.

Pneumoperitoneum was introduced by placing a Veress needle into the abdomen and insufflating with CO_2 to a pressure of 15 mmHg. The camera trocar was placed superior to the umbilicus and the *0°/30°* lens was inserted under direct visualization. The abdominal cavity was examined for any sign of injury, adhesions, and identification of anatomic landmarks. The remainder of the trocars were placed, which included a 12 mm port in the *right/left* lower quadrant medial to the anterior-superior iliac spine, two 8 mm ports at the left and right rectus margin slightly caudal to the camera port, and an 8 mm port medial to the *left/right* anterior-superior iliac spine. The robot was then docked.

The uterus was identified and a *1-0 polyester (Ethibond)/Gore-tex* stay suture was passed though the fundus and brought out through the abdominal wall for upward traction. Both ureters were visualized coursing along the peritoneal surface of the broad ligament.

The sigmoid colon was retracted laterally and the peritoneum overlying the sacral promontory was carefully opened to expose the anterior longitudinal ligament. The tissue over the sacral periosteum was carefully dissected, taking care not to injure the presacral vessels.

A *large Breisky retractor/lucite vaginal probe* was inserted transvaginally to assist with intrapelvic vaginal exposure. An inverted-U shaped peritoneal incision was made in the pouch of Douglas. The rectum was freed from the posterior vaginal wall by dividing the rectovaginal septum with the dissection continued toward the perineal body and laterally on both sides to the levator fascia. The peritoneum overlying the vesicovaginal space was sharply incised. The anterior dissection was carried distally toward the bladder neck using a combination of blunt and sharp dissection with care to avoid the ureters.

The incision over the sacral promontory was extended inferiorly to join the posterior dissection. A lightweight polypropylene Y-shaped mesh was fashioned with two 6 cm arms, and brought into the pelvis through the assistant port. The anterior and posterior arms of the mesh were each fixed to the vagina with three rows of interrupted *1-0 Ethibond/Gore-tex* sutures, avoiding entry into the vaginal lumen.

The tension on the mesh was adjusted while retracting the vaginal vault in the direction of the sacral promontory. The tail of the mesh was attached to the anterior longitudinal ligament overlying the sacral promontory with two *2-0 Ethibond/Gore-tex* sutures placed longitudinally to avoid injuring the presacral vessels. Excess mesh was excised.

A vaginal exam confirmed excellent support and the absence of intravaginal sutures.

Having completed the sacrocolpopexy, the peritoneum was closed with a purse-string 2-0 poliglecaprone (Monocryl) suture to retroperitonealize the Y-mesh.

The operative field was inspected for bleeding or injury. The insufflation pressure was reduced, again confirming the absence of bleeding. The robot was undocked and removed. The trocars and weighted vaginal retractor were withdrawn under direct visualization.

The anterior fascia at the umbilical site was carefully closed with a 1-0 polydioxanone (PDS) suture, and a total of __ml of local anesthetic (*specify*) injected subcutaneously at the port sites. The skin incisions were closed with 4-0 poliglecaprone (Monocryl) sutures and reinforced with sterile adhesive strips. Sterile dressings were applied and the patient repositioned supine.

At the end of the procedure, all counts were correct.

The patient tolerated the procedure well and was taken to the recovery room in satisfactory condition.

Estimated blood loss: Approximately _____ml

The sigmoid colon was retracted laterally and the peritoneum overlying the sacral promontory was carefully opened to expose the anterior longitudinal ligament. The tissue over the sacral periosteum was carefully dissected, taking care not to rupture the presacral vessels.

100

Robotic-Assisted Laparoscopic Bladder Diverticulectomy

Indications

- Symptomatic bladder diverticulum (recurrent infections, irritative, or obstructive voiding symptoms, hematuria, bladder calculi, etc.)
- Select intradiverticular bladder tumors

Essential Steps

1) Mobilize the bladder.
2) Identify the diverticulum and its relationship to the ureteral orifices.
3) Resect the diverticulum circumferentially.
4) Close the bladder in two layers.
5) Place a drain.

Note These Variations

- Access into the peritoneal cavity may be obtained with a Veress needle, with the open Hasson technique, or with direct vision optical trocars.
- The surgeon may elect for an extraperitoneal approach, which is especially beneficial in patients with prior abdominal surgery or vascular/anatomic variations. The potential space should be adequately developed prior to inserting instruments.
- Intraoperative identification and dissection of the diverticulum may be facilitated with the balloon of a council catheter advanced over a guidewire or a Fogarty occlusion catheter within the diverticulum.
- Diverticula located laterally or posteriorly may require concomitant ureteral reimplantation. In such cases, bladder mobilization can be facilitated by ligating the superior vesical pedicle.
- Ureteral stent(s) may be inserted to aid in identification of the ureter(s) during the mobilization and dissection of the diverticulum.
- The need for fascial closure of port sites depends on trocar size and design, patient characteristics, and surgeon preference. Fascial closures may be performed by a hand-sutured technique or with assistance of devices, under direct visualization, in order to minimize the risk of visceral injury.

Operative Dictations in Urologic Surgery, First Edition. Noel A. Armenakas, John A. Fracchia, and Ron Golan.
© 2019 John Wiley & Sons Ltd. Published 2019 by John Wiley & Sons Ltd.

Complications

- Bleeding
- Infection
- Ureteral injury/obstruction
- Urine leak/urinoma
- Intraabdominal organ injury
- Ileus
- Lymphocele
- Recurrent diverticulum

Template Operative Dictation

Preoperative diagnosis: *Symptomatic bladder diverticulum/Intradiverticular bladder tumor*

Postoperative diagnosis: Same

Procedure: Robotic-assisted laparoscopic bladder diverticulectomy

Indications: The patient is a _____ -year-old *male/female* with a *symptomatic bladder diverticulum/intradiverticular bladder tumor* presenting for a robotic-assisted laparoscopic diverticulectomy.

Description of Procedure: The indications, alternatives, benefits, and risks were discussed with the patient and informed consent was obtained.

The patient was brought onto the operating room table, placed supine, and secured with a strap. All pressure points were carefully padded and pneumatic compression devices placed on the lower extremities.

After the administration of intravenous antibiotics and general endotracheal anesthesia, the patient was repositioned in dorsal lithotomy using well-padded universal (Allen) stirrups. The arms were carefully tucked at the patient's side and secured with padding. The chest was secured in place with foam padding and cloth tape, and the table positioned in 30° Trendelenburg. The patient's abdomen, genitalia, and upper thighs were prepped and draped in the standard sterile manner.

The radiographic images were in the room.

A time-out was completed, verifying the correct patient, surgical procedure, and positioning, prior to beginning the procedure.

A 16 Fr urethral catheter was inserted to drain the bladder.

Pneumoperitoneum was introduced by placing a Veress needle into the abdomen and insufflating with CO_2 to a pressure of 15 mmHg. The camera trocar was placed superior to the umbilicus and the *0/30°* lens was inserted under direct visualization. The abdominal cavity was examined for any sign of injury, adhesions, and identification of anatomic landmarks. The remainder of the trocars were placed, which included a 12 mm port in the *right/left* lower quadrant medial to the anterior-superior iliac spine, two 8 mm ports at the left and right rectus margin slightly caudal to the camera port, and an 8 mm port medial to the *right/left* anterior-superior iliac spine. A 5 mm assistant port was placed in the *right/left* upper quadrant. The robot was then docked.

An incision was made in the peritoneum along the anterior abdominal wall above the level of the bladder. The urachus and median umbilical ligaments were incised using a combination of sharp dissection and electrocautery. The space of Retzius was developed distally toward the endopelvic fascia.

The urethral catheter was removed and replaced with a flexible cystoscope, which was advanced under direct vision into the urinary bladder. The bladder was thoroughly inspected. The bladder wall was *minimally/moderately/significantly/not* trabeculated, with a normal appearing mucosa. Both ureteral orifices were in the normal anatomic position with clear urinary efflux noted bilaterally. The diverticulum was identified on the _____*(location)*_____ wall. The region of interest was transilluminated and visualized laparoscopically, and the extravesical surface was circumferentially marked using electrocautery.

The cystoscope was removed, the urethral catheter was reinserted, and the bladder was drained entirely. The diverticulum was circumferentially excised at its ostium, placed in a specimen retrieval bag, and set aside. Meticulous hemostasis was obtained with electrocautery.

The bladder was closed in two layers with 2-0 polyglactin (Vicryl) sutures. Once the reconstruction was complete, a new ____ Fr urethral catheter was inserted. The bladder was irrigated with sterile normal saline, confirming a watertight closure.

> ***If a lymphadenectomy is performed***: A bilateral pelvic lymph node dissection was performed, beginning on the *right/left*. The iliac vessels were exposed from just above the common iliac bifurcation to the femoral canal. The ureters were identified over the common iliac bifurcation. The nodal dissection was started along the medial aspect of the *right/left* external iliac artery by incising the perivascular fibroareolar sheath. The lymph node packet was gently mobilized medially, and small vessels and lymphatic branches were fulgurated or ligated with surgical clips to maintain meticulous hemo- and lymphostasis. The obturator neurovascular bundle was identified posteriorly and preserved. The borders of dissection were the common iliac artery bifurcation cranially, the node of Cloquet caudally, the genitofemoral nerve laterally, and the obturator nerve posteriorly. A polymer ligating clip (e.g. Hem-o-lok) was used to secure the distal and proximal extent of the lymph node packet. The nodal packet was removed and sent to pathology for evaluation.
>
> The contralateral lymph node dissection was performed in a similar manner and the nodal packet sent to pathology for evaluation.

The operative field was inspected for bleeding or injury. The insufflation pressure was reduced, again confirming the absence of bleeding.

Pneumoperitoneum was reestablished and a surgical drain (e.g. Jackson-Pratt) was placed through a laparoscopic port into the pelvis and secured at the skin.

The robot was undocked and removed from the operative field.

The trocars were withdrawn under direct visualization. The periumbilical incision was extended and the specimen retrieval bag was removed. The anterior fascia at the umbilical site was carefully closed with a 1-0 polydioxanone (PDS) suture, and a total of __ml of local anesthetic (*specify*) injected subcutaneously at the port sites. The skin incisions

were closed with 4-0 poliglecaprone (Monocryl) sutures and reinforced with sterile adhesive strips. Sterile dressings were applied and the patient repositioned supine.

At the end of the procedure, all counts were correct.

The patient tolerated the procedure well and was taken to the recovery room in satisfactory condition.

Estimated blood loss: Approximately _____ml

101

Robotic-Assisted Laparoscopic Partial Cystectomy

Indications

- Select solitary urothelial cell carcinomas without associated carcinoma *in situ*, where an adequate surgical margin can be obtained
- Urachal adenocarcinoma

Essential Steps

1) Explore the pelvis to assess bladder mobility and evaluate the abdominal contents for visible metastatic disease.
2) Mobilize the bladder.
3) Identify the bladder tumor site and its relationship to the ureteral orifices.
4) Resect the tumor circumferentially, obtaining wide margins. In cases of urachal adenocarcinoma, the median umbilical ligament, umbilicus, and dome of the bladder should be sent *en bloc*.
5) Close the bladder in two layers.
6) Perform a bilateral pelvic lymph node dissection.
7) Place a drain.

Note These Variations

- Access into the peritoneal cavity may be obtained with a Veress needle, with the open Hasson technique, or with direct vision optical trocars.
- Tumors located laterally or posteriorly may require concomitant ureteral reimplantation. In such cases, bladder mobilization can be facilitated by ligating the superior vesical pedicle.
- The timing of the lymph node dissection within the procedure, and extent of the dissection, may vary by surgeon preference and patient disease.
- Cystoscopy and intraoperative ultrasonography may be performed to delineate the extent of the tumor.
- The need for fascial closure of port sites depends on trocar size and design, patient characteristics, and surgeon preference. Fascial closures may be performed by a

Operative Dictations in Urologic Surgery, First Edition. Noel A. Armenakas, John A. Fracchia, and Ron Golan.
© 2019 John Wiley & Sons Ltd. Published 2019 by John Wiley & Sons Ltd.

hand-sutured technique or with assistance of devices, under direct visualization in order to minimize the risk of visceral injury.

Complications

- Bleeding
- Infection
- Intraabdominal organ injury
- Ureteral injury/obstruction
- Urine leak/urinoma
- Lymphocele
- Ileus
- Tumor spillage/implantation

Template Operative Dictation

Preoperative diagnosis: *Invasive localized bladder cancer/Urachal adenocarcinoma*
Postoperative diagnosis: Same
Procedure: Robotic-assisted laparoscopic partial cystectomy
Indications: The patient is a _____ -year-old *male/female* with a *clinical stage T* ___ *urothelial cell carcinoma/urachal adenocarcinoma* presenting for a robotic-assisted laparoscopic partial cystectomy.
Description of Procedure: The indications, alternatives, benefits, and risks were discussed with the patient and informed consent was obtained.

The patient was brought onto the operating room table, placed supine, and secured with a strap. All pressure points were carefully padded and pneumatic compression devices were placed on the lower extremities.

After the administration of intravenous antibiotics and general endotracheal anesthesia, the patient was repositioned in dorsal lithotomy using well-padded universal (Allen) stirrups. The arms were carefully tucked at the patient's side and secured with padding. The chest was secured in place with foam padding and cloth tape, and the table positioned in 30° Trendelenburg. The patient's abdomen, genitalia, and upper thighs were prepped and draped in the standard sterile manner.

The radiographic images were in the room.

A time-out was completed, verifying the correct patient, surgical procedure, and positioning, prior to beginning the procedure.

A 16 Fr urethral catheter was inserted to drain the bladder.

Pneumoperitoneum was introduced by placing a Veress needle into the abdomen and insufflating with CO_2 to a pressure of 15 mmHg. The camera trocar was placed superior to the umbilicus and the *0°/30°* lens was inserted under direct visualization. The abdominal cavity was examined for any sign of injury, adhesions, and identification of anatomic landmarks. The remainder of the trocars were placed, which included a 12 mm port in the *right/left* lower quadrant medial to the anterior-superior iliac spine, two 8 mm ports at the left and right rectus margin slightly caudal to the camera port,

and an 8 mm port medial to the *right/left* anterior-superior iliac spine. A 5 mm assistant port was placed in the *right/left* upper quadrant. The robot was then docked.

An incision was made in the peritoneum along the anterior abdominal wall above the level of the bladder. The urachus and medial umbilical ligaments were incised using a combination of sharp dissection and electrocautery. The space of Retzius was developed distally toward the endopelvic fascia.

The urethral catheter was removed and replaced with a flexible cystoscope, which was advanced under direct vision into the urinary bladder. The bladder was thoroughly inspected and both ureteral orifices visualized in the normal anatomic position with clear efflux noted bilaterally. The tumor was identified on the ____*(location)*____. The region of interest was transilluminated and visualized laparoscopically, and the extravesical surface was circumferentially marked using electrocautery. No additional lesions were noted.

The cystoscope was removed, the urethral catheter was reinserted, and the bladder was drained entirely prior to excision of the tumor in order to minimize spillage. The full-thickness bladder tumor site was sharply excised with a wide margin. The resected tissue was placed in a specimen retrieval bag. Additional biopsies from the margins of the resection were obtained and sent to pathology for frozen section. Meticulous hemostasis was obtained with electrocautery.

The bladder wall was closed in two layers with 2-0 polyglactin (Vicryl) sutures. Once the reconstruction was complete, a new ____ Fr urethral catheter was inserted. The bladder was irrigated with sterile normal saline, confirming a watertight closure.

> ***If a lymphadenectomy is performed***: A bilateral pelvic lymph node dissection was performed, beginning on the *left/right*. The iliac vessels were exposed from just above the common iliac bifurcation to the femoral canal (node of Cloquet). The ureters were identified over the common iliac bifurcation. The nodal dissection was started along the medial aspect of the *left/right* external iliac artery by incising the perivascular fibroareolar sheath. The lymph node packet was gently mobilized medially, and small vessels and lymphatic branches were fulgurated or ligated with surgical clips to maintain meticulous hemo- and lymphostasis. The obturator neurovascular bundle was identified posteriorly and preserved. The borders of dissection were the common iliac artery bifurcation cranially, the node of Cloquet caudally, the genitofemoral nerve laterally, and the obturator nerve posteriorly. A polymer ligating clip (e.g. Hem-o-lok) was used to secure the distal and proximal extent of the lymph node packet. The nodal packet was removed and sent to pathology for evaluation.

The contralateral lymph node dissection was performed in a similar manner and the nodal packet sent to pathology for evaluation.The operative field was inspected for bleeding or injury. The insufflation pressure was reduced, again confirming the absence of bleeding.

> ***If a surgical drain is placed***: Pneumoperitoneum was reestablished and a surgical drain (e.g. Jackson-Pratt) was placed through a laparoscopic port into the pelvis and secured at the skin.

Pneumoperitoneum was re-established and a surgical drain (e.g. Jackson-Pratt) was placed through a laparoscopic port into the pelvis and secured at the skin. The robot was undocked and removed from the operative field.

The trocars were withdrawn under direct visualization. The periumbilical incision was extended and the specimen retrieval bag was removed. The anterior fascia at the umbilical site was carefully closed with a 1-0 polydioxanone (PDS) suture, and a total of __ml of local anesthetic (*specify*) injected subcutaneously at the port sites. The skin incisions were closed with 4-0 poliglecaprone (Monocryl) sutures and reinforced with sterile adhesive strips. Sterile dressings were applied and the patient repositioned supine.

At the end of the procedure, all counts were correct.

The patient tolerated the procedure well and was taken to the recovery room in satisfactory condition.

Estimated blood loss: Approximately _____ml

102

Robotic-Assisted Laparoscopic Radical Cystectomy (Female)

Indications

- Invasive urothelial cell carcinoma, primary intravesical squamous cell, bladder adenocarcinoma or sarcoma, refractory bladder carcinoma *in situ*
- Intravesical extension of tumors from adjacent organs precluding bladder preservation
- Persistent refractory intravesical bleeding (rare)

Essential Steps

1) Explore the pelvis to assess bladder mobility and evaluate the abdominal contents for visible metastatic disease.
2) Identify the ureters at their crossing over the common iliac arteries and carefully dissect them proximally and distally, preserving the periureteral tissue.
3) Develop the lateral pelvic and perivesical space with care to avoid injury to the pedicles.
4) Clip and divide the ureters and tag the transected distal end with a suture.
5) Ligate the lateral and posterior vascular pedicles to the bladder.
6) Incise the vagina at the apex and continue the dissection towards the bladder neck.
7) Mobilize the bladder off the anterior abdominal wall.
8) Open the endopelvic fascia bilaterally, and ligate and divide the dorsal venous complex.
9) Dissect the entire urethra. In patients undergoing an orthotopic diversion, the anterior vaginal wall and urethra should be preserved and dissection in those areas limited to avoid injury to the rhabdosphincteric complex.
10) Close the vaginal cuff.
11) Retrieve the bladder, ureter, cervix, anterior vaginal wall, and urethra *en bloc* and obtain meticulous hemostasis.
12) Perform a thorough pelvic lymph node dissection.
13) Tunnel the left ureter posterior to the sigmoid colon to the right side.
14) Perform a urinary diversion.

Operative Dictations in Urologic Surgery, First Edition. Noel A. Armenakas, John A. Fracchia, and Ron Golan.
© 2019 John Wiley & Sons Ltd. Published 2019 by John Wiley & Sons Ltd.

Note These Variations

- Preoperative bowel preparation and oral antibiotics varies by surgeon preference and institutional guidelines.
- Access into the peritoneal cavity may be obtained with a Veress needle, the open Hasson technique, or direct vision optical trocars.
- The timing of the lymph node dissection within the procedure, and extent of the dissection, may vary by surgeon preference and patient disease. Organ preservation of the ovaries, uterus, fallopian tubes, and anterior vaginal wall may be performed, depending on tumor stage and patient preference.
- Surgeon preference may dictate the configuration of bowel for an orthotopic neobladder or continent catheterizable pouch. A suprapubic catheter may be placed percutaneously for additional drainage from a continent diversion.
- The urinary diversion may be performed intra- or extracorporeally, depending on surgeon preference, patient habitus, and type of diversion to be performed. When an orthotopic neobladder is performed, a urethral margin may be sent to pathology for frozen section evaluation. In cases of a neobladder created extracorporeally, the neobladder-urethral anastomosis may be performed with robotic-assistance, or anastomotic sutures may be placed prior to undocking the robot to facilitate an open neobladder-urethral anastomosis.
- If the reason for cystectomy is refractory vesical bleeding, a pelvic lymphadenectomy is not routinely performed.
- The need for fascial closure of port sites depends on trocar size and design, patient characteristics, and surgeon preference. Fascial closures may be performed by a hand-sutured technique or with assistance of devices, under direct visualization, in order to minimize the risk of visceral injury.

Complications

- Bleeding
- Infection
- Ileus/bowel obstruction/leak
- Ureteral injury/obstruction
- Urine leak/urinoma
- Intraabdominal organ injury
- Nerve injury
- Lymphocele

Template Operative Dictation

Preoperative diagnosis: Bladder cancer
Postoperative diagnosis: Same
Procedure: Robotic-assisted laparoscopic anterior pelvic exenteration

Indications: The patient is a _____ -year-old female with clinical stage T__ *urothelial cell/squamous cell/adeno*carcinoma of the bladder presenting for a robotic-assisted laparoscopic anterior pelvic exenteration.

Description of Procedure: The indications, alternatives, benefits, and risks were discussed with the patient and informed consent was obtained.

The patient was brought onto the operating room table, placed supine, and secured with a safety strap. All pressure points were carefully padded and pneumatic compression devices were placed on the lower extremities.

After the administration of intravenous antibiotics and general endotracheal anesthesia, the patient was repositioned in dorsal lithotomy using well-padded universal (Allen) stirrups. The arms were carefully tucked at the patient's side and secured with padding. The chest was secured in place with foam padding and cloth tape, and the table positioned in 30° Trendelenburg. The patient's abdomen, genitalia, and upper thighs were prepped and draped in the standard sterile manner.

The radiographic images were in the room.

A time-out was completed, verifying the correct patient, surgical procedure, and positioning, prior to beginning the procedure.

A 16 Fr urethral catheter was inserted and the bladder drained.

Pneumoperitoneum was introduced by placing a Veress needle into the abdomen and insufflating with CO_2 to a pressure of 15 mmHg. The camera trocar was placed 5 cm cephalad to the umbilicus and the *0°/30°* lens was inserted under direct visualization. The abdominal cavity was examined for any sign of injury, adhesions, and identification of anatomic landmarks. The remainder of the trocars were placed, which included a 12 mm port in the *right/left* lower quadrant medial to the anterior-superior iliac spine, two 8 mm ports at the left and right rectus margin slightly caudal to the camera port, and an 8 mm port medial to the *right/left* anterior-superior iliac spine. A 5 mm assistant port was placed in the *right/left* upper quadrant. The robot was then docked.

The parietal peritoneum was incised along the white line of Toldt and the *right/left* colon reflected medially, exposing the psoas and iliac vessels. The ureter was identified at the common iliac bifurcation and dissected distally to the ureterovesical junction, ligating and dividing the obliterated umbilical artery and superior vesical pedicle as the plane between the bladder and pelvic sidewall was developed. The ureter was dissected cephalad to the level of the aortic bifurcation with care to preserve periureteral tissue.

A similar dissection was performed on the contralateral side.

The distal end of each ureter was clipped, divided, and tagged with a long 3-0 chromic suture to facilitate later identification. A distal margin from each ureter was sent for frozen-section analysis.

The uterus was retracted anteriorly with the fourth robotic arm. The infundibulopelvic ligaments and ovarian pedicles were bilaterally clipped and divided, as were the uterine artery pedicles. The posterior bladder pedicles were secured bilaterally with polymer ligating clips (e.g. Hem-o-lok) and sharply divided. An intravaginally placed povidone-iodine (Betadine) -soaked sponge stick was used to identify the apex of the vagina, which was transversely incised distal to the cervix. The plane of dissection was carried distally toward the bladder neck.

An incision was sharply made in the peritoneum along the anterior abdominal wall above the level of the bladder. The urachus and median umbilical ligaments were incised

using a combination of sharp dissection and electrocautery. The space of Retzius was developed to the level of the endopelvic fascia.

The urethra was isolated and sharply divided along with the anterior vaginal wall. The specimen – including bladder, ureter, cervix, anterior vaginal wall, and urethra – were extracted *en bloc* through the vaginal defect and sent to pathology for evaluation. Vaginal reconstruction was accomplished with a horizontal closure using a running 1-0 polyglactin (Vicryl) suture, and the vaginal wall suspended from Cooper's ligament to prevent subsequent prolapse. Pneumoperitoneum was reestablished. The pelvis was irrigated and hemostasis obtained. Patent venous sinuses were oversewn with 0 polyglactin (Vicryl) suture.

A bilateral pelvic lymph node dissection was performed, beginning on the *right/left*. The iliac vessels were exposed from just above the common iliac bifurcation to the femoral canal. The ureters were identified at the common iliac bifurcation. The nodal dissection was started along the medial aspect of the external iliac artery by incising the perivascular fibroareolar sheath. The lymph node packet was gently mobilized medially, and small vessels and lymphatic branches were fulgurated or ligated with surgical clips to maintain meticulous hemo- and lymphostasis. The obturator neurovascular bundle was identified posteriorly and preserved. The borders of dissection were the common iliac artery bifurcation cranially, the node of Cloquet caudally, the genitofemoral nerve laterally, and the obturator nerve posteriorly. A polymer ligating clip (e.g. Hem-o-lok) was used to secure the distal and proximal extent of the lymph node packet. The nodal packet was removed and sent to pathology for evaluation.

The contralateral lymph node dissection was performed in a similar manner, and the nodal packet was sent to pathology for evaluation.

A plane posterior to the sigmoid mesentery at the level of the aortic bifurcation was developed by elevating the sigmoid anteriorly, and the left ureter was tunneled without angulation to the right side.

The operative field was inspected for bleeding or injury and irrigated with warm sterile saline.

The insufflation pressure was reduced, again confirming the absence of bleeding.

Add the appropriate urinary diversion; see Section I, subsection Urinary Diversion

Estimated blood loss: Approximately _____ml

103

Robotic-Assisted Laparoscopic Radical Cystectomy (Male)

Indications

- Invasive urothelial cell carcinoma, primary intravesical squamous cell, adenocarcinoma, sarcoma, refractory bladder carcinoma *in situ*
- Intravesical extension of tumors from adjacent organs precluding bladder preservation
- Persistent refractory intravesical bleeding (rare)

Essential Steps

1) Explore the pelvis to assess bladder mobility and evaluate the abdominal contents for visible metastatic disease.
2) Identify the ureters at their crossing over the common iliac arteries and carefully dissect them proximally and distally, preserving the periureteral tissue.
3) Develop the lateral paravesical space with care to avoid injury to the pedicles.
4) Identify and divide the bilateral superior vesical arteries.
5) Clip and divide the ureters with a pre-placed suture to facilitate later identification.
6) Expose and develop the plane between the bladder and rectum.
7) Ligate the lateral and posterior vascular pedicles to the bladder.
8) Mobilize the bladder off the anterior abdominal wall.
9) Open the endopelvic fascia bilaterally.
10) Ligate and divide the dorsal venous complex.
11) Transect the urethra distal to the prostatic apex.
12) Perform a thorough pelvic lymph node dissection.
13) Tunnel the left ureter posterior to the sigmoid colon to the right side.
14) Perform a urinary diversion.
15) Place a drain.

Note These Variations

- Preoperative bowel preparation and oral antibiotics varies by surgeon preference and institutional guidelines.
- Access into the peritoneal cavity may be obtained with a Veress needle, with the open Hasson technique, or with direct vision optical trocars.

Operative Dictations in Urologic Surgery, First Edition. Noel A. Armenakas, John A. Fracchia, and Ron Golan.
© 2019 John Wiley & Sons Ltd. Published 2019 by John Wiley & Sons Ltd.

- The timing of the lymph node dissection within the procedure, and extent of the lymphadenectomy, may vary by surgeon preference and patient disease.
- The urinary diversion may be performed intra- or extracorporeally, depending on surgeon preference, patient habitus, and type of diversion to be performed. When a neobladder is performed, a urethral margin may be sent to pathology for frozen-section evaluation. In cases of a neobladder created extracorporeally, the neobladder-urethral anastomosis may be performed with robotic assistance, or anastomotic sutures may be placed prior to undocking the robot to facilitate an open neobladder-urethral anastomosis.
- Surgeon preference may dictate the configuration of bowel for an orthotopic neobladder or continent catheterizable pouch. A suprapubic catheter may be placed percutaneously for additional drainage from an orthotopic neobladder.
- When planning to perform an orthotopic neobladder, additional length of the urethral stump and the puboprostatic ligaments should be preserved. Nerve-sparing in these individuals may improve postoperative continence and erectile function. If the reason for cystectomy is refractory vesical bleeding, a pelvic lymphadenectomy is not routinely performed.
- The need for fascial closure of port sites depends on trocar size and design, patient characteristics, and surgeon preference. Fascial closures may be performed by a hand-sutured technique or with assistance of devices, under direct visualization in order to minimize the risk of visceral injury.

Complications

- Bleeding
- Infection
- Ileus/bowel obstruction/leak
- Ureteral injury/obstruction
- Urine leak/urinoma
- Intraabdominal organ injury
- Nerve injury
- Lymphocele

Template Operative Dictation

Preoperative diagnosis: Bladder cancer
Postoperative diagnosis: Same
Procedure: Robotic-assisted laparoscopic radical cystoprostatectomy
Indications: The patient is a _____ -year-old male with clinical stage T__ *urothelial cell/ squamous cell/adeno* carcinoma of the bladder presenting for a robotic-assisted laparoscopic radical cystoprostatectomy.
Description of Procedure: The indications, alternatives, benefits, and risks were discussed with the patient and informed consent was obtained.

The patient was brought onto the operating room table, placed supine, and secured with a safety strap. All pressure points were carefully padded and pneumatic compression devices were placed on the lower extremities.

After the administration of intravenous antibiotics and general endotracheal anesthesia, the patient was repositioned in dorsal lithotomy using well-padded universal (Allen) stirrups. The arms were carefully tucked at the patient's side and secured with padding. The chest was secured in place with foam padding and cloth tape, and the table positioned in 30° Trendelenburg. The patient's abdomen, genitalia, and upper thighs were prepped and draped in the standard sterile manner.

The radiographic images were in the room.

A time-out was completed, verifying the correct patient, surgical procedure, and positioning, prior to beginning the procedure.

A 16 Fr urethral catheter was inserted and the bladder drained.

Pneumoperitoneum was introduced by placing a Veress needle into the abdomen and insufflating with CO_2 to a pressure of 15 mmHg. The camera trocar was placed 5 cm cephalad to the umbilicus and the *0°/30°* lens was inserted under direct visualization. The abdominal cavity was examined for any sign of injury, adhesions, and identification of anatomic landmarks. The remainder of the trocars were placed, which included a 12 mm port in the *right/left* lower quadrant medial to the anterior-superior iliac spine, two 8 mm ports at the left and right rectus margin slightly caudal to the camera port, and an 8 mm port medial to the *right/left* anterior-superior iliac spine. A 5 mm assistant port was placed in the *right/left* upper quadrant. The robot was then docked.

The parietal peritoneum was incised along the white line of Toldt and the *right/left* colon reflected medially, exposing the psoas and iliac vessels. The ureter was identified at the common iliac bifurcation and dissected distally to the ureterovesical junction, ligating and dividing the obliterated umbilical artery and superior vesical pedicle as the plane between the bladder and pelvic sidewall was developed. The ureter was dissected cephalad to the level of the aortic bifurcation with care to preserve periureteral tissue.

A similar dissection was performed on the contralateral side.

The distal end of each ureter was clipped, divided, and tagged with a long 3-0 chromic suture to facilitate later identification. A distal margin from each ureter was sent for frozen section evaluation.

The posterior peritoneal reflection between the bladder and rectum was incised, and the bladder retracted anteriorly while the prerectal space below Denonvillier's fascia was carefully developed posterior to the seminal vesicles toward the prostatic apex. The posterior and lateral pedicles were clipped and sharply divided bilaterally.

An incision was made in the peritoneum along the anterior abdominal wall above the level of the bladder. The urachus and medial umbilical ligaments were incised using a combination of sharp dissection and electrocautery. The space of Retzius was developed to the level of the endopelvic fascia. The prostate was defatted, and the superficial dorsal venous complex was coagulated with electrocautery and divided. The endopelvic fascia was sharply opened bilaterally, and the levator muscle fibers were swept postero-laterally allowing for visualization of the deep dorsal vein complex and apex of the prostate. The puboprostatic ligaments were sharply divided with care to preserve the dorsal vein complex.

> *If a nerve sparing procedure is performed*: The plane between the prostatic capsule and prostatic fascia was developed and the nerve-sparing dissection plane defined. This plane was extended distally using a combination of sharp and blunt dissection, freeing the neurovascular bundle. The use of electrocautery was minimized to prevent thermal damage to the neurovascular bundle.

The dorsal vein complex was sharply divided. An occluding clip was placed on the urethra and the urethra sharply divided distally to prevent spillage. A urethral margin was sent to pathology for frozen-section evaluation. The pelvis was irrigated and hemostasis obtained. Patent venous sinuses of the transected dorsal venous complex were oversewn with 0 polyglactin (Vicryl) sutures. The bladder and prostate were placed in a specimen retrieval bag and set aside.

A bilateral pelvic lymph node dissection was performed, beginning on the *right/left.* The iliac vessels were exposed from just above the common iliac bifurcation to the femoral canal (node of Cloquet). The ureters were identified at the common iliac bifurcation. The nodal dissection was started along the medial aspect of the external iliac artery by incising the perivascular fibroareolar sheath. The lymph node packet was gently mobilized medially, and small vessels and lymphatic branches were fulgurated or ligated with surgical clips to maintain meticulous hemo- and lymphostasis. The obturator neurovascular bundle was identified posteriorly and preserved. The borders of dissection were the common iliac artery bifurcation cranially, the node of Cloquet caudally, the genitofemoral nerve laterally, and the obturator nerve posteriorly. A polymer ligating clip (e.g. Hem-o-lok) was used to secure the distal and proximal extent of the lymph node packet. The nodal packet was removed and sent to pathology for evaluation.

The contralateral lymph node dissection was performed in a similar manner and the nodal packet was sent to pathology for evaluation.

A plane posterior to the sigmoid mesentery at the level of the aortic bifurcation was developed by elevating the sigmoid anteriorly, and the left ureter was tunneled without angulation to the right side.

The operative field was inspected for bleeding or injury and irrigated with warm sterile saline. The insufflation pressure was reduced, again confirming the absence of bleeding.

Add the appropriate urinary diversion; see Section I, subsection Urinary Diversion

Estimated blood loss: Approximately _____ml

104

Robotic-Assisted Laparoscopic Vesicovaginal Fistula Repair

Indications

- Vesicovaginal fistula

Essential Steps

1) Perform cystoscopy to intubate the fistula with a stent.
2) Dissect the plane between the bladder and vagina to identify the fistulous tract, with care to avoid the ureters.
3) Excise the fistulous tract from the bladder and vagina.
4) Close the vagina in a single layer and the bladder in two layers.
5) Anchor an interposition flap between the bladder and vaginal suture lines.
6) Place a drain.

Note These Variations

- Access into the peritoneal cavity may be obtained with a Veress needle, with the open Hasson technique, or with direct vision optical trocars.
- The use of ureteral stents is optional depending upon the location of the vesicovaginal fistula.
- An extraperitoneal approach may offer avoidance of intraperitoneal contents. During the procedure there may be a decreased need to retract the bowel and lower the risk of elevated intraperitoneal pressures, but there may be less working space and proper port placement is critical.
- A transvesical approach through a separate cystotomy may be utilized to identify the fistulous tract and its relationship to the ureteral orifices.
- A suprapubic cystotomy catheter can be inserted in addition to the urethral catheter to optimize drainage and assist in the subsequent voiding trial.
- The need for fascial closure of port sites depends upon trocar size and design, patient characteristics, and surgeon preference. Fascial closures may be performed by a hand-sutured technique or with assistance of devices, under direct visualization in order to minimize the risk of visceral injury.

Operative Dictations in Urologic Surgery, First Edition. Noel A. Armenakas, John A. Fracchia, and Ron Golan.
© 2019 John Wiley & Sons Ltd. Published 2019 by John Wiley & Sons Ltd.

Complications

- Bleeding
- Infection
- Intraabdominal organ injury
- Ureteral injury/obstruction
- Ileus
- Recurrent/persistent fistula

Template Operative Dictation

Preoperative diagnosis: Vesicovaginal fistula
Postoperative diagnosis: same
Procedure: Robotic-assisted laparoscopic vesicovaginal fistula repair
Indications: The patient is a ___-year-old female with a vesicovaginal fistula presenting for robotic-assisted laparoscopic vesicovaginal fistula repair.
Description of Procedure: The indications, alternatives, benefits, and risks were discussed with the patient and informed consent was obtained.

The patient was brought onto the operating room table, placed supine and secured with a safety strap. All pressure points were carefully padded and pneumatic compression devices were placed on the lower extremities.

After the administration of intravenous antibiotics and general endotracheal anesthesia, the patient was repositioned in dorsal lithotomy using well-padded universal (Allen) stirrups. The arms were tucked at the patient's side and secured with padding. The chest was secured in place with foam padding and cloth tape, and the table positioned in 30° Trendelenburg. The patient's abdomen, genitalia, and upper thighs were prepped and draped in the standard sterile manner.

A time-out was completed, verifying the correct patient, surgical procedure, and positioning, prior to beginning the procedure.

The radiographic images were in the room.

A *17/22* Fr rigid cystoscope was inserted per meatus and advanced under direct vision into the urinary bladder. Cystoscopy was performed using the 30° and 70° lenses. The bladder was thoroughly inspected and both ureteral orifices were visualized in the normal anatomic position with clear efflux noted bilaterally. A 0.038 in. (Sensor) guidewire with a hydrophilic tip was advanced through the *right/left* ureteral orifice to the collecting system under fluoroscopic guidance. A 5 Fr open-ended catheter was advanced over the guidewire and positioned in the renal pelvis. The guidewire was then removed. *The contralateral ureter was similarly intubated.*

The fistula was visualized at the ____*(location)*____ and was intubated with an 8 Fr *Foley/infant feeding tube//5 Fr open-ended catheter* which was brought out through the vagina. The cystoscope was removed under direct vision.

A 16 Fr urethral catheter was inserted to drain the bladder and the ureteral catheter(s) secured to this.

Pneumoperitoneum was introduced by placing a Veress needle into the abdomen and insufflating with CO_2 to a pressure of 15 mmHg. The camera trocar was placed superior

to the umbilicus and the *0°/30°* lens was inserted under direct visualization. The abdominal cavity was examined for any sign of injury, adhesions, and identification of anatomic landmarks. The remainder of the trocars were placed, which included a 12 mm port in the *right/left* lower quadrant medial to the anterior-superior iliac spine, two 8 mm ports at the left and right rectus margin slightly caudal to the camera port, and an 8 mm port medial to the *right/left* anterior-superior iliac spine. A 5 mm assistant port was placed in the *right/left* upper quadrant. The robot was then docked.

The peritoneum overlying the vesicovaginal space was sharply incised. A weighted retractor was inserted intravaginally to aid in the identification and dissection of the anterior vaginal plane. Upon visualizing the stent traversing the fistulous tract, the dissection was continued circumferentially to completely separate the fistulous tract from the vagina. The fistula was widely excised obtaining healthy margins of bladder and vagina. The excised tissue was sent to pathology for evaluation. The vaginal defect was closed in a single layer using a running 2-0 polyglactin (Vicryl) suture.

The bladder defect was closed in two layers using 2-0 Vicryl sutures. Once the reconstruction was complete, a 16 Fr urethral catheter was inserted into the bladder. The bladder was irrigated with sterile normal saline, confirming a watertight closure. The operative field was inspected for bleeding or injury. The insufflation pressure was reduced, again confirming the absence of bleeding.

Pneumoperitoneum was reestablished and *an omental interposition flap/peritoneal flap/mesenteric fat/peri-colic fat* was mobilized and interposed between the bladder and vaginal suture line. It was anchored to the vagina overlying the site of repair using a 2-0 Vicryl suture.

> **If a surgical drain is placed:** A surgical drain (e.g. Jackson-Pratt) was placed through a laparoscopic port into the pelvis and secured at the skin.

The robot was undocked and removed. The trocars and weighted vaginal retractor were withdrawn under direct visualization. The anterior fascia at the umbilical site was carefully closed with a 1-0 polydioxanone (PDS) suture, and a total of __ml of local anesthetic (*specify*) injected subcutaneously at the port sites. The skin incisions were closed with 4-0 poliglecaprone (Monocryl) sutures and reinforced with sterile adhesive strips. Sterile dressings were applied and the patient repositioned supine.

At the end of the procedure, all counts were correct.

The patient tolerated the procedure well and was taken to the recovery room in satisfactory condition.

Estimated blood loss: Approximately _____ml

Kidney

105

Laparoscopic Living Donor Nephrectomy

Indications

- Elective kidney donation

Essential Steps

1) Incise the white line of Toldt to reflect the colon medially.
2) Mobilize adjacent organs and divide the surrounding renal attachments.
3) Identify and skeletonize the renal hilum. Clip and divide the adrenal, gonadal, or lumbar vein(s), when necessary.
4) Mobilize the kidney within Gerota's fascia and free the adrenal off the superior pole.
5) Identify and divide the ureter at the level of the pelvic brim with care to preserve the peri-ureteral tissue.
6) Obtain vascular control and divide the renal artery(ies) followed by the renal vein(s).
7) Inspect for bleeding or adjacent organ injury.

Note These Variations

- Preoperative planning with blood and urine testing along with imaging are critical in identifying appropriate candidates and in selecting the laterality of the kidney for donation.
- Access into the peritoneal cavity may be obtained with a Veress needle, with the open Hasson technique, or with direct vision optical trocars.
- Intravenous resuscitation with Ringer's lactate solution or sodium chloride should be carefully managed by the anesthesiology and surgical team. Intravenous mannitol may be administered prior to the nephrectomy.
- A retroperitoneal approach for the nephrectomy may be undertaken. This is especially beneficial in patients with prior abdominal surgery or vascular/anatomic variations. The potential retroperitoneal space should be adequately developed prior to inserting instruments.
- This procedure may vary with regards to port placement and instruments. Hand-assistance may be utilized to improve tactile feedback for dissection, retraction, and

Operative Dictations in Urologic Surgery, First Edition. Noel A. Armenakas, John A. Fracchia, and Ron Golan.
© 2019 John Wiley & Sons Ltd. Published 2019 by John Wiley & Sons Ltd.

hemostatic control. Robotic assistance may be utilized to improve visualization, dexterity, and surgical ergonomics.

- The specimen may be retrieved through a periumbilical, Pfannenstiel, modified Gibson, or paramedian incision.
- The need for fascial closure of port sites depends on trocar size and design, patient characteristics, and surgeon preference. Fascial closures may be performed by a hand-sutured technique or with assistance of devices, under direct visualization in order to minimize the risk of visceral injury.

Complications

- Bleeding
- Infection
- Intraabdominal organ injury
- Pneumothorax
- Ileus

Template Operative Dictation

Preoperative diagnosis: Kidney donor
Postoperative diagnosis: Same
Procedure: Laparoscopic *left/right* donor nephrectomy
Indications: The patient is a ___ -year-old *male/female* presenting for a laparoscopic donor nephrectomy.
Description of Procedure: The indications, alternatives, benefits, and risks were discussed with the patient and informed consent was obtained.

The patient was brought onto the operating room table, placed supine, and secured with a safety strap. All pressure points were carefully padded and pneumatic compression devices were placed on the lower extremities.

After the administration of intravenous antibiotics and general endotracheal anesthesia, a 16 Fr urethral catheter was inserted to drain the bladder. The patient was repositioned in the *right/left* lateral decubitus position at a 45° angle with the lower leg flexed 90° and the upper leg extended. An axillary roll was positioned to protect the brachial plexus and a gel pad placed to support the back. Multiple pillows were used to pad beneath and between both the upper and lower extremities to ensure adequate cushioning. The patient was secured in place across the hips, chest, and legs with foam padding and cloth tape, and the table was flexed. The patient was prepped and draped in the usual sterile manner.

The radiographic images were in the room.

A time-out was completed, verifying the correct patient, surgical procedure, site, and positioning, prior to beginning the procedure.

Pneumoperitoneum was introduced by placing a Veress needle into the abdomen and insufflating with CO_2 to a pressure of 15 mmHg. The camera trocar was placed periumbically and the *0°/30°* lens was inserted under direct visualization. The abdominal cavity

was examined for any sign of injury, adhesions, and identification of anatomic landmarks. The remainder of the trocars were placed, which included a 10 mm port placed in the anterior axillary line caudal to the umbilicus and a 5 mm port placed in the midline cephalad to the umbilicus. (*If retraction is required*: An additional assistant port was inserted to retract the *liver/spleen.*)

The parietal peritoneum was incised along the white line of Toldt and the colon reflected medially, exposing Gerota's fascia.

> **On the right**: The hepatic flexure was mobilized by dividing the triangular and coronary ligaments, allowing for retraction of the liver. The duodenum was kocherized and the inferior vena cava was visualized. The retroperitoneal fascia overlying the renal vessels was carefully separated, exposing the underlying renal vein. The renal vein was carefully dissected and mobilized.

> **On the left**: The splenorenal and splenophrenic ligaments were incised to mobilize the spleen. The tail of the pancreas was mobilized medially. The gonadal vein and ureter were identified and the dissection carried cephalad toward the renal vein. The renal vein was carefully dissected and mobilized. The gonadal, adrenal, and lumbar veins were visualized entering the renal vein, clipped, and sharply divided.

The kidney was circumferentially mobilized using the laparoscopic electrothermal bipolar tissue sealing device (e.g. LigaSure). Special attention was given to the cranial connections to the adrenal gland, which were carefully divided and freed from the superior pole of the kidney.

The renal artery*(ies) was/were* identified deep to the vein, carefully dissected, mobilized, and divided using the vascular stapling device. Having interrupted the renal vascular inflow, the renal vein was similarly stapled and divided. Inferiorly, the ureter was divided between clips at the level of the iliac vessels. The kidney was carefully placed into a specimen retrieval bag. Meticulous hemostasis was maintained throughout the procedure.

The periumbilical incision was extended and the specimen extracted. The specimen was placed into a sterile container and transferred in order to be processed for the recipient.

The anterior fascia at the umbilical site was carefully closed with a 1-0 polydioxanone (PDS) suture and pneumoperitoneum was reestablished. The renal fossa and remainder of the operative field were inspected for bleeding or injury. The insufflation pressure was reduced, again confirming the absence of bleeding.

The trocars were withdrawn under direct visualization. A total of ___ml of local anesthetic (*specify*) were injected subcutaneously at the port sites. The skin incisions were closed with 4-0 poliglecaprone (Monocryl) sutures and reinforced with sterile adhesive strips. Sterile dressings were applied and the patient repositioned supine.

At the end of the procedure, all counts were correct.

The patient tolerated the procedure well and was taken to the recovery room in satisfactory condition.

Estimated blood loss: Approximately _____ml

106

Laparoscopic Radical Nephrectomy

Indications

- Select solid renal masses
- Renal tumors with local extension
- Cytoreductive surgery for metastatic disease

Essential Steps

1) Incise the white line of Toldt to reflect the colon medially.
2) Mobilize adjacent organs and divide the surrounding renal attachments.
3) Identify and obtain early vascular control of the renal hilum. In addition, identify and divide the adrenal, gonadal, or lumbar vein(s), when necessary.
4) Mobilize Gerota's fascia circumferentially and free the adrenal off the superior pole of the kidney.
5) Identify and divide the ureter.
6) Inspect for bleeding or adjacent organ injury.

Note These Variations

- Access into the peritoneal cavity may be obtained with a Veress needle, with the open Hasson technique, or with direct vision optical trocars.
- A retroperitoneal approach for the nephrectomy may be undertaken. This is especially beneficial in patients with prior abdominal surgery or vascular/anatomic variations. The potential retroperitoneal space should be adequately developed prior to inserting instruments.
- This procedure may vary with regards to port placement and instruments. Hand-assistance may be utilized to improve tactile feedback for dissection, retraction, and hemostatic control. Robotic assistance may be utilized to improve visualization, dexterity, and surgical ergonomics.
- The ipsilateral adrenal gland may be removed *en bloc* in patients with upper pole tumors or tumors involving the adrenal.

Operative Dictations in Urologic Surgery, First Edition. Noel A. Armenakas, John A. Fracchia, and Ron Golan.
© 2019 John Wiley & Sons Ltd. Published 2019 by John Wiley & Sons Ltd.

- The specimen may be retrieved through a periumbilical, Pfannenstiel, modified Gibson, or paramedian incision.
- The need for fascial closure of port sites depends on trocar size and design, patient characteristics, and surgeon preference. Fascial closures may be performed by a hand-sutured technique or with assistance of devices, under direct visualization, in order to minimize the risk of visceral injury.

Complications

- Bleeding
- Infection
- Intraabdominal organ injury
- Pneumothorax
- Ileus

Template Operative Dictation

Preoperative diagnosis: Renal tumor
Postoperative diagnosis: Same
Procedure: Laparoscopic *right/left* radical nephrectomy
Indications: The patient is a ___-year-old *male/female* with a *right/left* renal tumor presenting for a laparoscopic radical nephrectomy.
Description of Procedure: The indications, alternatives, benefits, and risks were discussed with the patient and informed consent was obtained.

The patient was brought onto the operating room table, placed supine, and secured with a safety strap. All pressure points were carefully padded and pneumatic compression devices were placed on the lower extremities.

After the administration of intravenous antibiotics and general endotracheal anesthesia, a 16 Fr urethral catheter was inserted to drain the bladder. The patient was repositioned in the *left/right* lateral decubitus position at a 45° angle with the lower leg flexed 90° and the upper leg extended. An axillary roll was positioned to protect the brachial plexus and a gel pad placed to support the back. Multiple pillows were used to pad beneath and between both the upper and lower extremities to ensure adequate cushioning. The patient was secured in place across the hips, chest, and legs with foam padding and cloth tape, and the table was flexed. The patient was prepped and draped in the standard sterile manner.

The radiographic images were in the room.

A time-out was completed, verifying the correct patient, surgical procedure, site, and positioning, prior to beginning the procedure.

Pneumoperitoneum was introduced by placing a Veress needle into the abdomen and insufflating with CO_2 to a pressure of 15 mmHg. The camera trocar was placed periumbically and the *0°/30°* lens was inserted under direct visualization. The abdominal cavity was examined for any sign of injury, adhesions, and identification of anatomic landmarks. The remainder of the trocars were placed, which included a 10 mm port placed

in the anterior axillary line caudal to the umbilicus and a 5 mm port placed in the midline cephalad to the umbilicus. (*If retraction is required*: An additional assistant port was inserted to retract the *liver/spleen*.)

The parietal peritoneum was incised along the white line of Toldt and the colon reflected medially, exposing Gerota's fascia.

> ***On the right***: The hepatic flexure was mobilized by dividing the triangular and coronary ligaments of the liver. This allowed for further retraction of the liver. The duodenum was kocherized and the inferior vena cava was visualized. The retroperitoneal fascia overlying the renal vessels was carefully separated, exposing the underlying renal vein. The renal vein was carefully dissected and mobilized.

> ***On the left***: The splenorenal and splenophrenic ligaments were incised to mobilize the spleen. The tail of the pancreas was mobilized medially. The gonadal vein and ureter were identified and the dissection carried cephalad toward the renal vein. The renal vein was carefully dissected and mobilized. The gonadal, adrenal, and lumbar veins were visualized entering the renal vein, clipped, and sharply divided.

The main renal artery*(ies) was/were* identified deep to the vein, carefully dissected, mobilized, and divided using the vascular stapling device. Having interrupted the renal vascular inflow, the renal vein was similarly stapled and divided. Using the laparoscopic electrothermal bipolar tissue sealing device (e.g. LigaSure), Gerota's fascia was mobilized circumferentially, maintaining meticulous hemostasis. Special attention was given to the cranial connections to the adrenal gland, which were carefully divided using the LigaSure, completely freeing the adrenal off the superior pole of the kidney. Inferiorly, the ureter was identified and divided between clips.

The kidney was placed in a specimen retrieval bag and set aside. The renal fossa and remainder of the operative field were inspected for bleeding or injury. The insufflation pressure was reduced, again confirming the absence of bleeding.

The trocars were removed under direct visualization. The periumbilical incision was extended and the specimen retrieval bag was removed. The specimen was sent to pathology for evaluation.

The anterior fascia at the umbilical site was carefully closed with a 1-0 polydioxanone (PDS) suture, and a total of __ ml of local anesthetic (*specify*) injected subcutaneously at the port sites. The skin incisions were closed with 4-0 poliglecaprone (Monocryl) sutures and reinforced with sterile adhesive strips. Sterile dressings were applied and the patient repositioned supine.

At the end of the procedure, all counts were correct.

The patient tolerated the procedure well and was taken to the recovery room in satisfactory condition.

Estimated blood loss: Approximately _____ml

107

Laparoscopic Renal Cyst Decortication

Indications

- Symptomatic renal cyst
- Renal cyst causing urinary obstruction

Essential Steps

1) Mobilize the renal attachments to allow for visualization of the renal cyst(s).
2) Aspirate the renal cyst and debride its walls; these may be sent to pathology for evaluation or culture.
3) Evaluate for entry into the collecting system and repair if identified. Obtain hemostasis with electrocauterization of the resection margins and resection bed.
4) Irrigate the surgical field.
5) Place a drain.

Note These Variations

- Access into the peritoneal cavity may be obtained with a Veress needle, the open Hasson technique, or with direct vision optical trocars.
- A retroperitoneal approach for the cyst decortication may be undertaken. This is especially beneficial in patients with prior abdominal surgery or vascular/anatomic variations. The retroperitoneal space should be adequately developed prior to inserting instruments.
- This procedure may vary with regards to port placement and instruments. Hand-assistance may be utilized to improve tactile feedback for dissection, retraction, and hemostatic control. Robotic assistance may be utilized to improve visualization, dexterity, and surgical ergonomics.
- An open-ended ureteral catheter may be inserted in a retrograde manner into the collecting system prior to decortication if the renal cyst is abutting the collecting system in order to assist with identification of entry into the collecting system.
- The need for fascial closure of port sites depends on trocar size and design, patient characteristics, and surgeon preference. Fascial closures may be performed by a

Operative Dictations in Urologic Surgery, First Edition. Noel A. Armenakas, John A. Fracchia, and Ron Golan.
© 2019 John Wiley & Sons Ltd. Published 2019 by John Wiley & Sons Ltd.

hand-sutured technique or with assistance of devices, under direct visualization, in order to minimize the risk of visceral injury.

Complications

- Bleeding
- Infection
- Intraabdominal organ injury
- Pneumothorax
- Urine leak/urinoma
- Ileus

Template Operative Dictation

Preoperative diagnosis: Symptomatic renal cyst
Postoperative diagnosis: Same
Procedure: Laparoscopic *right/left* renal cyst decortication
Indications: The patient is a ___-year-old *male/female* with a symptomatic *right/left* renal cyst presenting for laparoscopic renal cyst decortication.
Description of Procedure: The indications, alternatives, benefits, and risks were discussed with the patient and informed consent was obtained.

The patient was brought onto the operating room table, placed supine, and secured with a safety strap. All pressure points were carefully padded and pneumatic compression devices were placed on the lower extremities.

After the administration of intravenous antibiotics and general endotracheal anesthesia, a 16 Fr urethral catheter was inserted to drain the bladder. The patient was repositioned in the *left/right* lateral decubitus position at a 45° angle with the lower leg flexed 90° and the upper leg extended. An axillary roll was positioned to protect the brachial plexus and a gel pad placed to support the back. Multiple pillows were used to pad beneath and between both the upper and lower extremities to ensure adequate cushioning. The patient was secured in place across the hips, chest, and legs with foam padding and cloth tape and the table was flexed. The patient was prepped and draped in the standard sterile manner.

The radiographic images were in the room.

A time-out was completed, verifying the correct patient, surgical procedure, site, and positioning, prior to beginning the procedure.

Pneumoperitoneum was introduced by placing a Veress needle into the abdomen and insufflating with CO_2 to a pressure of 15 mmHg. The camera trocar was placed periumbically and the *0/30°* lens was inserted under direct visualization. The abdominal cavity was examined for any sign of injury, adhesions, and identification of anatomic landmarks. The remainder of the trocars were placed, which included a 10 mm port placed in the anterior axillary line caudal to the umbilicus and a 5 mm port placed in the midline cephalad to the umbilicus. (*If retraction is required*: An additional assistant port was inserted to retract the *liver/spleen*.)

The parietal peritoneum was incised along the white line of Toldt and the colon reflected medially, exposing Gerota's fascia.

> ***On the right***: The hepatic flexure was mobilized by dividing the triangular and coronary ligaments, allowing for retraction of the liver. The duodenum was kocherized and the inferior vena cava was visualized.
>
> ***On the left***: The splenorenal and splenophrenic ligaments were incised to mobilize the spleen. The tail of the pancreas was mobilized medially.

The plane between Gerota's fascia and the kidney was developed, and the renal cyst(s) *was/were* visualized. Intraoperative ultrasound was used to facilitate identification of the cyst and its margins. The fluid within the cyst(s) was aspirated and sent for culture and cytology. Approximately ___ml of *clear/cloudy/purulent* appearing fluid were aspirated. The walls of the renal cyst were sharply excised and sent to pathology for evaluation. Hemostasis was obtained along the base and margins of the cyst with electrocautery.

> ***If there is concern for entry into the collecting system***: A collecting system defect was identified and closed using 3-0 chromic sutures in a figure-of-eight fashion.

The site of decortication and remainder of the operative field were irrigated with sterile normal saline and inspected for bleeding or injury. The insufflation pressure was reduced, again confirming the absence of bleeding.

Pneumoperitoneum was reestablished and a surgical drain (e.g. Jackson-Pratt) was placed through a laparoscopic port into the perirenal space and secured at the skin. The trocars were withdrawn under direct visualization.

The anterior fascia at the umbilical site was carefully closed with a 1-0 polydioxanone (PDS) suture, and a total of __ml of local anesthetic (*specify*) injected subcutaneously at the port sites. The skin incisions were closed with 4-0 poliglecaprone (Monocryl) sutures and reinforced with sterile adhesive strips. Sterile dressings were applied and the patient repositioned supine.

At the end of the procedure, all counts were correct.

The patient tolerated the procedure well and was taken to the recovery room in satisfactory condition.

Estimated blood loss: Approximately _____ml

108

Laparoscopic Simple Nephrectomy

Indications

- Nonmalignant renal disease (i.e. infection, nonfunctioning kidney, medically refractory renovascular hypertension, end-stage renal disease)

Essential Steps

1) Incise the white line of Toldt to reflect the colon medially.
2) Mobilize adjacent organs and divide the surrounding renal attachments.
3) Identify and obtain early vascular control of the renal hilum. In addition, identify and divide the adrenal, gonadal, or lumbar vein(s), when necessary.
4) Mobilize the kidney circumferentially within Gerota's fascia and free the adrenal off the superior pole.
5) Identify and divide the ureter.
6) Inspect for bleeding or surrounding organ injury.

Note These Variations

- Access into the peritoneal cavity may be obtained with a Veress needle, the open Hasson technique, or direct vision optical trocars.
- A retroperitoneal approach for the nephrectomy may be undertaken. This is especially beneficial in patients with prior abdominal surgery or vascular/anatomic variations. The potential retroperitoneal space should be adequately developed prior to inserting instruments.
- This procedure may vary with regards to port placement and instruments. Hand-assistance may be utilized to improve tactile feedback for dissection, retraction, and hemostatic control. Robotic-assistance may be utilized to improve visualization, dexterity, and surgical ergonomics.
- With severe renal scarring and/or inflammation, subscapsular renal dissection may be required.

Operative Dictations in Urologic Surgery, First Edition. Noel A. Armenakas, John A. Fracchia, and Ron Golan.
© 2019 John Wiley & Sons Ltd. Published 2019 by John Wiley & Sons Ltd.

- The specimen may be retrieved through a periumbilical, Pfannenstiel, modified Gibson, or paramedian incision.
- The need for fascial closure of port sites depends on trocar size and design, patient characteristics, and surgeon preference. Fascial closures may be performed by a hand-sutured technique or with assistance of devices, under direct visualization, in order to minimize the risk of visceral injury.

Complications

- Bleeding
- Infection
- Intraabdominal organ injury
- Pneumothorax
- Ileus

Template Operative Dictation

Preoperative diagnosis: _____
Postoperative diagnosis: Same
Procedure: Laparoscopic *right/left* simple nephrectomy
Indications: The patient is a ___-year-old *male/female* with ____ presenting for a laparoscopic simple nephrectomy.
Description of Procedure: The indications, alternatives, benefits, and risks were discussed with the patient and informed consent was obtained.

The patient was brought onto the operating room table, placed supine, and secured with a safety strap. All pressure points were carefully padded and pneumatic compression devices were placed on the lower extremities.

After the administration of intravenous antibiotics and general endotracheal anesthesia, a 16 Fr urethral catheter was inserted to drain the bladder. The patient was repositioned in the *left/right* lateral decubitus position at a 45° angle with the lower leg flexed 90° and the upper leg extended. An axillary roll was positioned to protect the brachial plexus and a gel pad placed to support the back. Multiple pillows were used to pad beneath and between both the upper and lower extremities to ensure adequate cushioning. The patient was secured in place across the hips, chest, and legs with foam padding and cloth tape, and the table was flexed. The patient was prepped and draped in the standard sterile manner.

The radiographic images were in the room.

A time-out was completed, verifying the correct patient, surgical procedure, site, and positioning, prior to beginning the procedure.

Pneumoperitoneum was introduced by placing a Veress needle into the abdomen and insufflating with CO_2 to a pressure of 15 mmHg. The camera trocar was placed periumbically and the *0°/30°* lens was inserted under direct visualization. The abdominal cavity was examined for any sign of injury, adhesions, and identification of anatomic landmarks. The remainder of the trocars were placed, which included a 12 mm port placed in the

anterior axillary line caudal to the umbilicus and a 5 mm port placed in the midline between the xiphoid and umbilicus. (*If retraction is required*: An additional assistant port was inserted to retract the *liver/spleen*.)

The parietal peritoneum was incised along the white line of Toldt and the colon reflected medially, exposing Gerota's fascia.

> ***On the right*:** The hepatic flexure was mobilized by dividing the triangular and coronary ligaments, allowing for retraction of the liver. The duodenum was kocherized and the inferior vena cava was visualized. The retroperitoneal fascia overlying the renal vessels was carefully separated, exposing the underlying renal vein. The renal vein was carefully dissected and mobilized.
>
> ***On the left*:** The splenorenal and splenophrenic ligaments were incised to mobilize the spleen. The tail of the pancreas was mobilized medially. The gonadal vein and ureter were identified and the dissection carried cephalad toward the renal vein. The renal vein was carefully dissected and mobilized. The gonadal, adrenal, and lumbar veins were visualized entering the renal vein, clipped, and sharply divided.

The main renal artery*(ies) was/were* identified deep to the vein, carefully dissected, mobilized, and divided using the vascular stapling device. Having interrupted the renal vascular inflow, the renal vein was similarly stapled and divided. Using the laparoscopic electrothermal bipolar tissue sealing device (e.g. LigaSure), Gerota's fascia was incised and the kidney mobilized circumferentially, maintaining meticulous hemostasis. Special attention was given to the cranial connections to the adrenal gland, which were carefully divided and freed from the superior pole of the kidney. Inferiorly, the ureter was identified and divided between clips.

The kidney was placed in a specimen retrieval bag and set aside. The renal fossa and remainder of the operative field were inspected for bleeding or injury. The insufflation pressure was reduced, again confirming the absence of bleeding.

> ***If a surgical drain is placed*:** Pneumoperitoneum was reestablished and a surgical drain (e.g. Jackson-Pratt) was placed through a laparoscopic port into the perirenal space and secured at the skin with a 2-0 silk suture.

The trocars were withdrawn under direct visualization. The periumbilical incision was extended and the specimen retrieval bag was removed. The specimen was sent to pathology for evaluation.

The anterior fascia at the umbilical site was carefully closed with a 1-0 polydioxanone (PDS) suture, and a total of __ ml of local anesthetic (*specify*) was injected subcutaneously at the port sites. The skin incisions were closed with 4-0 poliglecaprone (Monocryl) sutures and reinforced with sterile adhesive strips. Sterile dressings were applied and the patient repositioned supine.

At the end of the procedure, all counts were correct.

The patient tolerated the procedure well and was taken to the recovery room in satisfactory condition.

Estimated blood loss: Approximately _____ml

109

Robotic-Assisted Laparoscopic Nephroureterectomy

Indications

- Carcinoma of the upper urinary tract

Essential Steps

1) Incise the white line of Toldt to reflect the colon medially.
2) Mobilize adjacent organs and divide the surrounding renal attachments.
3) Identify and obtain early vascular control of the renal hilum. In addition, identify and divide the adrenal, gonadal, or lumbar vein(s), when necessary.
4) Mobilize Gerota's fascia circumferentially and free the adrenal off the superior pole of the kidney.
5) Identify and clip the ureter distal to the tumor to prevent tumor spillage during mobilization.
6) Mobilize the distal ureter to its insertion in the bladder.
7) Place stay sutures around the ureterovesical junction prior to making a circumferential incision of the bladder cuff.
8) Repair the cystotomy in a two-layer closure.
9) Place a drain.

Note These Variations

- Access into the peritoneal cavity may be obtained with a Veress needle, the open Hasson technique, or with direct vision optical trocars.
- This procedure may vary with regards to port placement and instruments. The robot may need to redocked and/or the patient repositioned between the kidney component and the distal ureterectomy/bladder cuff component. Alternatively, surgeons may elect for an open or endoscopic approach for the distal component.
- A transvesical approach may be taken whereby a separate cystotomy is made to facilitate intravesical dissection of the distal ureter and bladder cuff.
- A lymph node dissection is performed at the discretion of the surgeon and can include retroperitoneal and/or pelvic lymph nodes.

Operative Dictations in Urologic Surgery, First Edition. Noel A. Armenakas, John A. Fracchia, and Ron Golan.
© 2019 John Wiley & Sons Ltd. Published 2019 by John Wiley & Sons Ltd.

- A single intravesical instillation of Mitomycin C may be given immediately prior to surgery to decrease the risk of bladder recurrence.
- The need for fascial closure of port sites depends on trocar size and design, patient characteristics, and surgeon preference. Fascial closures may be performed by a hand-sutured technique or with assistance of devices, under direct visualization in order to minimize the risk of visceral injury.

Complications

- Bleeding
- Infection
- Intraabdominal organ injury
- Pneumothorax
- Urine leak/urinoma
- Ileus
- Lymphocele

Template Operative Dictation

Preoperative diagnosis: Upper urinary tract carcinoma
Postoperative diagnosis: Same
Procedure: Robotic-assisted *right/left* laparoscopic nephroureterectomy
Indications: The patient is a ____-year-old *male/female* with a _____cm *pelvis/ calyceal/ureteral* tumor presenting for a *right/left* robotic-assisted laparoscopic nephroureterectomy.
Description of Procedure: The indications, alternatives, benefits, and risks were discussed with the patient and informed consent was obtained.

The patient was brought onto the operating room table, placed supine, and secured with a safety strap. All pressure points were carefully padded and pneumatic compression devices were placed on the lower extremities.

After the administration of intravenous antibiotics and general endotracheal anesthesia, a 16 Fr urethral catheter was inserted to drain the bladder. The patient was repositioned in the *left/right* lateral decubitus position at a 45° angle with the lower leg flexed 90° and the upper leg extended. An axillary roll was positioned to protect the brachial plexus and a gel pad placed to support the back. Multiple pillows were used to pad beneath and between both the upper and lower extremities to ensure adequate cushioning. The patient was secured in place across the hips, chest, and legs with foam padding and cloth tape, and the table was flexed. The patient was prepped and draped in the standard sterile manner.

The radiographic images were in the room.

A time-out was completed, verifying the correct patient, surgical procedure, site, and positioning, prior to beginning the procedure.

Pneumoperitoneum was introduced by placing a Veress needle into the abdomen and insufflating with CO_2 to a pressure of 15 mmHg. The camera trocar was placed along

the *right/left* lateral edge of the rectus sheath slightly cephalad to the umbilicus and the *0/30°* lens was inserted under direct visualization. The abdominal cavity was examined for any sign of injury, adhesions, and identification of anatomic landmarks. The remainder of the robotic trocars were placed along the lateral edge of the rectus sheath, which included an 8 mm port below the costal margin, and two 8 mm ports caudal to the camera port. A 12 mm assistant port was placed in the midline above the umbilicus. (*If retraction is required*: An additional assistant port was inserted to retract the *liver/ spleen.*) The robot was then docked.

The parietal peritoneum was incised along the white line of Toldt and the colon reflected medially, exposing Gerota's fascia.

> **On the right**: The hepatic flexure was mobilized by dividing the triangular and coronary ligaments, allowing for retraction of the liver. The duodenum was kocherized and the inferior vena cava was visualized. The retroperitoneal fascia overlying the renal vessels was carefully separated, exposing the underlying renal vein. The renal vein was carefully dissected and mobilized.
>
> **On the left**: The splenorenal and splenophrenic ligaments were incised to mobilize the spleen. The tail of the pancreas was mobilized medially. The gonadal vein and ureter were identified and the dissection carried cephalad toward the renal vein. The renal vein was carefully dissected and mobilized. The gonadal, adrenal, and lumbar veins were visualized entering the renal vein, clipped, and sharply divided.

The main renal artery*(ies) was/were* identified deep to the vein, carefully dissected, mobilized and divided using the vascular stapling device. Having interrupted the renal vascular inflow, the renal vein was similarly stapled and divided. Using the laparoscopic electrothermal bipolar tissue sealing device (e.g. LigaSure), Gerota's fascia was mobilized circumferentially, maintaining meticulous hemostasis. Special attention was given to the cranial connections to the adrenal gland, which were carefully divided using the LigaSure, completely freeing the adrenal off the superior pole of the kidney. A clip was placed across the ureter distal to the tumor, and the ureter was further mobilized caudally.

> **If a perihilar or retroperitoneal lymphadenectomy is performed**: A perihilar and retroperitoneal lymphadenectomy including the *paracaval/retrocaval/para-aortic* lymph nodes was performed. The lymph node packet was gently mobilized medially, and small vessels and lymphatic branches were fulgurated or ligated with surgical clips to maintain meticulous hemo- and lymphostasis. A polymer ligating clip (e.g. Hem-o-lok) was used to secure the distal and proximal extents of the lymph node packet. The nodal packets were removed and sent to pathology for evaluation.

For the distal ureterectomy and bladder cuff excision, the robotic instruments were removed and the robot was redocked in the appropriate orientation. The distal ureter was further dissected to the level of the bladder. Gentle traction on the ureter confirmed the site of the intramural ureter and ureterovesical junction. Two 2-0 polyglactin (Vicryl) stay sutures were placed adjacent to this site and a circumferential incision

made through the mucosa, thereby freeing the full-thickness bladder cuff. The kidney and ureter were placed in the specimen retrieval bag and set aside. The cystotomy was closed with the previously placed stay sutures, and oversewn in a second layer using 2-0 Vicryl. The bladder was irrigated with sterile normal saline, confirming a water-tight closure.

> ***If a pelvic lymphadenectomy is performed:*** An ipsilateral pelvic lymph node dissection was performed. The nodal dissection was started along the medial aspect of the external iliac artery by incising the perivascular fibroareolar sheath. The lymph node packet was gently mobilized medially, and small vessels and lymphatic branches were fulgurated or ligated with surgical clips to maintain meticulous hemo- and lymphostasis. The obturator neurovascular bundle was identified posteriorly and preserved. The dissection was carried laterally to the genitofemoral nerve and medially to the ipsilateral ureter. The cranial and caudal limits of dissection were the common iliac bifurcation and femoral canal (node of Cloquet), respectively. A polymer ligating clip (e.g. Hem-o-lok) was used to secure the distal and proximal extents of the lymph node packet. The nodal packet was removed and sent to pathology for evaluation.

The operative field was inspected for bleeding or injury. The insufflation pressure was reduced, again confirming the absence of bleeding.

Pneumoperitoneum was reestablished and a surgical drain (e.g. Jackson-Pratt) was placed through a laparoscopic port into the pelvis and secured at the skin with a 2-0 silk suture.

The robot was undocked and removed from the operative field.

The trocars were withdrawn under direct visualization. The periumbilical incision was extended and the specimen retrieval bag was removed. The entire specimen was sent to pathology for evaluation.

The anterior fascia at the umbilical site was carefully closed with a 1-0 polydioxanone (PDS) suture, and a total of __ml of local anesthetic (*specify*) injected subcutaneously at the port sites. The skin incisions were closed with 4-0 poliglecaprone (Monocryl) sutures and reinforced with sterile adhesive strips. Sterile dressings were applied and the patient repositioned supine.

At the end of the procedure, all counts were correct.

The patient tolerated the procedure well and was taken to the recovery room in satisfactory condition.

Estimated blood loss: Approximately _____ml

110

Robotic-Assisted Laparoscopic Partial Nephrectomy

Indications

- Localized tumor that does not invade the renal hilum and is amenable to a partial nephrectomy
- Bilateral renal tumors
- Tumor in a solitary kidney

Essential Steps

1) Incise the white line of Toldt to reflect the colon medially.
2) Mobilize adjacent organs and divide the surrounding renal attachments.
3) Identify and skeletonize the renal hilum in order to provide exposure to the vessels.
4) Identify the mass and score a circumferential margin.
5) Clamp the renal artery and monitor duration of ischemia time.
6) Excise the mass.
7) Reconstruct the renal defect in multiple layers, including the collecting system if entry is noted.
8) Inspect the defect for hemostasis after unclamping of the vessel(s).
9) Place a drain.

Note These Variations

- Access into the peritoneal cavity may be obtained with a Veress needle, with the open Hasson technique, or with direct vision optical trocars.
- Resection may be performed with clamping of both the renal artery and vein, only the main renal artery, a segmental renal artery, or off-clamp entirely. Cooling of the renal unit is performed at the surgeon's discretion.
- A retroperitoneal approach for the partial nephrectomy may be undertaken. This is especially beneficial in patients with prior abdominal surgery or vascular/anatomic variations. The potential retroperitoneal space should be developed prior to inserting instruments.

Operative Dictations in Urologic Surgery, First Edition. Noel A. Armenakas, John A. Fracchia, and Ron Golan.
© 2019 John Wiley & Sons Ltd. Published 2019 by John Wiley & Sons Ltd.

- This procedure may vary with regards to port placement and instruments. This procedure may also be performed laparoscopically, and hand assistance may be utilized to improve tactile feedback for dissection, retraction, and hemostatic control.
- An open-ended ureteral catheter may be inserted in a retrograde manner prior to resection if the renal mass is abutting the collecting system, in order to assist with identification of entry into the collecting system.
- There are a number of ways to obtain renal hemostasis within the resection bed, including the use of electrocauterization, argon beam coagulation, sutures, absorbable bolsters, hemostatic agents and tissue sealants.
- Administration of mannitol in order to limit acute tubular injury is performed at the surgeon's discretion.
- The need for fascial closure of port sites depends on trocar size and design, patient characteristics, and surgeon preference. Fascial closures may be performed by a hand-sutured technique or with assistance of devices, under direct visualization in order to minimize the risk of visceral injury.

Complications

- Bleeding
- Infection
- Intraabdominal organ injury
- Pneumothorax
- Urine leak/urinoma
- Ileus
- Renal infarct/loss of renal function

Template Operative Dictation

Preoperative diagnosis: Renal mass
Postoperative diagnosis: Same
Procedure: Robotic-assisted laparoscopic *right/left* partial nephrectomy
Indications: The patient is a ___-year-old *male/female* with a *right/left* renal mass presenting for a robotic-assisted laparoscopic partial nephrectomy.
Description of Procedure: The indications, alternatives, benefits, and risks were discussed with the patient and informed consent was obtained.

The patient was brought onto the operating room table, placed supine, and secured with a safety strap. All pressure points were carefully padded and pneumatic compression devices were placed on the lower extremities.

After the administration of intravenous antibiotics and general endotracheal anesthesia, a 16 Fr urethral catheter was inserted in the bladder. The patient was repositioned in the *left/right* lateral decubitus position at a 45° angle with the lower leg flexed 90° and the upper leg extended. An axillary roll was positioned to protect the brachial plexus and a gel pad placed to support the back. Multiple pillows were used to pad beneath and between both the upper and lower extremities to ensure adequate cushioning. The

patient was secured in place across the hips, chest, and legs with foam padding and cloth tape, and the table was flexed. The patient was prepped and draped in the standard sterile manner.

The radiographic images were in the room.

A time-out was completed, verifying the correct patient, surgical procedure, site, and positioning, prior to beginning the procedure.

Pneumoperitoneum was introduced by placing a Veress needle into the abdomen and insufflating with CO_2 to a pressure of 15 mmHg. The camera trocar was placed along the *right/left* lateral edge of the rectus sheath slightly cephalad to the umbilicus and the *0°/30°* lens was inserted under direct visualization. The abdominal cavity was examined for any sign of injury, adhesions, and identification of anatomic landmarks. The remainder of the robotic trocars were placed along the lateral edge of the rectus sheath, which included an 8 mm port below the costal margin, and two 8 mm ports caudal to the camera port. A 12 mm assistant port was placed in the midline above the umbilicus. (*If retraction is required*: An additional assistant port was inserted to retract the *liver/ spleen.*) The robot was then docked.

The parietal peritoneum was incised along the white line of Toldt and the colon reflected medially, exposing Gerota's fascia.

> ***On the right***: The hepatic flexure was mobilized by dividing the triangular and coronary ligaments, allowing for retraction of the liver. The duodenum was kocherized and the inferior vena cava was visualized. The retroperitoneal fascia overlying the renal vessels was carefully separated, exposing the underlying renal vein. The main renal artery was identified deep to the vein and carefully dissected.
>
> ***On the left***: The splenorenal and splenophrenic ligaments were incised to mobilize the spleen. The tail of the pancreas was mobilized medially. The gonadal vein and ureter were identified and the dissection carried cephalad toward the renal vein. The adrenal and lumbar veins were visualized entering the renal vein. The main renal artery was identified deep to the vein and carefully dissected.

The renal mass was identified at the ____*(location)*____ and the overlying Gerota's fascia and fat removed. Intraoperative ultrasound was used to facilitate identification of the mass and its margins. A circumferential margin around the mass was scored with electrocauterization and 25 g of mannitol were administered intravenously. The laparoscopic bulldog clamp(s) *was/were* placed on the renal artery(*ies*)/*and renal vein*, and a timer tracking the ischemia time was started. The renal mass was sharply excised and placed aside in a specimen retrieval bag. Additionally, a deep margin specimen was obtained and sent to pathology for frozen section.

> ***If concern for entry into collecting system***: A collecting system defect was identified and closed using figure-of-eight 3-0 chromic sutures.

Suture ligation was performed using interrupted 3-0 chromic sutures to control transected parenchymal vessels in the resection bed. A hemostatic sealant (e.g. FloSeal) was

instilled into the resection bed, and the renal parenchyma was reconstructed using 2-0 polyglactin (Vicryl) sutures secured with polymer ligating clips (e.g. Hem-o-lok) over an absorbable hemostatic bolster (e.g. Surgicel). The bulldog clamp was then released under direct visualization.

There was a total ischemia time of ___ minutes.

Gerota's fascia was reapproximated using interrupted 2-0 Vicryl sutures.

The operative field was inspected for bleeding or injury. The insufflation pressure was reduced, again confirming the absence of bleeding.

Pneumoperitoneum was reestablished and a surgical drain (e.g. Jackson-Pratt) was placed through a laparoscopic port into the perirenal space, away from the repair, and secured at the skin.

The robot was undocked and removed from the operative field.

The trocars were removed under direct visualization. The periumbilical incision was extended and the specimen retrieval bag was removed. The specimen was sent to pathology for evaluation.

The anterior fascia at the umbilical site was carefully closed with a 1-0 polydioxanone (PDS) suture, and a total of __ml of local anesthetic (*specify*) injected subcutaneously at the port sites. The skin incisions were closed with 4-0 poliglecaprone (Monocryl) sutures and reinforced with sterile adhesive strips. Sterile dressings were applied and the patient repositioned supine.

At the end of the procedure, all counts were correct.

The patient tolerated the procedure well and was taken to the recovery room in satisfactory condition.

Estimated blood loss: Approximately _____ml

111

Robotic-Assisted Laparoscopic Pyelolithotomy

Indications

- Large stone burden or body habitus precluding percutaneous or ureteroscopic stone access and/or extraction.

Essential Steps

1) Mobilize the proximal ureter toward the renal pelvis with minimal ureteral handling and judicious use of electrocautery to preserve adventitial vessels.
2) Incise the renal pelvis or ureter and extract the stone(s).
3) Perform a nephroureteroscopy to evaluate for fragments, and retrieve any additional calculi with basket stone extraction or laser lithotripsy within the ureter or collecting system.
4) Repair the renal pelvis or ureteral defect over an indwelling double-J ureteral stent.
5) Place a drain.

Note These Variations

- Access into the peritoneal cavity may be obtained with a Veress needle, the open Hasson technique or with direct vision optical trocars.
- This procedure may vary with regards to port placement and instruments. This procedure may also be performed laparoscopically, and hand assistance may be utilized to improve feedback for dissection, retraction and hemostatic control.
- A retroperitoneal approach for the pyelolithotomy may be undertaken. This is especially beneficial in patients with prior abdominal surgery or vascular/anatomic variations. The potential retroperitoneal space should be adequately developed prior to inserting instruments.
- A nephrolithotomy may be performed concurrently whereby the parenchyma overlying the stone(s) is incised and the stone extracted *en bloc*. The defect may be closed in one or two layers, with or without the use of a hemostatic bolster or tissue sealants. The procedure may be performed with or without clamping of the renal hilum.

Operative Dictations in Urologic Surgery, First Edition. Noel A. Armenakas, John A. Fracchia, and Ron Golan.
© 2019 John Wiley & Sons Ltd. Published 2019 by John Wiley & Sons Ltd.

- Stones too large to remove through a laparoscopic port may be placed into a specimen retrieval bag and retrieved when the ports are removed.
- Antegrade or retrograde pyeloureteroscopy with laser lithotripsy and basket stone extraction may be utilized to remove remaining calculi, if present.
- The need for fascial closure of port sites depends on trocar size and design, patient characteristics, and surgeon preference. Fascial closures may be performed by a hand-sutured technique or with assistance of devices, under direct visualization in order to minimize the risk of visceral injury.

Complications

- Bleeding
- Infection
- Intraabdominal organ injury
- Pneumothorax
- Retained calculus(i)
- Urinary obstruction
- Anastomotic stricture

Template Operative Dictation

Preoperative diagnosis: Nephrolithiasis
Postoperative diagnosis: Same
Procedure: Robotic-assisted laparoscopic *right/left* pyelolithotomy and ureteral stent insertion
Indications: The patient is a ___-year-old *male/female* with *a ____ cm ureteral/renal* stone(s) presenting for a *right/left* robotic-assisted laparoscopic pyelolithotomy.
Description of Procedure: The indications, alternatives, benefits, and risks were discussed with the patient's family/guardian and informed consent was obtained.

The patient was brought onto the operating room table, placed supine, and secured with a safety strap. All pressure points were carefully padded and pneumatic compression devices were placed on the lower extremities.

After the administration of intravenous antibiotics and general endotracheal anesthesia, a 16 Fr urethral catheter was inserted to drain the bladder. The patient was repositioned in the *left/right* lateral decubitus position at a 45° angle with the lower leg flexed 90° and the upper leg extended. An axillary roll was positioned to protect the brachial plexus and a gel pad placed to support the back. Multiple pillows were used to pad beneath and between both the upper and lower extremities to ensure adequate cushioning. The patient was secured in place across the hips, chest, and legs with foam padding and cloth tape, and the table was flexed. The patient was prepped and draped in the standard sterile manner.

The radiographic images were in the room.

A time-out was completed, verifying the correct patient, surgical procedure, site, and positioning, prior to beginning the procedure.

If cystoscopy and ureteral stent insertion performed initially: A 22 Fr cystoscope with a 30° lens was inserted per meatus and advanced under direct

vision into the bladder. Urethroscopy revealed a normal urethra. There were no tumors, stones, or diverticula present. Both ureteral orifices were in the normal anatomic position. A 0.038 in. guidewire with a hydrophilic tip was advanced through the cystoscope and into the *right/left* ureteral orifice and advanced into the collecting system under fluoroscopic guidance. A 6 Fr ___ cm double-J stent was advanced over the guidewire and its proximal and distal ends positioned in the renal pelvis and bladder, respectively. The guidewire was removed and the distal curl visualized within the bladder. A 16 Fr urethral catheter was inserted to drain the bladder.

Pneumoperitoneum was introduced by placing a Veress needle into the abdomen and insufflating with CO_2 to a pressure of 15 mmHg. The camera trocar was placed periumbilically and the *0°/30°* lens was inserted under direct visualization. The abdominal cavity was examined for any sign of injury, adhesions, and identification of anatomic landmarks. The remainder of the robotic trocars were placed along the lateral edge of the rectus sheath, which included an 8 mm port below the costal margin, and two 8 mm ports caudal to the camera port. A 12 mm assistant port was placed in the midline above the umbilicus. (*If retraction is required*: An additional assistant port was inserted to retract the *liver/spleen*.) The robot was then docked.

The parietal peritoneum was incised along the white line of Toldt and the colon reflected medially, exposing Gerota's fascia.

> ***On the right***: The hepatic flexure was mobilized by dividing the triangular and coronary ligaments, allowing for retraction of the liver. The duodenum was kocherized and the inferior vena cava was visualized. The proximal ureter was identified and carefully dissected cephalad toward the renal pelvis while preserving periureteral tissue. The gonadal vein was identified and preserved. The retroperitoneal fascia overlying the renal vessels was carefully separated, exposing the underlying renal vein and artery.

> ***On the left***: The splenorenal and splenophrenic ligaments were incised to mobilize the spleen. The tail of the pancreas was mobilized medially. The proximal ureter was identified and carefully dissected cephalad toward the renal pelvis while preserving periureteral tissue. The retroperitoneal fascia overlying the renal vessels was carefully separated, exposing the underlying renal vein and artery.

The renal pelvis was visualized and sharply incised. The stones were extracted from the collecting system with the robotic instruments and placed into a specimen retrieval bag. Ultrasound was used to confirm removal of all stone fragments.

> ***If pyeloureteroscopy is performed***: A flexible *cystoscope/ureteroscope* was passed through the laparoscopic port and the remaining stone(s) visualized within the *collecting system/ureter*. A *200/365* μm laser fiber was passed through the scope adapter (e.g. UroLok) and advanced to the stone. The holmium:YAG laser was readied and the stone *fragmented/dusted* using a maximal energy of ____ Joules at a maximal rate of ____pulses/second. Fragments were extracted with a stone retrieval basket under direct visualization. Upon completion of the laser procedure, the ureter and collecting system were thoroughly inspected

confirming extraction of all visible stone fragments. The ureteroscope was removed slowly under direct vision, confirming an intact mucosa and the absence of residual stones.

***If a ureteral stent is placed upon completion of the case*:** A 6 Fr ___cm double-J stent was advanced over a guidewire in an antegrade manner with the distal end positioned in the bladder and the proximal end within the renal pelvis, and the wire removed.

Repair of the renal pelvis was performed with a running 4-0 polyglactin (Vicryl) suture. The operative field was inspected for bleeding or injury. The insufflation pressure was reduced, again confirming the absence of bleeding.

Pneumoperitoneum was reestablished and a surgical drain (e.g. Jackson-Pratt) was placed through a laparoscopic port into the perirenal space, away from the repair, and secured at the skin with a 2-0 silk suture.

The robot was undocked and removed from the operative field.

The trocars were withdrawn under direct visualization. The periumbilical incision was extended and the specimen retrieval bag was removed. The stone(s) *was/were* sent for chemical analysis and culture.

The anterior fascia at the umbilical site was carefully closed with a 1-0 polydioxanone (PDS) suture, and a total of __ml of local anesthetic (*specify*) injected subcutaneously at the port sites. The skin incisions were closed with 4-0 poliglecaprone (Monocryl) sutures and reinforced with sterile adhesive strips. Sterile dressings were applied and the patient repositioned supine.

At the end of the procedure, all counts were correct.

The patient tolerated the procedure well and was taken to the recovery room in satisfactory condition.

Estimated blood loss: Approximately _____ml

112

Robotic-Assisted Laparoscopic Pyeloplasty (Dismembered)

Indications

- Ureteropelvic junction obstruction

Essential Steps

1) Mobilize the proximal ureter toward the renal pelvis with minimal ureteral handling and judicious use of electrocautery to preserve adventitial vessels.
2) Define the ureteropelvic junction prior to incision and identify the etiology of the ureteral pelvic junction (e.g. crossing aberrant vessel, intrinsic narrowing, or scarring).
3) Divide and spatulate the ureter for a wide anastomosis.
4) Create a tension-free anastomosis.
5) Place a drain.

Note These Variations

- Access into the peritoneal cavity may be obtained with a Veress needle, with the open Hasson technique, or with direct vision optical trocars.
- A retroperitoneal approach for the pyeloplasty may be undertaken. This is especially beneficial in patients with prior abdominal surgery or vascular/anatomic variations. The potential retroperitoneal space should be adequately developed prior to inserting instruments.
- This procedure may vary with regards to port placement and instruments. This procedure may also be performed laparoscopically, and hand-assistance may be utilized to improve tactile feedback for dissection, retraction, and hemostatic control.
- For redo procedures, the ureter may initially be more easily identified distally and dissected proximally.
- A reductive pyeloplasty may be performed in the setting of a large, redundant pelvis.
- A retrograde pyelogram may be useful in identifying the relevant anatomy preoperatively. Antegrade or retrograde pyeloureteroscopy with laser lithotripsy and basket stone extraction may be utilized to remove calculi, if present.

Operative Dictations in Urologic Surgery, First Edition. Noel A. Armenakas, John A. Fracchia, and Ron Golan.
© 2019 John Wiley & Sons Ltd. Published 2019 by John Wiley & Sons Ltd.

- The need for fascial closure of port sites depends on trocar size and design, patient characteristics, and surgeon preference. Fascial closures may be performed by a hand-sutured technique or with assistance of devices, under direct visualization in order to minimize the risk of visceral injury.

Complications

- Bleeding
- Infection
- Intraabdominal organ injury
- Pneumothorax
- Urine leak/urinoma
- Ileus
- Recurrent ureteral pelvic junction obstruction/stricture

Template Operative Dictation

Preoperative diagnosis: Ureteropelvic junction obstruction
Postoperative diagnosis: Same
Procedure: Robotic-assisted laparoscopic dismembered *right/left* pyeloplasty and ureteral stent insertion
Indications: The patient is a ___-year-old *male/female* with a *right/left* ureteropelvic junction obstruction presenting for a robotic-assisted laparoscopic pyeloplasty.
Description of Procedure: The indications, alternatives, benefits, and risks were discussed with the patient and informed consent was obtained.

The patient was brought onto the operating room table, placed supine, and secured with a safety strap. All pressure points were carefully padded and pneumatic compression devices placed on the lower extremities.

After the administration of intravenous antibiotics and general endotracheal anesthesia, a 16 Fr urethral catheter was inserted to drain the bladder. The patient was repositioned in the *left/right* lateral decubitus position at a 45° angle with the lower leg flexed 90° and the upper leg extended. An axillary roll was positioned to protect the brachial plexus and a gel pad was placed to support the back. Multiple pillows were used to pad beneath and between both the upper and lower extremities to ensure adequate cushioning. The patient was secured in place across the hips, chest, and legs with foam padding and cloth tape and the table was flexed. The patient was prepped and draped in the standard sterile manner.

The radiographic images were in the room.

A time-out was completed, verifying the correct patient, surgical procedure, site, and positioning, prior to beginning the procedure.

Pneumoperitoneum was introduced by placing a Veress needle into the abdomen and insufflating with CO_2 to a pressure of 15 mmHg. The camera trocar was placed along the *right/left* lateral edge of the rectus sheath slightly cephalad to the umbilicus and the *0°/30°* lens was inserted under direct visualization. The abdominal cavity was examined

for any sign of injury, adhesions, and identification of anatomic landmarks. The remainders of the robotic trocars were placed along the lateral edge of the rectus sheath, which included an 8 mm port below the costal margin and one 8 mm port caudal to the camera port. A 5 mm assistant port was placed in the midline above the umbilicus. (*If retraction is required*: An additional assistant port was inserted to retract the *liver/spleen*.) The robot was then docked.

The parietal peritoneum was incised along the white line of Toldt and the colon reflected medially, exposing Gerota's fascia.

> **On the right**: The hepatic flexure was mobilized by dividing the triangular and coronary ligaments, allowing for retraction of the liver. The duodenum was kocherized and the inferior vena cava was visualized. The proximal ureter was identified and carefully dissected cephalad toward the renal pelvis while preserving periureteral tissue. The gonadal vein was identified and preserved. The retroperitoneal fascia overlying the renal vessels was carefully separated, exposing the underlying renal vein and artery.

> **On the left**: The splenorenal and splenophrenic ligaments were incised to mobilize the spleen. The tail of the pancreas was mobilized medially. The proximal ureter was identified and carefully dissected cephalad toward the renal pelvis while preserving periureteral tissue. The retroperitoneal fascia overlying the renal vessels was carefully separated, exposing the underlying renal vein and artery.

The hydronephrotic renal pelvis was visualized.

> **For a crossing vessel**: A vessel was identified crossing anterior to the ureteropelvic junction. The distended renal pelvis was transected sharply and a segment of the stenotic ureteropelvic junction sent to pathology for evaluation. The ureter was widely spatulated and transposed anterior to the crossing vessel.

> **For a stenotic ureteropelvic junction**: The stenotic ureteropelvic junction segment was identified, excised and sent to pathology for evaluation. The ureter was widely spatulated.

The tension-free anastomosis was performed starting posteriorly using interrupted 3-0 polyglactin (Vicryl) sutures. After placement of the posterior sutures, a 6 Fr ___ cm double-J stent was advanced over a guidewire in an antegrade manner with the distal end positioned in the bladder and the proximal end within the renal pelvis, and the guidewire removed. The anterior ureteropelvic anastomosis was completed in the identical fashion.

The operative field was inspected for bleeding or injury. The insufflation pressure was reduced, again confirming the absence of bleeding.

Pneumoperitoneum was reestablished and a surgical drain (e.g. Jackson-Pratt) was placed through a laparoscopic port into the perirenal space, away from the repair, and secured at the skin.

The robot was undocked and removed from the operative field.

The trocars were withdrawn under direct visualization.

The anterior fascia at the camera port site was carefully closed with a 1-0 polydioxanone (PDS) suture, and a total of ___ml of local anesthetic (*specify*) injected subcutaneously

at the port sites. The skin incisions were closed with 4-0 poliglecaprone (Monocryl) sutures and reinforced with sterile adhesive strips. Sterile dressings were applied and the patient repositioned supine.

At the end of the procedure, all counts were correct.

The patient tolerated the procedure well and was taken to the recovery room in satisfactory condition.

Estimated blood loss: Approximately _____ml

Lymphatics

113

Robotic-Assisted Laparoscopic Pelvic Lymph Node Dissection

Indications

- Prostate cancer
- Urethral cancer
- Bladder cancer
- Penile cancer with positive inguinal lymph nodes

Essential Steps

1) Identify and retract the ureters from their position anterior to the iliac vessels.
2) Perform a thorough bilateral pelvic lymph node dissection with the limits of dissection being the common iliac artery cranially, the genitofemoral nerve laterally, the ureter medially, the obturator nerve posteriorly, and the node of Cloquet caudally.
3) Maintain meticulous hemo- and lymphostasis using surgical clips and electrocautery.
4) Place a drain.

Note These Variations

- Access into the peritoneal cavity may be obtained with a Veress needle, with the open Hasson technique, or with direct vision optical trocars.
- An *extended* pelvic lymphadenectomy can be performed with the superior limit being the aortic bifurcation, also incorporating paraaortic and presacral lymph nodes.
- Ureteral stents may be placed cystoscopically prior to dissection to aid with identification of the ureters.
- The need for fascial closure of port sites depends on trocar size and design, patient characteristics, and surgeon preference. Fascial closures may be performed by a hand-sutured technique or with assistance of devices, under direct visualization in order to minimize the risk of visceral injury.

Operative Dictations in Urologic Surgery, First Edition. Noel A. Armenakas, John A. Fracchia, and Ron Golan.
© 2019 John Wiley & Sons Ltd. Published 2019 by John Wiley & Sons Ltd.

Complications

- Bleeding
- Infection
- Lymphocele
- Intraabdominal organ injury
- Nerve injury
- Ureteral injury
- Ileus

Template Operative Dictation

Preoperative diagnosis: *Prostate/bladder/urethral/penile* cancer
Postoperative diagnosis: Same
Procedure: Robotic-assisted laparoscopic *right/left/bilateral* pelvic lymph node dissection
Indications: The patient is a ___-year-old *male/female* with *prostate/bladder/urethral/penile* carcinoma presenting for a robotic-assisted pelvic lymph node dissection.
Description of Procedure: The indications, alternatives, benefits, and risks were discussed with the patient's family/guardian and informed consent was obtained.

The patient was brought onto the operating room table, placed supine, and secured with a safety strap. All pressure points were carefully padded and pneumatic compression devices were placed on the lower extremities.

After the administration of intravenous antibiotics and general endotracheal anesthesia, the patient was repositioned in dorsal lithotomy using well-padded universal (Allen) stirrups. The arms were carefully tucked at the patient's side and secured with padding. The chest was secured in place with foam padding and cloth tape, and the table was positioned in 30° Trendelenburg. The patient's abdomen, genitalia, and upper thighs were prepped and draped in the standard sterile manner.

The radiographic images were in the room.

A time-out was completed, verifying the correct patient, surgical procedure, and positioning, prior to beginning the procedure.

A 16 Fr urethral catheter was inserted to drain the bladder.

Pneumoperitoneum was introduced by placing a Veress needle into the abdomen and insufflating with CO_2 to a pressure of 15 mmHg. The camera trocar was placed superior to the umbilicus and the *0°/30°* lens was inserted under direct visualization. The abdominal cavity was examined for any sign of injury, adhesions, and identification of anatomic landmarks. The remainder of the trocars were placed, which included a 12 mm port in the *right/left* lower quadrant medial to the anterior–superior iliac spine, two 8 mm ports at the left and right rectus margin slightly caudal to the camera port, and an 8 mm port medial to the *right/left* anterior–superior iliac spine. A 5 mm assistant port was placed in the *right/left* upper quadrant. The robot was then docked.

The peritoneum lateral to the medial umbilical ligaments was incised and the dissection of peritoneum continued to expose the common iliac vessels. The median umbilical ligament and urachus were divided. The space of Retzius was developed

distally toward the endopelvic fascia and laterally toward the obturator fossa. The ureters were identified anteriorly at the bifurcation of the iliac vessels. The iliac vessels were exposed from just above the common iliac bifurcation to the femoral canal (node of Cloquet). The lymph nodes appeared *unremarkable/enlarged/matted*.

The nodal dissection was started along the medial aspect of the *right/left* external iliac artery by incising the perivascular fibroareolar sheath. The lymph node packet was gently mobilized medially, and small vessels and lymphatic branches were fulgurated or ligated with surgical clips to maintain meticulous hemo- and lymphostasis. The obturator neurovascular bundle was identified posteriorly and preserved. The dissection was carried laterally to the genitofemoral nerve and medially to the ipsilateral ureter. The cranial and caudal limits of dissection were the common iliac bifurcation and femoral canal (node of Cloquet), respectively. A polymer ligating clip (e.g. Hem-o-lok) was used to secure the distal and proximal extents of the lymph node packet. The nodal packet was removed and placed within a specimen retrieval bag.

The contralateral lymph node dissection was performed and the nodal packet placed within *the same/a separate* specimen retrieval bag.

The operative field was then inspected for bleeding or injury. The insufflation pressure was reduced, again confirming the absence of bleeding.

Pneumoperitoneum was reestablished and a surgical drain (e.g. Jackson-Pratt) was placed through a laparoscopic port into the pelvis and secured at the skin.

The robot was undocked and removed from the operative field.

The trocars were withdrawn under direct visualization. The periumbilical incision was extended and the specimen retrieval bag was removed. The anterior fascia at the umbilical site was carefully closed with a 1-0 polydioxanone (PDS) suture, and a total of __ml of local anesthetic (*specify*) injected subcutaneously at the port sites. The skin incisions were closed with 4-0 poliglecaprone (Monocryl) sutures and reinforced with sterile adhesive strips. Sterile dressings were applied and the patient repositioned supine.

At the end of the procedure, all counts were correct.

The patient tolerated the procedure well and was taken to the recovery room in satisfactory condition.

Estimated blood loss: Approximately _____ml

Prostate

114

Robotic-Assisted Laparoscopic Radical Prostatectomy with Bilateral Pelvic Lymph Node Dissection

Indications

- Prostate cancer

Essential Steps

1) Divide the medial umbilical ligaments and urachus, developing the space of Retzius as the bladder is mobilized off the anterior abdominal wall.
2) Defat the prostate to allow for better visualization of the puboprostatic ligament, superficial and deep dorsal venous complex, and the prostatovesical junction.
3) Identify the junction between the bladder neck and the base of the prostate by visualization by palpation using the robotic arms and/or manipulation of the urethral catheter balloon.
4) Transect the anterior bladder neck until the urethral catheter is visualized, then continue dissection of the posterior bladder neck until the vasa and seminal vesicles are exposed.
5) Dissect and divide the bilateral vasa and mobilize the seminal vesicles, maintaining meticulous hemostasis.
6) Incise Denonvillier's fascia and perform a posterior dissection toward the apex of the prostate.
7) Divide the bilateral pedicles using a combination of hemostatic clips and sharp dissection.
8) Transect the dorsal venous complex and urethra distal to the prostatic apex. The dorsal vein complex may be oversewn following division, or a suture ligature placed prior to division.
9) Complete the vesicourethral anastomosis. A Rocco stitch may be placed prior to relieve tension on the anastomosis.
10) Perform a pelvic lymph node dissection.
11) Place a drain.

Operative Dictations in Urologic Surgery, First Edition. Noel A. Armenakas, John A. Fracchia, and Ron Golan.
© 2019 John Wiley & Sons Ltd. Published 2019 by John Wiley & Sons Ltd.

Note These Variations

- Access into the peritoneal cavity may be obtained with a Veress needle, with the open Hasson technique, or with direct vision optical trocars.
- An initial posterior approach may be taken whereby the dissection begins with identification and exposure of the vasa deferentia and seminal vesicles followed by the posterior dissection of the prostate. The anterior dissection is then performed.
- An extraperitoneal approach may offer avoidance of intraperitoneal contents. During the procedure there may be a decreased need to retract the bowel and a lower risk of elevated intraperitoneal pressures, but there may be less working space. Proper port placement is critical.
- Depending on the patient's disease characteristics, baseline potency, and patient preferences, preservation of the neurovascular bundles may be complete, partial, or foregone entirely. The fascial plane for nerve sparing may be intrafascial or interfascial.
- The timing of the lymph node dissection within the procedure, and extent of the dissection, may vary by surgeon preference and patient disease.
- Prior to performing the urethrovesical anastomosis, a Rocco stitch may be placed within the posterior peri-vesical and peri-urethral tissue to approximate the bladder neck and cut edge of urethra. Additionally, large bladder necks may be reconstructed either anteriorly or posteriorly using a "tennis racket" configuration.
- The need for fascial closure of port sites depends on trocar size and design, patient characteristics, and surgeon preference. Fascial closures may be performed by a hand-sutured technique or with assistance of devices, under direct visualization, in order to minimize the risk of visceral injury.

Complications

- Bleeding
- Infection
- Rectal/ureteral injury
- Obturator nerve injury
- Urine leak/urinoma
- Lymphocele
- Ileus
- Erectile dysfunction
- Bladder neck stenosis/urethral stricture
- Urinary incontinence

Template Operative Dictation

Preoperative diagnosis: Prostate cancer
Postoperative diagnosis: Same
Procedure: Robotic-assisted laparoscopic radical prostatectomy, bilateral pelvic lymph node dissection

Indications: The patient is a ___-year-old male with a clinical stage T ____, Gleason score ____ prostate cancer presenting for robotic-assisted laparoscopic radical prostatectomy and bilateral pelvic lymph node dissection.

Description of Procedure: The indications, alternatives, benefits, and risks were discussed with the patient and informed consent was obtained.

The patient was brought onto the operating room table, placed supine, and secured with a safety strap. All pressure points were carefully padded and pneumatic compression devices were placed on the lower extremities.

After the administration of intravenous antibiotics and general endotracheal anesthesia, the patient was repositioned in dorsal lithotomy using well-padded universal (Allen) stirrups. The arms were carefully tucked at the patient's side and secured with padding. The chest was secured in place with foam padding and cloth tape, and the table positioned in 30° Trendelenburg. The patient's abdomen, genitalia, and upper thighs were prepped and draped in the standard sterile manner.

A time-out was completed, verifying the correct patient, surgical procedure, and positioning, prior to beginning the procedure.

A 16 Fr urethral catheter was inserted to drain the bladder.

Pneumoperitoneum was introduced by placing a Veress needle into the abdomen and insufflating with CO_2 to a pressure of 15 mmHg. The camera trocar was placed superior to the umbilicus and the *0°/30°* lens was inserted under direct visualization. The abdominal cavity was examined for any sign of injury, adhesions, and identification of anatomic landmarks. The remainder of the trocars were placed, which included a 12 mm port in the *right/left* lower quadrant medial to the anterior-superior iliac spine, two 8 mm ports at the left and right rectus margin slightly caudal to the camera port, and an 8 mm port medial to the *right/left* anterior-superior iliac spine. A 5 mm assistant port was placed in the *right/left* upper quadrant. The robot was then docked.

> ***If an anterior approach is performed:*** The urachus and median umbilical ligaments were incised and the bladder mobilized from the anterior bladder wall as the space of Retzius was developed below the pubis. The peritoneal incisions were carried laterally to the vasa deferentia, which were dissected and divided. The dissection of the fibroareolar tissue was carried distally to the endopelvic fascia. The prostate was defatted above the prostatovesicle junction, and the superficial dorsal venous complex was coagulated with electrocautery and divided. The endopelvic fascia was sharply opened bilaterally, and the levator muscle fibers were swept posterolaterally allowing for visualization of the deep dorsal venous complex and apex of the prostate. The puboprostatic ligaments were sharply divided with care taken to preserve the dorsal venous complex.

> The bladder was tented with the fourth arm, and the urethral catheter was manipulated by the assistant to further define the junction between the bladder and prostate. The anterior bladder neck was divided using electrocautery and sharp dissection until the urethral catheter was visualized. The urethral catheter balloon was deflated and pulled back into the prostatic urethra to facilitate posterior dissection of the bladder neck *and median lobe*. The posterior bladder neck was incised and the dissection carried posteriorly until the vasa and seminal vesicles were encountered. These were dissected using a combination of

electrocautery and sharp dissection. The posterior plane was incised in the midline and the plane *above/below* Denonvilliers' fascia bluntly developed between the prostate and rectum toward the apex of the prostate.

If a posterior approach is performed: The peritoneal reflection was inspected and the course of the vasa deferentia were visualized below the bladder. An incision was made in the peritoneum and the vasa were identified and dissected. The seminal vesicles were identified and dissected out using a combination of electrocauterization and sharp dissection.

For the anterior component of the dissection, the urachus and median umbilical ligaments were incised and the bladder was mobilized from the anterior bladder wall as the space of Retzius was developed below the pubis. The peritoneal incisions were carried laterally toward the vasa. The dissection of the fibroareolar tissue was then carried distally to the endopelvic fascia. The prostate was defatted and the superficial dorsal venous complex was coagulated with electrocautery and divided. The endopelvic fascia was sharply opened bilaterally, and the levator muscle fibers were swept posterolaterally, allowing for visualization of the deep dorsal venous complex and apex of the prostate. The puboprostatic ligaments were sharply divided with care to preserve the dorsal venous complex.

The bladder was tented with the fourth arm, and the urethral catheter was manipulated by the assistant to further define the junction between bladder and prostate. The anterior bladder neck was divided using cautery and sharp dissection until the urethral catheter was visualized. The urethral catheter balloon was then deflated and pulled back into the prostatic urethra to facilitate posterior dissection of the bladder neck *and median lobe*. The posterior bladder neck was incised and the dissection carried posteriorly until the previously dissected vasa and seminal vesicles were encountered. The plane posterior to the prostate was incised in the midline and the plane *above/below* Denonvilliers' fascia bluntly developed between the prostate and rectum towards the apex of the prostate.

The right and left pedicles were clipped with polymer ligating clips (e.g. Hem-o-lok) and divided in an antegrade manner with minimal use of electrocautery. The plane between the prostatic capsule and prostatic fascia was developed and the nerve-sparing dissection plane was defined. This plane was extended distally using a combination of sharp and blunt dissection, with the neurovascular bundle developed distal to the prostatic apex.

The dorsal venous complex and anterior urethra were sharply divided. The catheter was exposed and subsequently withdrawn to allow for visualization of the posterior urethra. The posterior urethra was sharply divided and the remaining pedicles and neurovascular bundles inspected for hemostasis or injury. Patent venous sinuses were oversewn with *a* 0 polyglactin (Vicryl) suture(s). The specimen was placed in a specimen retrieval bag and set aside.

A bilateral pelvic lymph node dissection was performed, beginning on the *right/left*. The nodal dissection was started along the medial aspect of the external iliac vein by incising the perivascular fibroareolar sheath. The lymph node packet was gently mobilized medially, and small vessels and lymphatic branches were fulgurated or ligated with

surgical clips to maintain meticulous hemo- and lymphostasis. The obturator neuro-vascular bundle was identified posteriorly and preserved. The borders of dissection were the common iliac artery bifurcation cranially, the node of Cloquet caudally, the genitofemoral nerve laterally, and the obturator nerve posteriorly. A polymer ligating clip (e.g. Hem-o-lok) was used to secure the distal and proximal extent of the lymph node packet. The nodal packet was removed and sent to pathology for evaluation.

The identical lymph node dissection was performed on the contralateral side.

The bladder neck was inspected and the ureteral orifices were identified bilaterally. The urethrovesical anastomosis was performed using a *double-armed/two* 2-0 poligle-caprone (Monocryl) suture(s) in a running fashion starting posteriorly and continuing clockwise and counterclockwise circumferentially. Advancement and withdrawal of the deflated urethral catheter combined with perineal pressure aided with identification of the distal urethral lumen. Once the reconstruction was complete, a new 18 Fr urethral catheter was inserted into the bladder and the balloon inflated with 10 ml sterile water. The bladder was irrigated with sterile normal saline, confirming a watertight closure. The operative field was inspected for bleeding or injury. The insufflation pressure was reduced and no bleeding was identified.

Pneumoperitoneum was reestablished and a surgical drain (e.g. Jackson-Pratt) was placed through a laparoscopic port into the pelvis and secured at the skin.

The robot was undocked and removed from the operative field.

The trocars were withdrawn under direct visualization. The periumbilical incision was extended and the specimen retrieval bag was removed. The specimen was sent to pathology for evaluation. The anterior fascia at the umbilical site was carefully closed with a 1-0 polydioxanone (PDS) suture, and a total of __ml of local anesthetic (*specify*) injected subcutaneously at the port sites. The skin incisions were closed with 4-0 poliglecaprone (Monocryl) sutures and reinforced with sterile adhesive strips. Sterile dressings were applied and the patient repositioned supine.

At the end of the procedure, all counts were correct.

The patient tolerated the procedure well and was taken to the recovery room in satis-factory condition.

Estimated blood loss: Approximately _____ml

115

Robotic-Assisted Laparoscopic Simple Prostatectomy

Indications

- Bladder outlet obstruction with prostate volume >100 g

Essential Steps

1) Divide the medial umbilical ligaments and urachus, developing the space of Retzius as the bladder is mobilized off the anterior abdominal wall.
2) Defat the prostate to allow for better visualization of the puboprostatic ligament, superficial and deep dorsal venous complex, and prostatovesical junction.
3) Identify the junction between the bladder neck and the base of the prostate by either visualization, by palpation using the robotic arms, and/or manipulation of the urethral catheter balloon.
4) Create a cystotomy to visualize the adenoma.
5) Place a traction suture in the adenoma to facilitate mobilization and exposure.
6) Perform a circumferential dissection along the avascular plane toward the prostatic apex, with care to preserve the external urinary sphincter.
7) Sharply transect the urethra distally under direct visualization.
8) Advance and reapproximate the bladder neck mucosa to the distal urethral mucosa.
9) Close the bladder in two layers.
10) Place a drain.

Note These Variations

- Access into the peritoneal cavity may be obtained with a Veress needle, the open Hasson technique, or with direct vision optical trocars.
- An extraperitoneal approach may offer avoidance of intraperitoneal contents. During the procedure there may be a decreased need to retract the bowel and a lower risk of elevated intraperitoneal pressures, but there may be less working space, and proper port placement is critical.
- The transcapsular approach involves creating a capsular incision distal to the prostatovesical junction. The adenoma is identified within the prostatic capsule and

Operative Dictations in Urologic Surgery, First Edition. Noel A. Armenakas, John A. Fracchia, and Ron Golan.
© 2019 John Wiley & Sons Ltd. Published 2019 by John Wiley & Sons Ltd.

circumferentially dissected. The adenoma is transected similar to the transvesical approach, and the urethral mucosa may be similarly advanced.

- The robotic tenaculum may be used to retract the adenoma in place of stay sutures. Frequent readjustments are often required to mobilize the adenoma.
- The need for fascial closure of port sites depends on trocar size and design, patient characteristics and surgeon preference. Fascial closures may be performed by a hand-sutured technique or with assistance of devices, under direct visualization, in order to minimize the risk of visceral injury.

Complications

- Bleeding
- Infection
- Urine leak/urinoma
- Intraabdominal organ injury
- Urinary incontinence
- Bladder neck contracture/urethral stricture

Template Operative Dictation

Preoperative diagnosis: Obstructive, clinically benign prostatic enlargement
Postoperative diagnosis: Same
Procedure: Robotic-assisted laparoscopic simple prostatectomy
Indications: The patient is a ___-old male with clinical bladder outlet obstruction presenting for robotic-assisted laparoscopic simple prostatectomy.
Description of Procedure: The indications, alternatives, benefits, and risks were discussed with the patient's family/guardian and informed consent was obtained.

The patient was brought onto the operating room table, placed supine, and secured with a safety strap. All pressure points were carefully padded and pneumatic compression devices were placed on the lower extremities.

After the administration of intravenous antibiotics and general endotracheal anesthesia, the patient was repositioned in dorsal lithotomy using well-padded universal (Allen) stirrups. The arms were carefully tucked at the patient's side and secured with padding. The chest was secured in place with foam padding and cloth tape, and the table was positioned in 30° Trendelenburg. The patient's abdomen, genitalia, and upper thighs were prepped and draped in the standard sterile manner.

A time-out was completed, verifying the correct patient, surgical procedure, and positioning, prior to beginning the procedure.

A 16 Fr urethral catheter was inserted to drain the bladder.

Pneumoperitoneum was introduced by placing a Veress needle into the abdomen and insufflating with CO_2 to a pressure of 15 mmHg. The camera trocar was placed superior to the umbilicus and the *0°/30°* lens was inserted under direct visualization. The abdominal cavity was examined for any sign of injury, adhesions, and identification of anatomic landmarks. The remainder of the trocars were placed, which included

a 12 mm port in the *right/left* lower quadrant medial to the anterior–superior iliac spine, two 8 mm ports at the left and right rectus margin slightly caudal to the camera port, and an 8 mm port medial to the *right/left* anterior–superior iliac spine. A 5 mm assistant port was placed in the *right/left* upper quadrant. The robot was then docked.

The urachus and medial umbilical ligaments were incised and the bladder was mobilized from the anterior bladder wall as the space of Retzius was developed below the pubis. The dissection was carried distally to the endopelvic fascia. The prostate was defatted and the superficial dorsal venous complex was coagulated with electrocautery and divided. The bladder was tented with the fourth arm, and the urethral catheter was manipulated by the assistant to further define the junction between the bladder and prostate.

If a transvesical approach is performed: A *horizontal/vertical* cystotomy was made *proximal to the prostatovesical junction/at the bladder dome*, exposing the bladder mucosa, and underlying prostatic adenoma as well as the bilateral ureteral orifices. A stay suture was placed through the mucosa and underlying adenoma to facilitate mobilization, and an incision was made in the mucosa to expose the adenoma. The adenoma was retracted anteriorly, posteriorly, and laterally to identify the avascular plane between the adenoma and the prostatic capsule as the dissection was carried distally toward the prostatic apex. Perforating vessels were carefully cauterized. At the apex, care was taken to avoid the sphincteric complex. The adenoma was freed from the capsule, placed in a specimen retrieval bag, and set aside.

If a transcapsular approach is performed: A *horizontal/vertical* incision was made in the capsule distal to the prostatovesical junction. A stay suture was placed through the adenoma to facilitate mobilization. The adenoma was retracted anteriorly, posteriorly, and laterally to identify the avascular plane between the adenoma and the prostatic capsule as the dissection was carried distally towards the prostatic apex. Perforating vessels were carefully cauterized. At the apex, care was taken to avoid the sphincteric complex. The adenoma was freed from the capsule, placed in a specimen retrieval bag and set aside.

Bleeding vessels were oversewn within the prostatic capsule with 2-0 polyglactin (Vicryl) sutures. The bladder neck mucosa was advanced and approximated to the distal urethral mucosa using 3-0 poliglecaprone (Monocryl). A 24 Fr three-way urethral catheter was inserted into the bladder and the balloon inflated to _____ cc with sterile water. The *bladder/capsule* was closed in *one/two* layer(s) with *a* 2-0 Vicryl suture(s). The bladder was irrigated with sterile normal saline, confirming a watertight closure. The operative field was inspected for bleeding or injury. The insufflation pressure was reduced and no bleeding was identified.

Pneumoperitoneum was reestablished and a surgical drain (e.g. Jackson-Pratt) was placed through a laparoscopic port into the pelvis and secured at the skin.

The robot was undocked and removed from the operative field.

The trocars were withdrawn under direct visualization. The periumbilical incision was extended and the specimen retrieval bag was removed. The specimen was sent to

pathology for evaluation. The anterior fascia at the umbilical site was carefully closed with a 1-0 polydioxanone (PDS) suture, and a total of __ml of local anesthetic (*specify*) injected subcutaneously at the port sites. The skin incisions were closed with 4-0 Monocryl sutures and reinforced with sterile adhesive strips. Sterile dressings were applied and the patient repositioned supine.

At the end of the procedure, all counts were correct.

The patient tolerated the procedure well and was taken to the recovery room in satisfactory condition.

Estimated blood loss: Approximately _____ml

NOTES

NOTES

SECTION VI   PEDIATRIC SURGERY

116

Ablation of Posterior Urethral Valves

Indications

- Urinary outlet obstruction with a distended bladder and radiographic evidence of posterior urethral valves

Essential Steps

1) Distend the bladder and use manual suprapubic compression to assist in visualizing the urethral leaflets.
2) Resect the valves at the 5 o'clock and 7 o'clock positions.

Note These Variations

- Alternatively, a pediatric cystoscope with a 2 Fr or 3 Fr endoscopic monopolar electrode (Bugbee) can be used.
- A 5 Fr or 8 Fr pediatric feeding tube can be placed transurethrally for 24–48 hours postoperatively.

Complications

- Persistent obstruction
- Urethral injury/stricture
- Urinary Incontinence

Template Operative Dictation

Preoperative diagnosis: Posterior urethral valves
Postoperative diagnosis: Same
Procedure: Ablation of posterior urethral valves

Operative Dictations in Urologic Surgery, First Edition. Noel A. Armenakas, John A. Fracchia, and Ron Golan.
© 2019 John Wiley & Sons Ltd. Published 2019 by John Wiley & Sons Ltd.

Indications: The patient is a _____-old male with a clinical diagnosis of posterior urethral valves presenting for valve ablation.

Description of Procedure: The indications, alternatives, benefits, and risks were discussed with the patient's *family/guardian* and informed consent was obtained.

The patient was brought onto the operating room table, positioned supine with the hips abducted (frog leg) and secured with a safety strap. All pressure points were carefully padded.

After the administration of intravenous antibiotics and general endotracheal anesthesia, the genitalia were prepped and draped in the standard sterile manner.

A time-out was completed, verifying the correct patient, surgical procedure, and positioning, prior to beginning the procedure.

1.5% glycine was used for irrigation.

The fossa navicularis was gently calibrated and an 8.5 Fr pediatric resectoscope was carefully introduced into the proximal urethra. Urethroscopy was performed and the obstructing sail-like valve leaflets were visualized at the verumontanum. Suprapubic manual compression of the bladder confirmed ballooning of the valves. The bladder was distended with warm irrigating solution and was noted to be *normal/trabeculated*.

The resectoscope with a *loop/diathermy knife/hook* was positioned at the posterior urethra, and a cutting power setting of 20 watts was used to disrupt and ablate the leaflets at the 5 o'clock and 7 o'clock positions. Bleeding was controlled with judicious fulguration.

After redistending the bladder, the resectoscope was removed under direct vision, confirming thorough destruction of the valves and the absence of any bleeding or urethral trauma. Manual suprapubic pressure was applied ensuring a forceful stream. A diaper was placed.

At the end of the procedure, all counts were correct.

The patient tolerated the procedure well and was taken to the recovery room in satisfactory condition.

Estimated blood loss: Approximately _____ ml

117

Meatal Advancement and Glanuloplasty (MAGPI Repair)

Indications

- Distal hypospadias (meatus at corona)

Essential Steps

1) Inject the glans with 1% lidocaine containing 1:100000 epinephrine to assist in hemostasis.
2) Induce an artificial erection to exclude the presence of a chordee.
3) Make a vertical incision from the meatus to the distal end of the glanular groove.
4) Advance the meatus as far distally as possible, using a transverse Heineke-Mikulicz-type closure.
5) Approximate the glans wings in three layers.
6) Complete the penile skin closure with a circumcision or foreskin reconstruction.

Note These Variations

- In cases where there is a deep and wide glanular groove, a glans approximation procedure should be considered.
- A 5 Fr or 8 Fr infant feeding tube may be left postoperatively for bladder drainage to reduce the incidence of urinary retention.
- A hemostatic sealant (e.g. fibrin glue) can be used in conjunction with the anastomotic sutures to reinforce the repair.

Complications

- Bleeding
- Infection
- Dehiscence
- Meatal stenosis/retraction
- Urethral stricture

Operative Dictations in Urologic Surgery, First Edition. Noel A. Armenakas, John A. Fracchia, and Ron Golan.
© 2019 John Wiley & Sons Ltd. Published 2019 by John Wiley & Sons Ltd.

Template Operative Dictation

Preoperative diagnosis: Distal hypospadias
Postoperative diagnosis: Same
Procedure: Meatal advancement and glanuloplasty (MAGPI repair)
Indications: The patient is a _____-old boy with distal hypospadias presenting for a meatal advancement and glanuloplasty (MAGPI repair).
Description of Procedure: The indications, alternative, benefits, and risks were discussed with the patient's *family/guardian* and informed consent was obtained.

The patient was brought onto the operating room table, positioned supine, and secured with a safety strap. All pressure points were carefully padded.

After the administration of intravenous antibiotics and general anesthesia, the external genitalia, lower abdomen, and perineum were prepped and draped in the standard sterile manner.

A time-out was completed, verifying the correct patient, surgical procedure, and positioning, prior to beginning the procedure.

A 4-0 polypropylene (Prolene) stay suture was placed through the anterior mid glans for traction. The corona and dorsal web of glanular tissue were infiltrated with 1% lidocaine containing 1 : 100000 epinephrine to aid in hemostasis. Additional 4-0 polyglactin (Vicryl) sutures were placed ventrolaterally in each glans wing to facilitate the dissection.

Using optical magnification with surgical loupes, a transverse ventral penile skin incision was made approximately 8 mm from the coronal sulcus. This was taken down beneath the dartos fascia to the level of the penoscrotal junction, taking care not to injure the urethra wall.

A tourniquet (e.g. 0.25 in. Penrose drain) was used to constrict the penile base and an artificial erection induced using injectable sterile saline through a 15 gauge butterfly needle placed into the *right/left* corpus cavernosum. There was no chordee visualized and the tourniquet was removed.

A vertical incision was made from the dorsal edge of the meatus to the distal end of the glanular groove. The resultant widening meatal "V" incision was sutured to the glans groove using interrupted 6-0 Vicryl sutures, completing the transverse Heineke-Mikulicz type closure to advance the meatus.

The proximal end of the meatus was elevated with a skin hook toward the tip of the glans, drawing the glans wings together. Several interrupted 6-0 Vicryl sutures were used to close the deep glans tissue. Additional buried subcutaneous sutures were placed to minimize tension. Lastly, the two midline edges were closed with 6-0 Vicryl vertical mattress sutures, ensuring an orthotopic neomeatus.

The excess preputial skin was excised and meticulous hemostasis achieved using electrocautery. The penile skin was closed with interrupted 6-0 Vicryl sutures.

A sterile adhesive penile dressing was applied. A double diaper was placed taking care not to occlude the urethral meatus.

At the end of the procedure, all counts were correct.

The patient tolerated the procedure without difficulty and was transported to the recovery room in satisfactory condition.

Estimated blood loss: Approximately _____ml

118

Megaureter Repair

Indications

- Pain, ureteral obstruction and/or urinary tract infection attributable to the megaureter
- Initially compromised renal function (<40%) on renal scan and/or decreasing (>10%) renal function on repeat scans
- Progressive hydroureteronephrosis

Essential Steps

1) Fill the bladder through a urethral catheter.
2) Expose the bladder through a small transverse abdominal incision, sweep the peritoneum superiorly, and make a vertical anterior cystotomy.
3) Position a self-retaining ring retractor to facilitate exposure of the ureteral orifices.
4) Pass a 5 Fr infant feeding tube into the ureter and secure it at the ureteral orifice with a purse-string suture.
5) Circumscribe the ureteral orifice and free the intramural ureter.
6) Dissect the ureter extravesically above the area of dilation, preserving the vascular ureteral adventitia.
7) Taper the dilated ureter laterally over a 12 Fr red rubber catheter, if necessary.
8) Create a submucosal tunnel from the native ureteral orifice to the new ureteral hiatus and carefully pull the ureter through this. The ratio of tunnel length to ureteral width should be 5 : 1.
9) Confirm that the ureter lies appropriately within the newly created submucosal tunnel and check for ureteral obstruction or kinking.
10) Create a spatulated ureterovesical anastomosis with absorbable interrupted sutures.
11) Close the bladder in two layers.
12) Place a drain.

Operative Dictations in Urologic Surgery, First Edition. Noel A. Armenakas, John A. Fracchia, and Ron Golan.
© 2019 John Wiley & Sons Ltd. Published 2019 by John Wiley & Sons Ltd.

Note These Variations

- In infants with poor renal function, consider performing an end cutaneous ureterostomy initially, proceeding to definitive reconstruction if the renal function adequately improves.
- In cases where the ureteral dilation and tortuosity extends more proximally (e.g. with prune belly syndrome), exposure is best achieved using a vertical abdominal incision.
- Alternatively, the ureter can be tapered by infolding and imbricating.
- The placement of a ureteral stent is optional.

Complications

- Bleeding
- Infection
- Urine leak/urinoma
- Persistent or recurrent ureteral reflux
- Ureteral obstruction/stricture
- Urinary retention
- Recurrent urinary tract infections
- Difficulty with subsequent ureteral catheterization

Template Operative Dictation

Preoperative diagnosis: *Right/left* megaureter
Postoperative diagnosis: Same
Procedure: *Right/left* megaureter repair
Indications: The patient is a ___-old *male/female* with evidence of an ____ *obstructed/refluxing right/left* megaureter presenting for surgical correction.
Description of Procedure: The indications, alternatives, benefits, and risks were discussed with the patient's *family/guardian* and informed consent was obtained.

The patient was brought onto the operating room table, positioned supine, with the hips abducted, and secured with a safety strap. All pressure points were carefully padded.

After the administration of intravenous antibiotics and *general endotracheal* anesthesia, the abdomen and external genitalia were prepped and draped in the standard sterile manner.

A time-out was completed, verifying the correct patient, procedure, site, and positioning, prior to beginning the procedure.

A ___Fr urethral catheter was inserted into the bladder, filled with ____ ml sterile normal saline and clamped.

[*Note:* Bladder volume in children (cc) = (age + 2) × 30].

A semilunar transverse incision was made along Langer's lines, one fingerbreadth above the symphysis pubis and carried down to the rectus abdominis aponeurosis. This was incised in a semilunar arc using electrocautery, avoiding the inguinal canals. The rectus abdominis muscles were separated at the midline and retracted laterally, taking

care not to injure the underlying inferior epigastric vessels. The anterior bladder wall and vesical neck were exposed and the peritoneum was swept cephalad. A self-retaining retractor (e.g. Balfour, Denis-Browne, Bookwalter) was appropriately positioned to optimize exposure, using padding on each retractor blade.

The anterior bladder wall was grasped with Allis clamps and a vertical midline cystotomy made using electrocautery. Upon entry into the bladder, four interrupted 3-0 chromic stay sutures were placed on each side of the cystotomy and the bladder drained using suction. The urethral catheter was removed. An additional figure-of-eight 3-0 chromic suture was placed at the apex to avoid caudal extension of the incision.

The *right/left* ureteral orifice was identified and easily cannulated with a 5 Fr infant feeding tube, which was secured to the adjacent ureteral wall with a 4-0 polyglactin (Vicryl) suture. Using gentle traction on the infant feeding tube, the ureteral orifice was elevated and circumscribed with *a hooked blade/electrocautery*. Tenotomy scissors were used to sharply dissect the inferior aspect of the ureter and completely liberate it from the detrusor in a circumferential fashion. The peritoneum was swept from the posterior bladder wall, under direct vision, using a fine gauze dissector (Kittner). Throughout the dissection, care was taken to preserve the ureteral adventitia.

Having completely freed the ureter intravesically, the ureter was passed through the bladder wall and the dissection continued extravesically. The distal ureter was carefully freed from the adjacent peritoneum, preserving the periureteral tissue and its blood supply. Proximal ureteral mobilization was continued above the area of dilation at the level of the *common/external* iliac bifurcation.

The dilated ureter measured over ___ Fr in diameter. The decision was made to excisionally taper the ureter in order to provide a distal segment that could be reimplanted in an antirefluxing manner. The ureter and its blood supply were carefully examined and the longitudinal vessels of the ureter on its medial aspect were visualized and preserved. The distal nondilated segment of ureter was transected and the 5 Fr ureteral infant feeding tube replaced with a 12 Fr red rubber catheter, which was advanced to the renal pelvis.

Small Babcock clamps were applied to the lateral aspect of the dilated ureter and approximately _____ cm of redundant ureteral wall *was/were* sharply excised and sent for pathologic evaluation. The ureteral wall was reapproximated over the red rubber catheter in two layers. The mucosa and muscularis were closed with a running locking 5-0 Vicryl suture and the muscularis and adventitia approximated with a running 5-0 Vicryl suture.

After completion of the ureteral tapering, the red rubber catheter was removed and a 4-0 Vicryl traction suture was placed in the distal ureteral wall. The ureter was examined, confirming peristalsis and the absence of any injury or bleeding.

Attention was then directed intravesically. The mucosa superolateral to the contralateral ureteral orifice was incised and a submucosal tunnel created from the original native ureteral orifice to the new ectopic ureteral hiatus, using sharp and blunt dissection. The tapered ureter was pulled via its traction suture through the submucosal tunnel, and it was appropriately positioned without tension within the tunnel.

The ureter was spatulated ventrally and the edges trimmed to ensure an uncompromised blood supply. Dorsally the ureter was anchored to the trigone muscle and vesical mucosa with two interrupted 5-0 Vicryl sutures. The ureterovesical anastomosis was completed with similar sutures placed at the 9, 12, and 3 o'clock positions. Jets of

urine were seen exiting from both ureteral orifices, confirming the absence of obstruction or kinking.

Meticulous hemostasis was achieved throughout the procedure with electrocautery.

A 5 Fr infant feeding tube was placed through the neoureteral orifice and easily advanced into the renal pelvis. The tube was anchored to the adjacent bladder mucosa with a 4-0 plain catgut suture.

Upon completion of the reconstructive procedure a ___Fr urethral catheter was advanced into the bladder and connected to a drainage bag.

The midline cystotomy was closed in two layers using a running 4-0 chromic and interrupted 4-0 Vicryl sutures for the mucosal and muscularis layers, respectively. A watertight bladder closure was confirmed by irrigating the urethral catheter with sterile normal saline.

A surgical drain (e.g. Jackson-Pratt, 0.25 in. Penrose) was placed in the space of Retzius away from the cystotomy. The drain and infant feeding tube were brought out through a separate cutaneous incision and secured to the skin with a silk suture.

The self-retaining ring retractor was removed and the abdominal incision was closed using a running 3-0 chromic suture to approximate the rectus muscles and 3-0 polydioxanone (PDS) suture for the rectus aponeurosis. 3-0 chromic sutures were used on Scarpa's fascia and the skin approximated with a subcuticular 5-0 poliglecaprone (Monocryl) suture.

A sterile dressing was applied.

At the end of the procedure, all counts were correct.

The patient tolerated the procedure without difficulty and was transported to the recovery room in satisfactory condition.

Estimated blood loss: Approximately _____ml

119

Open Inguinal Hernia Repair

Indications

- Intermittent groin bulge with or without a reducible mass
- Incarcerated or symptomatic hernia

Essential Steps

1) Make an incision in the skin overlying the external inguinal ring.
2) Identify the external oblique fascia and the external inguinal ring.
3) Open the external ring toward the internal ring, identifying and avoiding the ilioinguinal nerve.
4) Dissect the hernia sac away from the spermatic cord vessels and vas deferens or the round ligament.
5) Perform a high ligation of the sac.
6) Reapproximate the external oblique fascia and Scarpa's fascia.

Note These Variations

- A concomitant hydrocelectomy in males may be performed whereby the testicle is delivered and the overlying tunica vaginalis is opened.
- Repair of the canal floor may be considered in the setting of a large hernia or in patients with connective tissue disorders.
- Depending on patient age, length of inguinal canal, and surgeon preference, a high ligation of the hernia sac may be performed without opening the external oblique aponeurosis.
- In older patients, a Lichtenstein tension-free hernioplasty with mesh can be performed.
- When indicated, contralateral exploration may be performed through open surgical exploration or laparoscopically.

Operative Dictations in Urologic Surgery, First Edition. Noel A. Armenakas, John A. Fracchia, and Ron Golan.
© 2019 John Wiley & Sons Ltd. Published 2019 by John Wiley & Sons Ltd.

Complications

- Bleeding
- Postoperative swelling (inguinal, scrotal, labial)
- Ilioinguinal nerve injury
- Testicular/vas deferens injury
- Bowel injury
- Recurrent hernia

Template Operative Dictation

Preoperative diagnosis: *Right/left/bilateral* inguinal hernia(s)
Postoperative diagnosis: Same
Procedure: *Right/left/bilateral* inguinal hernia repair
Indications: The patient is a ___-year-old *male/female* with *a right/left//bilateral* inguinal hernia(s).
Description of Procedure: The indications, alternatives, benefits, and risks were discussed with the patient's *family/guardian* and informed consent was obtained.

The patient was brought onto the operating room table, positioned supine, and secured with a safety strap. All pressure points were carefully padded and pneumatic compression devices were placed on the lower extremities.

After the administration of intravenous antibiotics and *general/regional anesthesia*, the lower abdomen and external genitalia were prepped and draped in the standard sterile manner.

A time-out was completed, verifying the correct patient, surgical procedure, site, and positioning, prior to beginning the procedure.

A 2 cm *right/left* inguinal skin incision was made between the ipsilateral pubic tubercle and the anterior superior iliac spine, following Langer's lines. Scarpa's fascia was divided with electrocautery and the aponeurosis of the external oblique visualized. The external inguinal ring was carefully opened toward the internal ring and the ilioinguinal nerve was identified, isolated and carefully retracted out of the operative field.

For males: The spermatic cord was elevated into the surgical field, confirming the presence of a hernia sac. The spermatic vessels and vas deferens were identified, and the hernia sac was meticulously dissected from the cord. No bowel contents or omentum were visualized within the sac.

For females: The hernia sac was visualized over the round ligament. The hernia sac was meticulously dissected from adjacent structures. No bowel contents or omentum were visualized within the sac.

> *If a diagnostic laparoscopy is performed:* The edges of the opened hernia sac were grasped and a laparoscopic trocar was inserted through the opening. The abdominal cavity was insufflated with CO_2 to a pressure of 8 mmHg. A *0°/30°/70°* degree lens was inserted to visualize the contralateral internal ring. ____*(describe)*____. The abdominal cavity was desufflated and the trocar withdrawn under direct visualization.

A high ligation of the sac was then performed with 4-0 polydioxanone (PDS). The *spermatic cord/round ligament* was replaced into its orthotopic position in the appropriate orientation. The inguinal canal was irrigated with sterile normal saline and thoroughly examined for bleeding. Meticulous hemostasis was achieved with electrocautery. The ilioinguinal nerve was inspected, noted to be intact and replaced in its normal anatomic position below the external oblique aponeurosis.

For bilateral hernias: An identical procedure was performed on the contralateral side.

The inguinal incision(s) *was/were* closed using a running 4-0 polyglactin (Vicryl) suture on the external oblique aponeurosis and a 4-0 chromic suture on Scarpa's fascia. The skin was approximated with a 5-0 subcuticular polyglecaprone (Monocryl) suture. The incision was reinforced with sterile adhesive strips and a sterile dressing applied.

At the end of the procedure all counts were correct.

The patient tolerated the procedure without difficulty and was taken to the recovery room in satisfactory condition.

Estimated blood loss: Approximately _____ml

120

Transurethral Incision of Ureterocele

Indications

- Ureterocele causing renal obstruction, obstruction of the bladder neck, vaginal mass (prolapse of an ectopic ureterocele)

Essential Steps

1) Visualize the ureterocele and have an array of instruments (pediatric cystoscope, Bugbee, resectoscope, loop, neodymium:YAG laser) readily available depending on the urethral size.
2) Incise the ureterocele transversely as distal as possible but proximal to the bladder neck to help reduce the incidence of subsequent vesicoureteral reflux.

Note These Variations

- In older children or adults, a resectoscope loop, bipolar electrode (Collins' knife) or laser fiber may be used to incise the ureterocele.
- For duplicated systems and ectopic ureters, open surgery (i.e. intravesical repair) may be required.

Complications

- Bleeding
- Infection
- Bladder/ureteral/rectal/vaginal injury
- Persistent obstruction
- Vesicoureteral reflux
- Urinary incontinence

Operative Dictations in Urologic Surgery, First Edition. Noel A. Armenakas, John A. Fracchia, and Ron Golan.
© 2019 John Wiley & Sons Ltd. Published 2019 by John Wiley & Sons Ltd.

Template Operative Dictation

Preoperative diagnosis: *Right/left/bilateral* ureterocele(s)
Postoperative diagnosis: Same
Procedure: Transurethral incision of ureterocele(s)
Indications: The patient is a ___-old *male/female* with a clinical diagnosis of a *right/ left/bilateral* ureterocele(s) presenting for ureterocele incision(s).
Description of Procedure: The indications, alternatives, benefits and risks were discussed with the patient's *family/guardian* and informed consent was obtained.

The patient was brought onto the operating room table, positioned supine with the hips abducted (frog leg) and secured with a safety strap. All pressure points were carefully padded.

After the administration of intravenous antibiotics and general endotracheal anesthesia, the genitalia were prepped and draped in the standard sterile manner.

A time-out was completed, verifying the correct patient, surgical procedure, site, and positioning, prior to beginning the procedure.

A 7.5 Fr rigid pediatric cystoscope with a 30° lens was inserted per meatus and advanced under direct vision into the urinary bladder. Urethroscopy revealed a normal urethra. The bladder was evaluated with both the 30° and 70° lenses. The media was clear, the bladder capacity was normal and the bladder wall noted to expand symmetrically in all dimensions. The bladder wall was *minimally/moderately/significantly/not* trabeculated with a normal appearing mucosa. There were no diverticula present.

The *right/left* ureterocele was clearly seen and the pinpoint ureteral meatus was identified. A 3 Fr endoscopic monopolar electrode (Bugbee) was introduced through the cystoscopic working port and positioned at the base of the ureterocele. Using cutting current, a full-thickness transverse incision was made distally in the ureterocele wall, away from the bladder neck.

A strong ureteral jet was evident from the incised ureterocele, confirming its patency. A urine specimen was collected and sent for urinalysis and culture.

> ***For bilateral ureteroceles***: The identical procedure was performed on the contralateral side, again confirming ureteral patency.

Minor bleeding areas were gently cauterized. The bladder was emptied and the cystoscope removed, under direct vision, confirming the absence of any injuries.

At the end of the procedure, all counts were correct.

The patient tolerated the procedure without difficulty and was taken to the recovery room in satisfactory condition.

Estimated blood loss: Approximately _____ml

121

Transverse Preputial Onlay Island Flap

Indications

- Mid-shaft hypospadias

Essential Steps

1) Inject the glans with 1% lidocaine containing 1:100000 epinephrine to assist in hemostasis.
2) Deglove the penis through a circumscribing incision below the urethral meatus.
3) Release any chordee and induce an artificial erection confirming a straight penis.
4) Incise the lateral margins of the urethral plate from below the hypospadiac meatus to the tip of the glans, separating the urethral plate from the corporal bodies and creating glans wings.
5) Isolate a transverse flap of inner prepuce, maintaining a well-vascularized dartos pedicle.
6) Rotate, invert, and suture the flap edges to lateral urethral plate, bilaterally.
7) Close the glans wings in two layers over the neourethra.
8) Complete the penile skin closure.

Note These Variations

- The neourethra alternatively can be fashioned as a tubular flap or by using the split prepuce technique.
- The glanular reconstruction can be performed using a glans cap approach, whereby a fine scissors is inserted flat against the corporal bodies and a wide subglanular tunnel is created by cutting distally to the tip of the glans. Excess glanular tissue is excised and a V-shaped orthotopic neomeatal opening fashioned.
- A hemostatic sealant (e.g. fibrin glue) can be used in conjunction with the anastomotic sutures to reinforce the repair.

Operative Dictations in Urologic Surgery, First Edition. Noel A. Armenakas, John A. Fracchia, and Ron Golan.
© 2019 John Wiley & Sons Ltd. Published 2019 by John Wiley & Sons Ltd.

Complications

- Bleeding
- Infection
- Dehiscence
- Meatal stenosis/retraction
- Urethrocutaneous fistula
- Urethral stricture

Template Operative Dictation

Preoperative diagnosis: Mid-shaft hypospadias
Postoperative diagnosis: Same
Procedure: Transverse preputial onlay island flap
Indications: The patient is a _____-old male with a distal hypospadias presenting for a tubularized incised plate repair.
Description of Procedure: The indications, alternatives, benefits, and risks were discussed with the patient's *family/guardian* and informed consent was obtained.

The patient was brought onto the operating room table, positioned supine, and secured with a safety strap. All pressure points were carefully padded.

After the administration of intravenous antibiotics and general endotracheal anesthesia, the patient's external genitalia, lower abdomen, and perineum were prepped and draped in the standard sterile manner.

A time-out was completed, verifying the correct patient, surgical procedure, and positioning, prior to beginning the procedure.

A 4-0 polypropylene (Prolene) traction suture was placed through the anterior mid glans and the penis placed on stretch. The ventral perimeatal tissues were infiltrated with 1% lidocaine containing 1 : 100000 epinephrine to aid in hemostasis.

Using optical magnification with surgical loupes, a circumscribing penile skin incision was made 5 mm below the urethral meatus, preserving the urethral plate. The lateral margins of the urethral plate were marked and incised from below the hypospadiac meatus to the tip of the glans, separating the urethral plate from the corporal bodies and forming glans wings. The dissection was taken down to Buck's fascia, releasing any tethering. An artificial erection was induced using injectable sterile saline through a 25 gauge butterfly needle placed in the *right/left* corpus cavernosum to confirm the absence of a ventral chordee.

The penis was carefully degloved to the level of Buck's fascia using sharp and blunt dissection. Four-quadrant 5-0 chromic stay sutures were placed in the inner prepuce for traction. A rectangular segment 1.0 cm wide and _____cm long was marked on the inner preputial surface, incised laterally and distally, and carefully dissected from the underlying skin. The dissection was continued proximally, just below the subdermal plexus to the penoscrotal junction, creating a robust well-vascularized dartos pedicle. Meticulous hemostasis was achieved using the microbipolar cautery.

The flap was rotated ventrally, inverted over the urethral plate, and trimmed appropriately. The pedicle edge of the flap was sutured to the lateral border of the urethral plate in one layer using a running 7-0 polydioxanone (PDS) suture. The hypospadiac

meatus was minimally debrided and spatulated ventrally for approximately 3 mm. The proximal flap edge was sutured to this using interrupted 7-0 PDS sutures, creating a patent anastomosis. The urethra was stented with a 5 Fr infant feeding tube and the contralateral flap edge was sutured to the lateral border of the urethral plate in two layers with a running 7-0 PDS suture.

The glans wings were closed in two layers with interrupted 6-0 polyglactin (Vicryl) sutures ensuring an orthotopically situated patent neomeatus. The urethral stent was secured to the initially placed mid-glans suture.

After completion of the glans and urethral reconstructions, the preputial hood was excised and the penile skin closed with interrupted 6-0 Vicryl sutures. Prior to the skin closure, the penis was thoroughly inspected for bleeding and hemostasis confirmed.

A sterile penile dressing and plastic adhesive were applied. A double diaper was placed, taking care not to occlude the urethral meatus. The urethral stent was placed within the diapers.

At the end of the procedure, all counts were correct.

The patient tolerated the procedure without difficulty and was transported to the recovery room in satisfactory condition.

Estimated blood loss: Approximately _____ml

122

Tubularized Incised Plate Urethroplasty

Indications

- Distal or mid-shaft hypospadias

Essential Steps

1) Inject the glans with 1% lidocaine containing 1:100000 epinephrine to assist in hemostasis.
2) Deglove the penis through a circumscribing incision below the urethral meatus.
3) Induce an artificial erection. If a ventral chordee is present, a dorsal plication should be performed concurrently.
4) Create glans wings.
5) Make a midline incision through the entire urethral plate.
6) Tubularize the urethral plate over a stent.
7) Cover the repair with a ventrally based dartos flap.
8) Close the glans wings in two layers over the neourethra.
9) Complete the penile skin closure with a circumcision or foreskin reconstruction.

Note These Variations

- There are several alternate techniques for the correction of a distal hypospadias, including the MAGPI (meatal advancement and glanuloplasty) and Mathieu (meatal based flip-flap) procedures.
- If a circumcision will not be performed, the urethra can be exposed through a ventral penile skin incision and the penis dissected ventrally only. The foreskin should be reconstructed in three layers (dartos, inner prepuce, and skin) by reapproximating the preputial hood ventrally using 6-0 Vicryl sutures.
- In cases where the urethral plate is wide, a simple tubularized plate urethroplasty (Thiersch-Duplay) can be performed without incising the urethral plate (Snodgrass modification).
- A hemostatic sealant (e.g. fibrin glue) can be used in conjunction with the anastomotic sutures to reinforce the repair.

Operative Dictations in Urologic Surgery, First Edition. Noel A. Armenakas, John A. Fracchia, and Ron Golan.
© 2019 John Wiley & Sons Ltd. Published 2019 by John Wiley & Sons Ltd.

Complications

- Bleeding
- Infection
- Dehiscence
- Meatal stenosis/retraction
- Urethrocutaneous fistula
- Urethral stricture

Template Operative Dictation

Preoperative diagnosis: Distal hypospadias
Postoperative diagnosis: Same
Procedure: Tubularized incised plate repair
Indications: The patient is a _____-year-old male with distal hypospadias presenting for a tubularized incised plate repair.
Description of Procedure: The indications, alternatives, benefits, and risks were discussed with the patient's *family/guardian* and informed consent was obtained.

The patient was brought onto the operating room table, positioned supine, and secured with a safety strap. All pressure points were carefully padded.

After the administration of intravenous antibiotics and general endotracheal anesthesia, the patient's external genitalia, lower abdomen, and perineum were prepped and draped in the standard sterile manner.

A time-out was completed verifying the correct patient, surgical procedure, and positioning, prior to beginning the procedure.

A 4-0 polypropylene (Prolene) stay suture was placed through the anterior mid glans for traction. Additional 4-0 polyglactin (Vicryl) stay sutures were placed ventrolaterally in the foreskin to facilitate the dissection.

Using optical magnification with surgical loupes, a circumscribing penile skin incision was made approximately 3 mm below the urethral meatus, preserving the urethral plate. The penis was carefully degloved, using sharp and blunt dissection deep to the dartos fascia, taking care not to injure the underlying urethra.

A tourniquet (e.g. 0.25 in. Penrose drain) was used to constrict the penile base and an artificial erection induced using injectable sterile saline through a 25-gauge butterfly needle placed into the *right/left* corpus cavernosum. Having confirmed the absence of ventral penile chordee, the tourniquet was removed.

The junction of the proposed glans wings to the urethral plate was marked and infiltrated with 1% lidocaine containing 1:100000 epinephrine to aid in hemostasis. The glans wings were created using two parallel vertical glans incisions separating the urethral plate from the glans. The incisions were carried proximally to the hypospadiac meatus, dissecting the urethral plate from the corporeal bodies.

A midline full-thickness incision was made in the dorsal urethral plate extending from the meatus to the tip of the glans. The urethral plate was tubularized, from distal to proximal, over a *5/8* Fr infant feeding tube in two layers using running 7-0 Vicryl sutures. Care was taken to create an oval orthotopic neomeatus.

A dorsal based dartos flap was fashioned from the inner prepuce, buttonholed, and transposed ventrally to cover the entire neourethra.

The glans wings were closed in two layers with interrupted 6-0 Vicryl sutures, again ensuring an orthotopically situated neomeatus.

Meticulous hemostasis was achieved with the microbipolar electrocautery. The lateral foreskin traction sutures were removed and the urethral stent secured to the initially placed mid-glans suture.

Having completed the glans and urethral reconstructions, the preputial hood was excised and the penile skin closed with interrupted 6-0 Vicryl sutures. Prior to the skin closure the penis was thoroughly inspected for bleeding and hemostasis obtained.

A sterile penile dressing and adhesive were applied. A double diaper was placed, taking care not to occlude the urethral meatus. The urethral stent was placed within the diapers.

At the end of the procedure, all counts were correct.

The patient tolerated the procedure without difficulty and was transported to the recovery room in satisfactory condition.

Estimated blood loss: Approximately _____ml

123

Ureteral Reimplantation

Extravesical Technique

Indications

- Persistent high grade vesicoureteral reflux
- Recurrent upper urinary tract infections in patients on suppressive antibiotics or in poorly compliant patients

Essential Steps

1) Fill the bladder through a urethral catheter.
2) Expose the bladder through a small transverse abdominal incision, sweep the peritoneum superiorly and identify and ligate the ipsilateral obliterated hypogastric artery.
3) Mobilize the distal ureter to the ureterovesical junction. At that level, stay close to the ureter to avoid injury to the terminal nerve branches entering the bladder.
4) Create a trough by incising the serosal and muscular bladder layers for a distance of 3 to 4 cm. Avoid disrupting the ureteral orifice or bladder mucosa.
5) Complete the repair by loosely reapproximating the detrusor muscle over the distal ureter. The ratio of tunnel length to ureteral width should be 5:1.
6) Empty the bladder and check for ureteral obstruction or kinking.

Note These Variations

- Optical magnification, using surgical loupes, can be used to enhance visualization.
- The procedure can be further simplified by limiting mobilization of the intramural ureter, as described in the original Gregoir technique.

Complications

- Bleeding
- Infection
- Persistent/recurrent ureteral reflux

Operative Dictations in Urologic Surgery, First Edition. Noel A. Armenakas, John A. Fracchia, and Ron Golan.
© 2019 John Wiley & Sons Ltd. Published 2019 by John Wiley & Sons Ltd.

- Urinary retention
- Injury to the vas deferens/round ligament
- Ureteral obstruction
- Recurrent upper urinary tract infections

Template Operative Dictation

Preoperative diagnosis: *Right/left/bilateral* vesicoureteral reflux
Postoperative diagnosis: Same
Procedure: *Right/left/bilateral* extravesical ureteral reimplantation
Indications: The patient is a __-old *male/female* with ureteral reflux presenting for extravesical *right/left/bilateral* ureteral reimplantation.
Description of Procedure: The indications, alternatives, benefits, and risks were discussed with the patient's *family/guardian* and informed consent was obtained.

The patient was brought onto the operating room table, positioned supine with the hips abducted, and secured with a safety strap. All pressure points were carefully padded.

After the administration of intravenous antibiotics and general anesthesia, the patient's entire lower abdomen and external genitalia were prepped and draped in the standard sterile manner.

A time-out was completed, verifying the correct patient, procedure, site, and positioning, prior to beginning the procedure.

A ___Fr urethral catheter was inserted into the bladder, filled with _____ ml sterile normal saline and clamped, partially filling the bladder.

[*Note:* Bladder volume in children (cc) = (age + 2) × 30].

A small semilunar transverse incision was made along Langer's lines one fingerbreadth above the symphysis pubis and carried down to the rectus abdominis aponeurosis. Using electrocautery this was incised in a semilunar arc, avoiding the inguinal canals. The rectus abdominis muscles were separated at the midline and retracted laterally, taking care not to injure the underlying inferior epigastric vessels. The anterior bladder wall was exposed and the peritoneum was swept cephalad. A self-retaining ring retractor (e.g. Denis-Browne) was positioned within the true pelvis, using moist sponges on each retractor blade.

The *right/left* obliterated hypogastric artery was identified between the bladder and pelvic sidewall, dissected, and ligated with 3-0 silk ties. Using gentle inferomedial bladder retraction, the *right/left* ureter was identified medial to the origin of the obliterated umbilical artery. The ureter was carefully dissected laterally to the ureterovesical junction, preserving the medial blood supply while staying close to the ureteral wall to avoid inadvertent injury to the terminal nerve branches entering the bladder.

The ureter was encircled with a vessel loop and gently lifted. Using blunt and sharp circumferential dissection, the intramural ureter was carefully separated from the detrusor muscle. A 4 cm full-thickness vertical incision was made in the detrusor, maintaining an intact bladder mucosa and ureteral orifice. The incised detrusor was undermined on both sides, creating a trough wide enough to accommodate the ureter. The distal ureter was positioned within this and the bladder drained. The overlying detrusor flaps were approximated, from proximal to distal, using interrupted 3-0 polyglactin (Vicryl) sutures.

Retraction on the bladder was released and the bladder again partially distended with sterile normal saline. The ureter was inspected, confirming its straight course without kinking or compression. Meticulous hemostasis was achieved throughout the procedure using judicious electrocautery.

> ***For bilateral ureteral reimplantation:*** The identical procedure was performed on the contralateral side.

The self-retaining ring retractor was removed and the abdominal incision was closed using a running 3-0 chromic suture to approximate the rectus muscles and 3-0 polydioxanone (PDS) suture for the rectus aponeurosis. 4-0 chromic sutures were used on Scarpa's fascia and the skin approximated with a subcuticular 5-0 poliglecaprone (Monocryl) suture. A sterile dressing was applied. The urethral catheter was connected to a drainage bag.

At the end of the procedure, all counts were correct.

The patient tolerated the procedure without difficulty and was transported to the recovery room in satisfactory condition.

Estimated blood loss: Approximately _____ml

124

Ureteral Reimplantation

Suprahiatal Transvesical Advancement (Politano-Leadbetter Procedure)

Indications

- Persistent high-grade vesicoureteral reflux
- Recurrent upper urinary tract infections in patients on suppressive antibiotics, or in poorly compliant patients who have vesicourethral reflux

Essential Steps

1) Fill the bladder through a urethral catheter.
2) Expose the bladder through a small transverse abdominal incision, sweep the peritoneum superiorly and make a vertical anterior cystotomy.
3) Position a self-retaining ring retractor to facilitate exposure of the ureteral orifices.
4) Pass a 5 Fr infant feeding tube into the ureter and secure it at the ureteral orifice with a purse-string suture.
5) Circumscribe the ureteral orifice and adequately mobilize it preserving the vascular ureteral adventitia.
6) Make a new hiatus approximately 2.5 cm cephalad and medial to the native ureteral orifice, and close the bladder muscle behind the original hiatus.
7) Create a submucosal tunnel from the neoureteral hiatus to the native ureteral orifice and carefully pull the ureter through this, without tension. The ratio of tunnel length to ureteral width should be 5 : 1.
8) Confirm that the ureter lies appropriately within the newly created submucosal tunnel and check for ureteral obstruction or kinking.
9) Create a spatulated ureterovesical anastomosis with absorbable interrupted sutures.
10) Close the proximal mucosal incision, avoiding injury to the underlying ureter.
11) Close the bladder in two layers.
12) Place a drain in the pelvis.

Note These Variations

- Optical magnification, using surgical loupes, can be used to enhance visualization.
- For an ectopic (laterally placed) ureteral orifice, consider the infrahiatal advancement technique (Glenn-Anderson).

Operative Dictations in Urologic Surgery, First Edition. Noel A. Armenakas, John A. Fracchia, and Ron Golan.
© 2019 John Wiley & Sons Ltd. Published 2019 by John Wiley & Sons Ltd.

- In patients with a neurogenic or small capacity bladder, the transtrigonal (Cohen) technique is preferable.
- For redo procedures, a midline vertical abdominal incision can be used.
- The use of ureteral stents and pelvic drains are at the discretion of the surgeon.

Complications

- Bleeding
- Infection
- Urine leak
- Persistent or recurrent ureteral reflux
- Ureteral obstruction from angulation or compression
- Urinary retention
- Recurrent upper urinary tract infections

Template Operative Dictation

Preoperative diagnosis: *Right/left/bilateral* vesicoureteral reflux
Postoperative diagnosis: Same
Procedure: *Right/left/bilateral* ureteral reimplantation: suprahiatal transvesical technique
Indications: The patient is a __ -old *male/female* with ureteral reflux in need of surgical correction presenting for suprahiatal transvesical *right/left/bilateral* ureteral reimplantation.
Description of Procedure: The indications, alternatives, benefits, and risks were discussed with the patient's *family/guardian* and informed consent obtained.

The patient was brought onto the operating room table, positioned supine, with the hips abducted, and secured with a safety strap. All pressure points were carefully padded.

After the administration of intravenous antibiotics and general anesthesia, the lower abdomen and external genitalia were prepped and draped in the standard sterile manner.

A time-out was completed, verifying the correct patient, procedure, site, and positioning, prior to beginning the procedure.

A ___Fr urethral catheter was inserted into the bladder, filled with ____ ml sterile normal saline and clamped.

[*Note:* Bladder volume in children (cc) = (age + 2) × 30].

A small semilunar transverse incision was made along Langer's lines one finger-breadth above the symphysis pubis and carried down to the rectus abdominis aponeu-rosis. This was incised in a semilunar arc using electrocautery, avoiding the inguinal canals. The rectus abdominis muscles were separated at the midline and retracted later-ally, taking care not to injure the underlying inferior epigastric vessels. The anterior bladder wall and vesical neck were exposed and the peritoneum was swept cephalad. A self-retaining retractor (e.g. Balfour, Denis-Browne) was appropriately positioned to optimize exposure, using padding on each retractor blade.

The anterior bladder wall was grasped with Allis clamps and a vertical midline cystotomy made using electrocautery. Upon entrance into the bladder, four interrupted 3-0 chromic stay sutures were placed on each side of the cystotomy and the bladder drained using suction. The urethral catheter was removed. An additional figure-of-eight 3-0 chromic suture was placed at the apex to avoid caudal extension of the incision. Bladder blades, each padded with a moist sponge, were used to identify the ureteral orifices.

The *right/left* ureteral orifice was identified and easily cannulated with a 5 Fr infant feeding tube, which was secured to the adjacent ureteral wall with a purse-string 4-0 polyglactin (Vicryl) traction suture. Using gentle traction on the infant feeding tube, the ureteral orifice was elevated and circumscribed with *a hooked blade/electrocautery.* Tenotomy scissors were used to sharply dissect the inferior aspect of the ureter and completely liberate it from the detrusor in a circumferential fashion. The peritoneum was swept from the posterior bladder wall under direct vision using a fine gauze dissector (Kittner). Throughout the dissection, care was taken to preserve the ureteral adventitia and to avoid any injury to the ureter.

A blunt right-angle clamp was passed posteriorly through the hiatus tenting an area of bladder muscle and mucosa approximately 2.5 cm cephalad and medial to the native ureteral orifice. The tented area was sharply incised over the points of the right-angle clamp. A second right-angle clamp was passed inside-out of the neoureteral hiatus to grasp the ureteral traction suture and bring it into the bladder. A 2–3 mm incision was made in the inferior aspect of the neoureteral hiatus to eliminate any ureteral angulation. The bladder muscle behind the original hiatus was closed with 4-0 interrupted Vicryl sutures.

A submucosal tunnel was created from the new to the native ureteral orifice using sharp and blunt dissection. The ureteral infant feeding tube was removed and the ureter was pulled, via its traction suture, through the submucosal tunnel and positioned without tension comfortably within the tunnel.

The ureter was spatulated ventrally and the edges trimmed to ensure an intact blood supply. Dorsally, the ureter was anchored to the trigone muscle and vesical mucosa using interrupted 5-0 Vicryl sutures. The ureterovesical anastomosis was completed with similar sutures placed at the 9, 12, and 3 o'clock positions.

Urinary efflux was observed from the neoureteral orifice, which was then intubated with the 5 Fr infant feeding tube confirming the absence of ureteral obstruction or kinking, and the feeding tube was removed.

The proximal bladder mucosal incision was closed with interrupted 4-0 Vicryl sutures, avoiding the underlying ureter. Meticulous hemostasis was achieved throughout the procedure with electrocautery.

> **For bilateral ureteral reimplantation**: The identical procedure was performed on the contralateral side.

Upon completion of the reconstructive procedure, a ____Fr urethral catheter was placed into the bladder and connected to a drainage bag.

The midline cystotomy was closed in two layers using a running 4-0 chromic and interrupted 4-0 Vicryl sutures for the mucosal and muscularis layers, respectively. A watertight bladder closure was confirmed by irrigating the urethral catheter with sterile normal saline.

A surgical drain (e.g. Jackson-Pratt, 0.25 in. Penrose) was placed in the space of Retzius away from the cystotomy. The drain was brought out through a separate cutaneous incision and secured at the skin with a 3-0 silk suture.

The self-retaining ring retractor was removed and the pelvis irrigated with sterile normal saline. The abdominal incision was closed using a running 3-0 chromic suture to approximate the rectus muscles and 3-0 polydioxanone (PDS) suture for the rectus aponeurosis. 3-0 chromic sutures were used on Scarpa's fascia and the skin approximated with a subcuticular 5-0 poliglecaprone (Monocryl) suture.

A sterile dressing was applied.

At the end of the procedure, all counts were correct.

The patient tolerated the procedure without difficulty and was transported to the recovery room in satisfactory condition.

Estimated blood loss: Approximately _____ml

125

Ureteral Reimplantation

Transtrigonal Technique (Cohen Procedure)

Indications

- Persistent high grade vesicoureteral reflux
- Recurrent upper urinary tract infections in patients on suppressive antibiotics, or in poorly compliant patients who have vesicourethral reflux

Essential Steps

1) Fill the bladder through a urethral catheter.
2) Expose the bladder through a small transverse abdominal incision, sweep the peritoneum superiorly and make a vertical anterior cystotomy.
3) Position a self-retaining ring retractor to facilitate exposure of the ureteral orifices.
4) Pass a 5 Fr infant feeding tube into the ureter and secure it at the ureteral orifice with a purse-string suture.
5) Circumscribe the ureteral orifice and adequately mobilize it preserving the vascular ureteral adventitia.
6) Make a new hiatus superolateral to the contralateral ureteral orifice. For bilateral ureteral reimplantation, the more laterally displaced ureter should be positioned superolateral, and the contralateral ureter inferolateral to the native ureteral orifices.
7) Create a submucosal tunnel from the native ureteral orifice to the neoureteral hiatus and carefully pull the ureter through this, without tension. The ratio of tunnel length to ureteral width should be 5:1.
8) Confirm that the ureter lies appropriately within the newly created submucosal tunnel and check for ureteral obstruction or kinking.
9) Create a spatulated ureterovesical anastomosis with absorbable interrupted sutures.
10) Close the mucosa over the original ureteral orifices, avoiding injury to the underlying ureter.
11) Close the bladder in two layers.
12) Place a drain in the pelvis.

Operative Dictations in Urologic Surgery, First Edition. Noel A. Armenakas, John A. Fracchia, and Ron Golan.
© 2019 John Wiley & Sons Ltd. Published 2019 by John Wiley & Sons Ltd.

Note These Variations

- Optical magnification, using surgical loupes, can be used to enhance visualization.
- For redo procedures, a midline vertical abdominal incision may be used.
- The use of ureteral stents and pelvic drains are at the discretion of the surgeon.

Complications

- Bleeding
- Infection
- Urine leak
- Persistent or recurrent ureteral reflux
- Ureteral obstruction from angulation or compression
- Urinary retention
- Recurrent upper urinary tract infections
- Difficulty with subsequent ureteral catheterization

Template Operative Dictation

Preoperative diagnosis: *Right/left/bilateral* vesicoureteral reflux
Postoperative diagnosis: Same
Procedure: *Right/left/bilateral* ureteral reimplantation: transtrigonal technique
Indications: The patient is a __-year-old *male/female* with ureteral reflux in need of surgical correction presenting for transtrigonal *right/left/bilateral* ureteral reimplantation.
Description of Procedure: The indications, alternatives, benefits, and risks were discussed with the patient's *family/guardian* and informed consent was obtained.

The patient was brought onto the operating room table, positioned supine with the hips abducted, and secured with a safety strap. All pressure points were carefully padded.

After the administration of intravenous antibiotics and general anesthesia, the lower abdomen and external genitalia were prepped and draped in the standard sterile manner.

A time-out was completed verifying the correct patient, procedure, site, and positioning, prior to beginning the procedure.

A ___Fr urethral catheter was inserted into the bladder, filled with ____ ml sterile normal saline and clamped.

[*Note:* Bladder volume in children (cc) = (age + 2) × 30].

A small semilunar transverse incision was made along Langer's lines, one finger-breadth above the symphysis pubis and carried down to the rectus abdominis aponeurosis. This was incised in a semilunar arc using electrocautery, avoiding the inguinal canals. The rectus abdominis muscles were separated at the midline and retracted laterally, taking care not to injure the underlying inferior epigastric vessels. The anterior bladder wall and vesical neck were exposed and the peritoneum was swept cephalad. A self-retaining retractor (e.g. Balfour, Denis-Browne) was appropriately positioned to optimize exposure, using padding on each retractor blade.

The anterior bladder wall was grasped with Allis clamps and a vertical midline cystotomy made using electrocautery. Upon entrance into the bladder, four interrupted 3-0 chromic stay sutures were placed on each side of the cystotomy and the bladder drained using suction. The urethral catheter was removed. An additional figure-of-eight 3-0 chromic suture was placed at the apex to avoid caudal extension of the incision. Bladder blades, each padded with a moist sponge, were used for retraction to identify the ureteral orifices.

The *right/left* ureteral orifice was identified and easily cannulated with a 5 Fr infant feeding tube, which was secured to the adjacent ureteral wall with a purse-string 4-0 polyglactin (Vicryl) suture. Using gentle traction on the infant feeding tube, the ureteral orifice was elevated and circumscribed with *a hooked blade/electrocautery*. Tenotomy scissors were used to sharply dissect the inferior aspect of the ureter and completely liberate it from the detrusor in a circumferential fashion. The peritoneum was swept from the posterior bladder wall under direct vision using a fine gauze dissector (Kittner). Throughout the dissection, care was taken to preserve the ureteral adventitia and to avoid any injury to the ureter.

The mucosa superolateral to the contralateral ureteral orifice was incised and a submucosal tunnel created from the existing native ureteral orifice to the neoureteral hiatus using sharp and blunt dissection. The ureteral infant feeding tube was removed and the ureter was pulled via its traction suture through the submucosal tunnel and positioned, without tension, comfortably within the tunnel.

The ureter was spatulated ventrally and the edges trimmed to ensure an intact blood supply. Dorsally the ureter was anchored to the trigone muscle and vesical mucosa using interrupted 5-0 Vicryl sutures. The ureterovesical anastomosis was completed with similar sutures placed at the 9, 12, and 3 o'clock positions.

The original hiatus was closed with 4-0 interrupted Vicryl sutures, avoiding the underlying ureter.

Meticulous hemostasis was achieved throughout the procedure with electrocautery.

Urinary efflux was observed from the neoureteral orifice, which was then intubed with the 5 Fr infant feeding tube confirming the absence of ureteral obstruction or kinking, and the feeding tube was removed.

> **For bilateral ureteral reimplantation:** The *left/right* ureteral reimplant was performed in a similar fashion, except that the new ureteral hiatus was positioned at the inferior edge of the contralateral native ureteral orifice.

Upon completion of the reconstructive procedure, a ___Fr urethral catheter was placed into the bladder and connected to a drainage bag.

The midline cystotomy was closed in two layers using a running 4-0 chromic and interrupted 4-0 Vicryl sutures for the mucosal and muscularis layers, respectively. A watertight bladder closure was confirmed by irrigating the urethral catheter with sterile normal saline.

A surgical drain (e.g. Jackson-Pratt, 0.25 in. Penrose) was placed in the space of Retzius away from the cystotomy. The drain was brought out through a separate cutaneous incision and secured at the skin with a 3-0 silk suture.

The self-retaining ring retractor was removed and the pelvis irrigated with sterile normal saline. The abdominal incision was closed using a running 3-0 chromic suture

to approximate the rectus muscles and 3-0 polydioxanone (PDS) suture for the rectus aponeurosis. 3-0 chromic sutures were used on Scarpa's fascia and the skin approximated with a subcuticular 5-0 poliglecaprone (Monocryl) suture.

A sterile dressing was applied.

At the end of the procedure, all counts were correct.

The patient tolerated the procedure without difficulty and was transported to the recovery room in satisfactory condition.

Estimated blood loss: Approximately _____ml

NOTES

NOTES

SECTION VII MISCELLANEOUS PROCEDURES

126

Extracorporeal Shock Wave Lithotripsy

Indications

- Urolithiasis

Essential Steps

1) Confirm the location of the calculus(i) radiographically prior to the time out.
2) During the procedure, frequently image the calculus(i) in collimated mode to ensure adequate targeting.
3) Administer the allowable number of shocks to optimize stone fragmentation.

Note These Variations

- The maximum number of shock waves administered is dependent on stone location and the lithotripter manufacturer's recommendations.
- Middle and distal ureteral stones can often be treated with a higher number of shocks than intrarenal and proximal ureteral stones.
- Alternatively, sonography can be used for stone localization and treatment.

Complications

- Hematuria
- Renal parenchymal injury/hematoma
- Post-procedure pain (parenchymal insult, colic)
- Ureteral obstruction (impacted calculus(i), steinstrasse)
- Failure to fragment calculus(i)

Template Operative Dictation

Preoperative diagnosis: Urolithiasis *(indicate location)*
Postoperative diagnosis: Same

Operative Dictations in Urologic Surgery, First Edition. Noel A. Armenakas, John A. Fracchia, and Ron Golan.
© 2019 John Wiley & Sons Ltd. Published 2019 by John Wiley & Sons Ltd.

Procedure: *Right/Left* extracorporeal shock wave lithotripsy (ESWL)

Indications: The patient is a _____-year-old *male/female* with a _____mm *right/left// renal/ureteral* stone presenting for extracorporeal shock wave lithotripsy.

Description of Procedure: The indications, alternatives, benefits, and risks were discussed with the patient and informed consent obtained.

The patient was brought onto the lithotripsy table, positioned *supine/prone* and secured with a safety strap. All pressure points were carefully padded and pneumatic compression devices were placed on the lower extremities. *Fluoroscopy/sonography* confirmed the location of the calculus(i) as described in the pre-ESWL imaging report.

The radiographic images were in the room.

A time-out was completed, verifying the correct patient, surgical procedure, and exact location of the calculus(i) to be treated, prior to beginning the procedure.

After induction of *general anesthesia/managed anesthesia care*, the ESWL treatment head was appropriately positioned below the patient's *right/left* side. Limited *fluoroscopy/sonography* was used to confirm the radiographic placement of the calculus(i) within the imaging modality's cross hairs.

Treatment was begun at a low kilovoltage and slow rate. The power was progressively increased to a maximum setting of _____. The treatment was concluded at *2500/3000/*_____ shocks. The calculus(i) *was/were* imaged periodically throughout the course of treatment, confirming fragmentation.

The lithotripter's treatment head was lowered and the *flank/abdomen* examined confirming the absence of a visible hematoma.

The patient tolerated the procedure well and was taken to the recovery room in satisfactory condition.

Estimated blood loss: None

NOTES

NOTES

Index

Operative Dictations in Urologic Surgery, First Edition. Noel A. Armenakas, John A. Fracchia, and Ron Golan.
© 2019 John Wiley & Sons Ltd. Published 2019 by John Wiley & Sons Ltd.

Printed and bound by CPI Group (UK) Ltd, Croydon, CR0 4YY

27/10/2024

14580362-0003